THE ATI NCLEX-RN® REVIEW

COMPLETE SOURCE OF ESSENTIAL NCLEX® EXAM INFORMATION

16TH EDITION

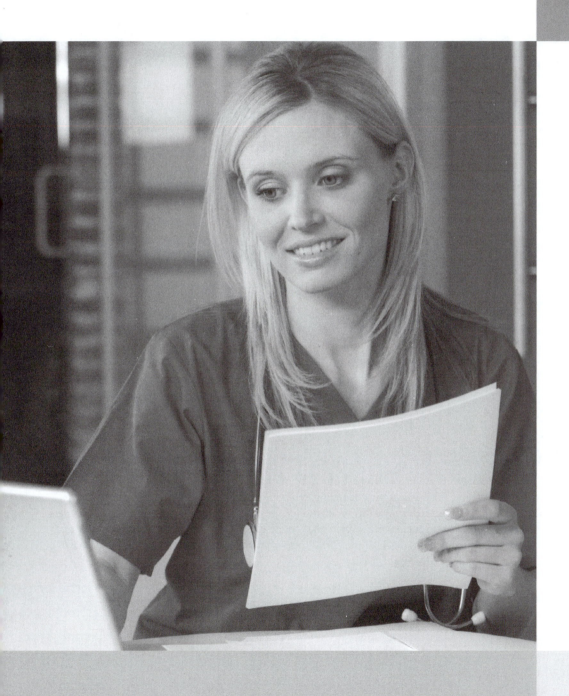

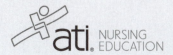

ati. NURSING EDUCATION

Assessment Technologies Institute®, LLC
7500 W. 160th St.
Stilwell, Kansas 66085
www.atitesting.com

ISBN 978-1-56533-526-4

6048

Printed in the United States of America

15 14 13 12 11   10 9 8 7 6 5 4 3 2 1

Important Notice to the Reader

Assessment Technologies Institute®, LLC, is the publisher of this publication. The publisher reserves the right to modify, change, or update the content of this publication at any time. The content of this publication, such as text, graphics, images, information obtained from the publisher's licensors, and other material contained in this publication are for informational purposes only. The content is not providing medical advice and is not intended to be a substitute for professional medical advice, diagnosis, or treatment. Always seek the advice of your primary care provider or other qualified healthcare provider for any questions you may have regarding a medical condition. Never disregard professional medical advice or delay seeking it because of something you have read in this publication. If you think you may have a medical emergency, go to your local emergency department or call 911 immediately.

The publisher does not recommend or endorse any specific tests, primary care providers, products, procedures, processes, opinions, or other information that may be mentioned in this publication. Reliance on any information provided by the publisher, the publisher's employees, or others contributing to the content at the invitation of the publisher is solely at the reader's own risk. Healthcare professionals need to use their own clinical judgment in interpreting the content of this publication, and details such as medications, dosages, and laboratory tests and results should always be confirmed with other resources.

This publication may contain health- or medical-related materials that are sexually explicit. If you find these materials offensive, you may not want to use this publication.

The publishers, editors, advisors, and reviewers make no representations or warranties of any kind or nature, including, but not limited to, the accuracy, reliability, completeness, currentness, timeliness, or the warranties of fitness for a particular purpose or merchantability, nor are any such representations implied with respect to the content herein (with such content to include text and graphics), and the publishers, editors, advisors, and reviewers take no responsibility with respect to such content. The publishers, editors, advisors, and reviewers shall not be liable for any actual, incidental, special, consequential, punitive, or exemplary damages (or any other type of damages) resulting, in whole or in part, from the reader's use of, or reliance upon, such content.

USER'S GUIDE AND ORGANIZATION

Congratulations, graduate! You have successfully completed your program of nursing studies and are now eligible to take the licensing exam created by the National Council of State Boards of Nursing (NCSBN®).

Understanding the organizational format of this review book will help guide you through a focused review in preparation for NCLEX®. Each unit focuses on a specific area of nursing care. Unit 1 offers practical information about the exam, including how to prepare, along with test-taking strategies. The next eight units review essential content for the exam:

- Fundamentals for Nursing
- Adult Medical-Surgical Nursing
- Mental Health Nursing
- Maternal and Newborn Nursing
- Nursing Care of Children
- Pharmacology
- Nursing Leadership and Management
- Community Health Nursing

Tables and graphics are provided throughout to simplify more challenging content.

The content provided in this book is organized by body systems and focuses on definitions, contributing factors, manifestations, and collaborative care, which includes nursing interventions, diagnostics, medications, therapeutic measures, client education, and referral. The information is presented in a manner that promotes analysis and application of knowledge and reinforces priority of care when managing client care.

Feedback is always welcome. Therefore, please send suggestions for improvement, any noted errors, and personal testimonials of effectiveness to: *comments@atitesting.com*.

Contributing NCLEX® Experts

Lawrette Axley, PhD, RN, CNE
Regional Live Review Manager
NCLEX® Specialist

Janel Crawford, MS, RN
Live Review Educator
NCLEX® Specialist

Melesia Henry, PhDc, MSN, RN
Regional Live Review Manager
NCLEX® Specialist

Stacey Kinney, MSN, RN
Live Review Educator
NCLEX® Specialist

Carol Isaac MacKusick, PhDc, MSN, RN, CNN
Live Review Educator
NCLEX® Specialist

Nancy Murren, MSN, RN
Live Review Educator
NCLEX® Specialist

Lynn Schneider, MSN, RN, FNP
Live Review Educator
NCLEX® Specialist

Heather Stranger, MS, RN, CNE
Live Review Educator
NCLEX® Specialist

Contents

UNIT FOUR ❖ Mental Health Nursing   91

UNIT FIVE ❖ Maternal and Newborn Nursing   115

UNIT SIX ❖ Nursing Care of Children   151

UNIT SEVEN ❖ Pharmacology 207

UNIT EIGHT ❖ Nursing Leadership and Management 241

UNIT NINE ❖ Community Health Nursing 251

UNIT ONE

Review of Test-Taking Strategies for the NCLEX-RN® Exam

Information About NCLEX®

A. General Information

1. The purpose of the NCLEX-RN® is to determine that a candidate is prepared to safely practice entry-level nursing.

2. The exam is designed to test essential nursing knowledge and a candidate's ability to apply that knowledge to clinical situations.

3. The new test plan will bring the exam in line with current nursing behaviors (the nursing process and decision making).

4. The exam is pass/fail, and no other score is given.

B. Computerized Adaptive Testing (CAT)

1. CAT is a system that selects test items for you based on your ability to answer previous items.

2. When a question is answered, CAT determines the next question based on its estimate that you will have a 50% chance of answering the question correctly.

3. Passing or failing is determined when you reach a point in the test when minimal competency has been demonstrated.

4. Use the mouse to move the cursor on the screen to a desired location.

5. Single-click the mouse to select an option as the answer.

6. A drop-down calculator is also featured. Double-click the mouse on the calculator icon, and the drop-down calculator will appear.

7. After confirming the selection, click on "next" to input the answer and proceed to the next screen.

8. You cannot go back to a previous question to change your answer.

C. Exam Schedule

1. The exam is given all year long.

2. The exam can be repeated every 45 days.

D. Number of Questions and Time Allowed

1. There is not a minimum amount of time for the exam, and the maximum time allowed is 6 hours. The average time for a candidate is 2.4 hours.

2. A candidate must answer a minimum of 75 test questions with a maximum of 265 test questions. The average candidate takes approximately 118 questions. There is no time limit per question.

3. The computer will automatically stop as soon as one of the following occurs:

    a. The candidate's measure of competency is determined to be above or below the passing standard.

    b. The candidate has answered all 265 test questions.

    c. The maximum amount of time (6 hr) has expired.

    d. It is not possible to skip questions or return to previous questions.

    e. The exam includes 15 unmarked experimental questions that do not impact the final score.

    f. There will be two optional breaks, one after 2 hours and another after 3.5 hours. Break time is part of the 6 hours.

The NCLEX-RN® Test Plan

A. The NCLEX-RN® test plan is revised every 3 years. The current 2010 test plan, available at www.ncsbn.org, identifies the major categories and nursing activities that guide the exam's content and questions.

B. NCLEX® questions are distributed and weighted according to the following client need categories in the 2010 test plan blueprint:

1. Safe and Effective Care Environment

    a. Management of Care: 16–22%

    b. Safety and Infection Control: 8–14%

2. Health Promotion and Maintenance: 6–12%

3. Psychosocial Integrity: 6–12%

4. Physiological Integrity

    a. Basic Care and Comfort: 6–12%

    b. Pharmacological and Parenteral Therapies: 13–19%

    c. Reduction of Risk Potential: 10–16%

    d. Physiological Adaptation: 11–17%

(*The above information is provided courtesy of the National Council of State Boards of Nursing, Inc., Test Plan April 2010.*)

C. The NCLEX-RN® Registration Process

1. Submit an application for licensure to the board of nursing in the state in which you want to be licensed. Be sure to follow your school's protocol to prevent delays in processing.

2. When the state board determines that you are eligible to test, it will send the information to the NCSBN.

3. Register with Pearson VUE either though the Internet or by mail.

4. Apply to Pearson VUE to take the NCLEX-RN® when you apply to your state's board of nursing so that Pearson VUE will already have your information when it receives your approval to test. You should have a confirmation of receipt of your application within 2 weeks. When the state board forwards the approval to test to the NCSBN, Pearson VUE will send you an authorization to test (ATT).

5. Schedule your test date as soon as possible after receiving your ATT. First-time candidates receive a test date within 30 days of their telephone request, and repeat test takers within 45 days. To schedule your test, call NCLEX® Candidates Services or go to www.pearsonvue.com/nclex.

NCLEX-RN® Item Types

A. Standard Multiple-Choice Question

1. Traditional NCLEX® question

2. Most common type of question on the exam

3. Has four options, only one of which is correct

! **Point to Remember:** Point to Remember: As of April 2003, the NCLEX® started including items other than standard multiple-choice questions. These items are known as alternate test items. The candidate should allow more time for answering alternate test items.

B. Fill-in-the-Blank

1. Fill-in-the-blank items are primarily calculation problems. The question may ask for an answer in a specific unit amount or a rounded decimal.

2. To answer these questions, a number should be typed into the answer box on the screen.

3. When answering the question, solve for the correct unit value.

4. Write out the calculations on material provided.

5. Bring up the drop-down calculator and double-check your work.

C. Drag-and-Drop/Ordered Response

1. Drag-and-drop/ordered response items list steps that must be placed in a correct sequence as indicated by the prompt.

2. To answer these questions, drag options in the left-hand column into the appropriate order of performance in the right-hand column.

3. There is only one correct sequence to maintain the client's safety at each step in the care continuum.

D. Multiple Response

1. Multiple-response items require test takers to choose more than one answer. Any number of the options may be correct, AND not all the options in a question can be correct.

2. To answer these questions, click on all the answers that apply.

3. Credit will only be given for completely correct answers. No partial credit is given.

4. Consider each response as a true-false question.

E. Hot Spot

1. Hot spot items use a "point-and-click" method that requires a test taker to choose the correct anatomical location on a figure.

2. Click on the area that constitutes the landmark to correctly answer the item.

3. Read the question carefully, then analyze the image.

4. The exam will allow the test taker to reclick on the image as many times as necessary.

! **Point to Remember:** It is very important to remember that the screen is NOT a mirror image. If the question asks for an answer on the right or left side of the body, make sure to click on the appropriate side.

F. Chart/Exhibit

1. Standard multiple-choice questions may also include chart exhibits that must be analyzed and understood to correctly answer the question. The chart/exhibit question cannot be answered without obtaining further information; this is where the chart comes in to play. On-screen tabs, similar to the tabs either in a client's chart or computerized medical record, will allow the test taker to select various client documents. For example, one tab may say "Medication Administration Record," another may be labeled "Vital Signs," and another "Laboratory Results." These documents will contain information that the test taker must analyze to correctly answer the question.

2. First, read the question carefully. Then, analyze the charts or exhibit. Use the mouse to click on each tab to open the document. When the tab is clicked, a separate window will open to display the data contained in the selected section of the client's chart. Analysis of the data in each of these documents provides the information necessary to answer the question.

G. Graphic Option

1. These items display images for each answer option.

2. The answers to these items are preceded by circles. Be sure to click on the circle to select the answer.

H. Audio

1. Audio items may test knowledge of audible breath and heart sounds, or examples of change-of-shift client reports or unit-transfer reports.

2. When an audio item is presented on NCLEX®, the candidate is prompted to apply headphones. Ear phones will be provided to accurately identify the audio sound. The volume of the audio may be adjusted and replayed as often as needed.

Preparing for and Answering Questions on the Exam

A. New nursing graduates should review content and questions daily until they take the exam. Adequate review depends on scores obtained on practice assessments, and NCLEX® preparation after a live review may take anywhere from 2 to 8 weeks.

B. For content review, use this NCLEX-RN® review book that outlines content. Use other nursing reference materials for more detailed information.

C. Your practice assessment score reports will identify and help direct review of content.

D. Begin with areas that are most difficult or least familiar.

E. When studying body systems and the associated diseases:

1. Define the disease in terms of the pathophysiological process that is occurring.

2. Identify the client's early and late manifestations.

3. Identify the most important or life-threatening complications.

4. Review the prescribed medical plan including ordered diagnostic and laboratory tests, expected lab value alterations, medications, and ordered treatments.

5. Identify and prioritize the nursing interventions associated with early and late manifestations.

6. Identify client teaching that the nurse should provide to the client/family to prevent or adapt to the disease process and/or clinical condition.

Interpreting ATI Assessment Scores

A. At the end of your NCLEX® review, you will be provided with codes and passwords to access a set of new assessments in the following content areas:

1. Fundamentals of Nursing
2. Medical-Surgical Nursing
3. Maternal Newborn Nursing
4. Nursing Care of the Child
5. Mental Health Nursing
6. Pharmacology
7. Leadership

B. Complete the ATI assessments to identify areas of weakness. Strive to achieve an assessment score of 60% correct or greater.

C. If you answer less than 60% correctly on an exam, or in a subcontent area within a practice exam, this is a signal that additional time needs to be spent reviewing content in this area.

Test-Taking Strategies

A. Reading Test Items

1. Because the amount of information in a test stem and distractors can be overwhelming, a useful approach is to break the analysis of the question into a series of steps.

2. Most questions on the NCLEX® are standard multiple-choice questions that have four options. The correct answer is the BEST answer. The other three options are distractors. Distractors are options made to look like correct answers. They are intended to distract you from selecting the correct answer.

3. Initially, read the case scenario and question stem and apply your knowledge of test-taking strategies.

4. Develop a set of possible answers.

5. Review the distractors one at a time.

6. Choose the correct answer or answers.

B. Identify the Issue in the Question

1. The issue in a question is the problem that is asked. The issue may be a:

    a. Medication: digoxin (Lanoxin)

    b. Nursing problem: a client who is at risk for infection or in pain

    c. Behavior: restlessness, agitation

    d. Disorder: diabetes mellitus, ulcerative colitis

    e. Procedure: glucose-tolerance test, cardiac catheterization

C. Identify the Client in the Question

1. The client in the question usually has a health problem.

2. The client may be a relative, significant other, or another member of the health care team with whom the nurse is interacting.

3. The correct answer to the question must relate to the client in the question.

D. Look for Key Words

1. Key words focus attention on important details such as:

    a. During the **early** period, which of the following nursing **procedures** is **best**?

    b. The nurse should **expect** to find which of the following characteristics in an **adult** who has **diabetes mellitus**?

    c. Which of the following nursing **actions** is **essential**?

    d. Which of the following nursing **actions** should the nurse take **first**?

E. Identify What the Stem Is Asking

1. Understand what the stem is asking before viewing the options.

2. If the question is not clear, rephrase it.

3. Determine whether the question has a true-response, a false-response, or a priority stem.

  a. True-response stem

    1) Requires an answer that is a true statement such as:

      a) Which of the following tasks should the nurse assign to assistive personnel?

      b) Which of the following manifestations should the nurse expect to assess?

      c) Which of the following is a therapeutic response by the nurse?

      d) The nurse evaluates that the client has a positive response to the medication when the client exhibits what?

  b. False-response stem

    1) Requires an answer that is a false statement such as:

      a) Which of the following nursing actions is inappropriate?

      b) Which of the following statements by the client indicates a need for further instruction?

      c) Which of the following describes incorrect placement of the hands during CPR?

      d) Which of the following actions will place the client at risk?

4. Eliminating incorrect options

  a. As you read each of the four to possibly six options, make a decision such as:

    1) This option is true (+).

    2) This option is false (−).

    3) I am not sure about this option (?).

  b. If the stem is a true-response stem:

    1) An option that is true (+) may be the correct answer.

    2) An option that is false (−) is a distractor. Eliminate this option.

    3) An option that you are not sure about (?) may be a correct answer.

  c. If the stem is a false-response stem:

    1) An option that is true (+) is a distractor. Eliminate this option.

    2) An option that is false (−) may be the correct answer.

    3) An option that you are not sure about (?) may be the correct answer.

  d. Avoid returning to options that have been eliminated.

    1) If one option is left, that is the answer.

    2) If one option is (+) and another (?), select the (+) option as the answer.

    3) If two (+) options remain, use strategies to select the best answer.

  e. Answering communication questions

  f. Because the ability to communicate is essential for safe practice, the NCLEX® includes communication questions.

  g. Identify the critical elements in all questions. Pay particular attention to identification of the client in the question. Remember that the answer must relate to the client.

  h. Identify the communication tools that enhance communication such as:

    1) Being silent: nonverbal communication

    2) Offering self: "Let me sit with you."

    3) Showing empathy: "You are upset."

    4) Focusing: "You say that . . ."

    5) Restatement: "You feel anxious?"

    6) Validation/clarification: "What you are saying is…?"

    7) Giving information: "Your room is 423."

  i. Learning to identify nontherapeutic communication blocks.

    1) Giving advice: "If I were you, I would…"

    2) Showing approval/disapproval: "You did the right thing."

    3) Using clichés and false reassurances: "Don't worry. It will be all right."

    4) Requesting an explanation: "Why did you do that?"

    5) Belittling feelings: "Everyone feels that way."

    6) Being defensive: "Every nurse on this unit is exceptional."

    7) Focusing on inappropriate issues or persons: "Have I said something wrong?"

    8) Placing the client's issues on hold: "Talk to your doctor about that."

  j. When answering communication questions, select an option that illustrates a therapeutic communication tool. Eliminate options that illustrate nontherapeutic communication blocks.

5. Answering questions that focus on priorities

  a. The majority of NCLEX® questions will be priority-setting questions, which ask the test taker to identify what comes first, is most important, or gets the highest priority.

  b. The NCLEX® will use distractors, which ask, "What will the nurse do FIRST"; for example:

    1) What is the nurse's initial response?

    2) A nurse should give immediate consideration to which of the following?

    3) Which of the following nursing actions should receive the highest priority?

    4) Which of the following actions should the nurse take first?

  c. Use guidelines to answer priority-setting questions.

    1) Maslow's Hierarchy of Needs indicates that physiological needs come first.

2) "ABC"—airway, breathing, circulation needs will frequently take priority.

3) The hierarchy indicates that when no physiological need is identified, safety should come first.

4) The nursing process indicates that assessment is a priority.

5) The communication theory indicates the need to focus on encouraging the client to verbalize feelings.

6) The teaching/learning theory emphasizes the importance of client motivation as the criterion for success.

SECTION 7

The Day of the Exam

A. Plan for everything!

B. Everything needed for the exam should be assembled the night before.

C. Identification: When candidates arrive at the test center, they will be required to present one form of acceptable identification and their valid authorization-to-test (ATT) form. The name on the ID must match, exactly, the name on the application sent to the Board of Registered Nursing. Please visit the NCSBN website for acceptable forms of ID—www.ncsbn.org.

D. Plan to arrive at the test site early.

E. Verify the route to the exam site, and take a test-drive several days prior.

F. Pay close attention to your physiological needs.

G. Dress in layers to accommodate your comfort in the testing center.

H. Get a good night's sleep the night before the exam.

I. Eat a nourishing meal that includes protein and long-acting carbohydrates.

J. Avoid stimulants and depressants.

K. Meet elimination needs prior to beginning the exam.

L. During the exam:

1. Listen to and carefully read the instructions.

2. Don't let yourself become distracted. Focus on answering one question at a time.

3. Think positive.

M. Manage your anxiety level.

1. Mild levels of anxiety increase effectiveness.

2. Avoid cramming the night before the exam.

3. Do something enjoyable and relaxing the night before the exam.

4. Learn and practice measures to manage your anxiety level during the exam, as needed.

   a. Take a few deep breaths.

   b. Tense and relax muscles.

   c. Visualize a peaceful scene.

   d. Visualize your success.

UNIT TWO

Fundamentals for Nursing

Fundamentals of nursing practice integrate principles and concepts essential to all categories of the NCLEX-RN®.

SECTION 1

Client Safety

Falls

A significant number of reported facility accidents are related to falls. The nurse is accountable for implementation of essential actions to reduce the risk associated with falls.

A. Contributing Factors

1. Identify clients "at risk" for falls:
   a. Older adult
   b. Impaired mobility
   c. Cognitive and/or sensory impairment
   d. Bowel and bladder dysfunction
   e. Side effects of medications

B. NURSING INTERVENTIONS

1. Complete a **falls risk assessment** upon admission and update as needed.
2. Communicate identified risks with the health care team.
3. Assign clients at risk for falls to a room close to the nurses' station and assess frequently.
4. Provide the client with nonskid footwear.
5. Keep the floor free of clutter and maintain an unobstructed path to the bathroom.
6. Orient the client to the setting (grab bars, call light), including how to use and locate all necessary items.
7. Maintain the bed in low position.
8. Instruct a client who is unsteady to use the call light for assistance before ambulating.
9. Answer call lights promptly to prevent clients who are at risk from trying to ambulate independently.
10. Provide adequate lighting (a night-light for necessary trips to the bathroom).
11. Determine the client's ability to use assistive devices (walkers, canes, etc.). Keep all items within reach.
12. Use chair or bed sensors for clients who are at risk.
13. Lock wheels on beds, wheelchairs, and gurneys to prevent rolling during transfers or stops.
14. Report and document all incidents per the facility's policy.

Restraints

A. Current client safety standards focus on reducing the need for client restraints. The type or technique of restraint or seclusion used must be the least restrictive intervention that will be effective to protect the client, staff members, or others from harm.

B. Definition: Restraints include human, mechanical, chemical, or physical devices that restrict freedom of movement or diminish the client's access to parts of the body.

 C. NURSING INTERVENTIONS

1. Implement non-pharmacologic measures such as distraction, frequent observation, or diversion activities.
2. Prior to application, review manufacturer's instructions for correct application.
3. Notify the health care provider immediately when restraints are implemented.
4. Remove the restraints and assess client every 2 hours.
5. Assess neurovascular and neurosensory status every 2 hours.
6. Leave the restraint loose enough to prevent injury.
7. Always tie the restraint to the bed frame (using loose knots that are easily removed).
8. Reassess the need for continued use.
9. Document
   a. Behaviors making restraint necessary
   b. Alternatives attempted and the client's response
   c. Type and location of the restraint and time applied
   d. Frequency and type of assessments
   e. Restraints should **NEVER**:
      1) Interfere with treatment
      2) Be used because of short staffing or staff convenience

Seizure Precautions

Seizures may have a sudden onset and include loss of consciousness, violent tonic-clonic movements, and risk of injury to the client (head injury, aspiration, and falls).

A. NURSING INTERVENTIONS

1. Assess the client's seizure history, noting frequency, presence of auras, and sequence of events.
2. Identify precipitating factors that may exacerbate or lead to seizures.
3. Review the client's medication history.
4. Place rescue equipment at the client's bedside, including oxygen, an oral airway, and suction equipment.
5. Establish IV or saline lock access for high-risk clients.
6. Inspect the client's environment for items that may cause injury in the event of a seizure. Remove any unnecessary items from the immediate environment.
7. At the onset of a seizure, position the client for safety and remain with the client.
8. If the client is sitting or standing, ease him to the floor. Protect the client's head. If the client is in bed, raise the side rails and pad for safety.
9. Roll the client to the side with his head flexed slightly forward.
10. Do not put anything in the client's mouth.
11. Loosen restrictive clothing.

12. Accurately document the event, including timing, precipitating behaviors or events, and a description of the event (movements, any injuries, mention of aura, postictal state).

13. Report the seizure to the provider.

SECTION 2
Environmental Safety

Fire

All staff must be instructed in fire response procedures.

A. NURSING INTERVENTIONS

1. Know the facility's fire drill and evacuation plan.

2. Keep emergency numbers near or on the phone at all times.

3. Know the location of all fire alarms, extinguishers, and exits, including oxygen shut-off valves.

4. Follow the fire response sequence in the facility (**RACE**):

   a. **R**escue: Protect and evacuate clients in immediate danger.

   b. **A**larm: Activate the alarm and report the fire.

   c. **C**ontain: Close doors or windows.

   d. **E**xtinguish: Use correct fire extinguisher to eliminate the fire.

      1) **Class A**: paper, wood, cloth, or trash
      2) **Class B**: flammable liquids and gases
      3) **Class C**: electrical fires

   e. Extinguish properly.

   f. **P**ull, **A**im, **S**queeze, **S**weep (**PASS**)

5. Considerations for home health setting

   a. Post "No Smoking" signs.

   b. Assess for risk (oxygen therapy, smoking, electrical equipment).

   c. Teach client to develop a plan of action in the event of a fire, including a route of exit and a location where family members will meet.

   d. Instruct client to keep fire extinguisher accessible.

   e. Review "Stop, Drop, and Roll."

Equipment

All staff should be alert for potential safety hazards

A. NURSING INTERVENTIONS

1. Electrical equipment must be grounded.

2. Do not overcrowd outlets.

3. The use of extension cords is not permitted in any client care areas.

4. Only use equipment for its intended purpose.

5. Regularly inspect equipment for frayed cords.

6. Disconnect all equipment prior to cleaning.

Chemical Agents and Radiation

Nurses must review institutional guidelines and follow all safety guidelines.

A. NURSING INTERVENTIONS

1. Determine type and amount of radiation used.

2. Place a sign on door: "Caution Radioactive Material."

3. Wear monitoring badge to record amount of exposure.

4. Wear appropriate protective equipment.

5. Dispose of items removed from the room in appropriate containers.

6. Never handle any type of radioactive agent with bare hands.

SECTION 3
Ergonomics and Client Positioning

Lifting and Transfer of Clients

Implement safe care using proper body mechanics when lifting, positioning, transporting, or assisting a client to reduce the risk of injury.

A. NURSING INTERVENTIONS

1. Assess client's mobility and strength.

2. Instruct client to assist when possible.

3. Use mechanical lift and assistive devices.

4. Avoid twisting the thoracic spine or bending at the waist.

5. Use major muscle groups and tighten abdominal muscles.

Client Transfer and Positioning

Maintain safe practices with patient transfer and ensure proper positioning of clients to maintain good body alignment.

A. NURSING INTERVENTIONS

1. Transferring clients from bed to chair or chair to bed

   a. Instruct the client how to assist when possible.

   b. Lower the bed to the lowest setting.

   c. Position the bed or chair so that the client is moving toward the strong side.

   d. Assist the client to stand, then pivot.

2. Repositioning clients in bed

   a. Raise the bed to waist level.

   b. Lower side rails.

   c. Use slide boards or draw sheets.

   d. Have the client fold his arms across his chest while lifting the head.

   e. Proceed in one smooth movement.

   f. Collaborate with other staff members for assistance.

Positioning Clients

Position	Description	Indications
Semi-Fowler's	Head of bed elevated to 30°	Gastric feedings, head injury, postoperative cranial surgery, respiratory illness with dyspnea, postoperative cataract removal, increased intracranial pressure
Fowler's	Head of bed elevated to 45°	Head injury, postoperative cranial surgery, postoperative abdominal surgery, respiratory illness with dyspnea, cardiac problems with dyspnea, bleeding esophageal varices, postoperative thyroidectomy, postoperative cataract removal, increased intracranial pressure
High-Fowler's	Head of bed elevated to 90°	Respiratory illness with dyspnea: emphysema, status asthmaticus, pneumothorax, cardiac problems with dyspnea, feeding, meal times, hiatal hernia, during and after meals
Supine (dorsal recumbent)	Lying on back, head, and shoulders; slightly elevated with a small pillow	Spinal cord injury (no pillow), urinary catheterization
Prone	Lying on abdomen, legs extended, and head turned to the side	Client who is immobilized or unconscious, post lumbar puncture 6 to 12 hr, post myelogram 12 to 24 hr (oil-based dye), postoperative tonsillectomy and adenoidectomy
Lateral (side-lying)	Lying on side with most of the body weight borne by the lateral aspect of the lower ilium	Post abdominal surgery, client who is unconscious, seizures (head to side), postoperative tonsillectomy and adenoidectomy, postoperative pyloric stenosis of the lower scapula and the lateral (right side), post liver biopsy (right side), rectal irrigations

Position	Description	Indications
Sims' (semi-prone)	Lying on left side with most of the body weight borne by the anterior aspect of the ilium, humerus, and clavicle	Client who is unconscious, enemas
Lithotomy	Lying on the back with hips and knees flexed at right angles and feet in stirrups	Perineal procedures, rectal procedures, vaginal procedures
Trendelenburg	Head and body lowered while feet are elevated	Shock
Modified Trendelenburg	Supine with the legs elevated	Prevent shock
Reverse Trendelenburg	Head elevated while feet are lowered	Cervical traction; also used to feed clients restricted to supine position, such as post cardiac catheterization
Elevate one or more extremities	Elevate legs/feet or arms/hands by adjusting or supporting with pillows	Thrombophlebitis, application of cast, edema, postoperative surgical procedure on extremity

SECTION 4

Assistive Devices for Ambulation

Definition: used to provide an extension of the upper extremities to help transmit body weight and provide support for the client (eg, canes, crutches, walkers)

A. Collaborative Care

1. Nursing Interventions
   a. Determine client's mobility status and ability to bear weight per provider's order
   b. Assess client for the need of a safety belt
   c. Instruct client to wear shoes with non-slip soles
   d. Assess client for risk of orthostatic hypotension
   e. Provide safe environment free of clutter

B. Client Education and Referral

1. Avoid rapid position changes to prevent orthostatic hypotension
2. Inspect rubber tips on the device for wear and replace as needed
3. Physical Therapy consult

C. Crutches

1. Assess client for correct fit of crutches: 2-3 finger widths between the axilla and top of the crutch

2. Position hands on crutch pads with elbows flexed (do not bear weight on axilla)

D. Non-weight bearing

1. Begin in the tripod position, maintain weight on the "unaffected" (weight-bearing) extremity

2. Advance both crutches and the affected extremity

3. Move the "unaffected" weight-bearing foot/leg forward (beyond the crutches)

4. Advance both crutches, and then the affected extremity

5. Continue sequence making steps of equal length

E. Weight bearing

1. Move crutches forward about one step's length

2. Move "affected" leg forward; level with the crutch tips

3. Move the "unaffected" leg forward

4. Continue sequence making steps of equal length

F. Walking up stairs

1. Hold to rail with one hand and crutches with the other hand.

2. Push down on the stair rail and the crutches and step up with the "unaffected" leg.

3. If not allowed to place weight on the "affected" leg, hop up with the "unaffected" leg.

4. Bring the "affected" leg and the crutches up beside the "unaffected" leg.

5. Remember, the "unaffected" leg goes up first and the crutches move with the "affected" leg.

G. Walking down stairs

1. Place the "affected" leg and the crutches down on the step below; support weight by leaning on the crutches and the stair rail.

2. Bring the "unaffected" leg down.

3. Remember the "affected" leg goes down first and the crutches move with the "affected" leg.

H. Cane

1. For correct size have the client wear shoes. The correct length is measured from the wrist to the floor.

2. Cane is used on the "unaffected" side to provide support to the opposite lower limb

3. Advance the cane simultaneously with the opposite affected lower limb

4. The "unaffected" lower limb should assume the first full weight-bearing step on level surfaces

I. Walker

1. For correct size have the client wear shoes. The client's wrists are even with the handgrips on the walker when arms are dangling downward

2. Advance the walker approximately 12 inches

3. Advance with the "affected" lower limb

4. Move unaffected limb forward

SECTION 5

Infection Control

All members of the health care team are accountable for adhering to measures to reduce the growth and transmission of infectious agents. According the Centers for Disease Control and Prevention (CDC), "hand hygiene" is the single most important practice in preventing health care associated infections (HAIs).

Medical Asepsis (Clean Technique)

Precise practices to reduce the number, growth, and spread of microorganisms

 A. NURSING INTERVENTIONS

1. Perform hand hygiene frequently.

2. Use personal protective equipment (PPE) as indicated.

3. Do not place items on the floor of client's room.

4. Do not shake linens.

5. Clean least soiled area first.

6. Place moist items in plastic bags.

7. Educate client and caregivers.

Surgical Asepsis (Sterile Technique)

Precise practices to eliminate all microorganisms from an object or area (surgical technique)

 A. NURSING INTERVENTIONS

1. Avoid coughing, sneezing, and talking directly over field.

2. Only dry sterile items touch the field (1-inch border is nonsterile).

3. Keep all objects above the waist.

4. Don sterile gloves to perform procedure.

Isolation Guidelines

A group of actions that include hand hygiene and the use of standard precautions intended to reduce the transmission of infectious organisms

Standard Precautions (Tier One)

Applies to all body fluids, non-intact skin, and mucous membranes

 A. PPE: Gloves, as needed use of mask, gown, and goggles

 B. NURSING INTERVENTIONS

1. Implement standard precautions for all clients.
2. Determine need for client-specific, disease-specific precautions.
3. Provide education to health care team, clients, and visitors.
4. Report communicable diseases (per CDC policy).
5. Handle all blood and body fluids as if contaminated.
6. Use PPE to reduce risk of transmission:
    a. Gown and gloves when touching blood or body fluids, non-intact skin, mucous membranes, or contaminated materials
    b. Masks and face and eye protection when anticipating splashing of body fluids
7. Consider room placement for client safety:
    a. Private room
    b. Cohort (patient must have same organism)
8. Clean equipment according to the facility's policy.
9. Discard all needles and sharps in the appropriate containers; do not recap.
10. Place contaminated linens in the appropriate receptacles per the facility's policy.
11. Clean spills with a solution of bleach and water (1:10 dilution).

Transmission-Based Precautions (Tier Two)

Transmission-based precautions are used in addition to standard precautions for clients who are known or suspected to be infected or colonized with infectious organisms.

A. Airborne Precautions

1. Diseases known to be transmitted by air for infectious agents smaller than 5 mcg (measles, varicella, pulmonary or laryngeal tuberculosis)
2. **PPE: Gloves, MASK** (N95 respirator for known or suspected TB)

 a. **NURSING INTERVENTIONS** (in addition to standard precautions)
1) Provide private room with monitored negative airflow (air exchange and air discharge through HEPA filter).
2) Keep door closed.
3) Respiratory protection:
    a) The nurse must be FIT tested for N95 respirator
    b) Apply a small, particulate mask to that client if leaving room for medical necessity

B. Droplet Precautions

1. Prevent the transmission of pathogens spread through close contact with mucous membranes or respiratory secretions
2. Protect against droplets larger than 5 mcg (streptococcal pharyngitis, pneumonia, scarlet fever, rubella, pertussis, mumps mycoplasma pneumonia, meningococcal pneumonia/sepsis, pneumonic plague)
3. **PPE: Gloves, MASK**

 a. **NURSING INTERVENTIONS** (in addition to standard precautions)
1) Private room preferred, may cohort with client who has infection with same organism.
2) Keep door closed.
3) Mask is required when working within 3 feet of the client.

C. Contact Precautions (includes enteric precautions)

1. Prevent transmission of infectious agents that are spread by direct or indirect contact with the client or the client's environment. These precautions are applied in the presence of wound drainage, fecal incontinence, or other bodily discharges that suggest an increased potential for environmental contamination and risk of transmission.
2. **PPE: Gloves, gown, as needed use of mask and goggles**

 a. **NURSING INTERVENTIONS** (in addition to standard precautions)
1) Private room preferred; may cohort with client who has infection with same organism
2) Gloves and gown worn by caregivers and visitors
3) Disposal of infectious dressing material into nonporous bag
4) Dedicated equipment for the patient or disinfect after each use
5) Client to leave room only for essential clinical reasons

3. Protective Isolation
    a. **Definition:** Used to protect clients who (a) have an increased susceptibility to infections, (b) are receiving chemotherapy, or (c) are immunosuppressed or neutropenic

    b. **NURSING INTERVENTIONS**
    1) Follow standard precautions.
    2) Institute maximum protection, which may include the use of sterile linens, food, and other supplies.
    3) Minimize exposure to microorganisms found on the outer layers of fresh flowers, fruits, and vegetables.
    4) Wear sterile gloves and gown/mask when in contact with client.
    5) Maximum protection will require ventilated/positive pressure room.

Order of PPE Application	Order of PPE Removal
Gown: Cover body from the bottom of the neck to the knees and wrists. Fasten securely behind the neck and at waist.	**Gloves**: Extend arms and slowly peel one glove downward, turning it inside out. With the ungloved hand, slide a finger under the inside portion of the remaining glove, turning inside out, and discard.
Mask: Secure with ties or elastic. Pinch the flexible bridge to secure at nose. Must extend below and under the chin.	**Goggles/face shield**: Grasp the ear pieces or headband only to remove.
Goggles/face shield: Verify fit is secure to prevent slipping off.	**Gown**: Unfasten neck, then waist ties; pull gown forward away from the body, folding it inside out and rolling it into a bundle for disposal.
Gloves: Use correct size for a snug fit. Must extend upward to completely cover the wrist portion of the gown.	**Mask**: Remove by only touching ties. Take care not to touch the front of the mask.

! c. **POINTS TO REMEMBER**

1) Perform frequent hand hygiene.
2) PPE is disposed of in the client's room.
3) Monitor clients for psychosocial needs related to isolation.
4) Only transport client outside of the room as medically necessary.
5) Extend isolation precautions for immunosuppressed clients.
6) CDC recognizes situations may occur necessitating the cohorting of clients; use the following guidelines:
   a) Avoid placing clients on Contact Precautions in the same room with patients who are immunocompromised, have open wounds, or have anticipated prolonged lengths of stay.
   b) Ensure clients are located > 3 feet apart from each other. (Use privacy curtain between beds to minimize opportunities for direct contact.)
   c) Change protective attire and perform hand hygiene between contact with clients in the same room, regardless of disease status.

Precautions Required for Specific Disease Process

Disease/Infectious Agent	Precautions	Duration of Precautions	Reservoir	Nursing Considerations
AIDS/HIV	Standard/contact precautions	Duration of illness	Blood and body fluids including breast milk	Hand hygiene; personal protective equipment if in contact with potentially contaminated materials
Chickenpox (varicella)	Standard/airborne/contact precautions	Until lesions crust over	Lesions, respiratory secretions	Pregnant women and persons who have not had chickenpox or the vaccine should not care for the client
Clostridium difficile	Standard/contact precautions	Duration of illness	Feces	Hand hygiene; personal protective equipment (enteric precautions) if in contact with potentially contaminated materials
Hepatitis A	Standard/contact precautions	Until 7 days after onset of jaundice	Feces	Contact precautions used, particularly for clients wearing diapers or who are incontinent; minimum of 1 week, depending on the client's age
Hepatitis B	Standard/contact precautions	Duration of illness	Blood and body fluids	Contact precautions for blood and body fluids; hand hygiene
Hepatitis C	Standard/contact precautions	Duration of illness	Blood and body fluids	Hand hygiene
Herpes simplex (recurrent oral, skin, genital)	Standard/contact precautions	Until lesions crust over	Fluid from lesions	Horizontal transmission from contact with skin, saliva, and secretions; vertical transmission from mother to child in utero or childbirth

(continues)

Precautions Required for Specific Disease Process (continued)

Disease/Infectious Agent	Precautions	Duration of Precautions	Reservoir	Nursing Considerations
Herpes zoster (shingles) disseminated or localized in clients who are immunocompromised	Standard/airborne/ contact precautions	Duration of illness or with visible lesions	Lesions	Persons who have not had chicken-pox or the vaccine should not provide care
Measles (Rubeola virus)	Standard/airborne precautions	Duration of illness	Respiratory secretions	Virus can live on infected surfaces for up to 2 hours
Meningococcal disease	Standard/droplet	Until therapy continuous 24 hours	Respiratory secretions	Post exposure prophylaxis is recommended to control outbreaks
Methicillin-resistant Staphylococcus aureus (MRSA)	Standard/contact precautions	Duration of illness	Body fluids and sites contaminated with MRSA	Gloves; personal protective equipment including a gown/mask if in contact with site of infection
Pneumonia Standard/droplet		Until culture is negative	Respiratory Secretions	Consider organism specific precautions as indicated
Respiratory syncytial virus	Standard/airborne/ contact precautions	Duration of illness	Respiratory secretions	Contact/droplet precautions; follow established guidelines for administration of Ribavirin
Rotavirus	Standard precautions	Duration of illness	Feces	Contact precautions used, particularly for children who are wearing diapers or incontinent; < 6 years old for duration of illness
Rubella	Standard/droplet	7 days after onset of rash	Respiratory Secretions	Non-immune pregnant women should not care for these clients
Salmonella	Standard/contact precautions	Duration of illness	Feces	Contact precautions used, particularly for children who are wearing diapers or incontinent; < 6 years old for duration of illness
Shigellosis (dysentery)	Standard/contact precautions	Duration of illness	Feces	Contact precautions used, particularly for children who are wearing diapers or incontinent; < 6 years old for duration of illness
Staphylococcus aureus (infection or colonization)	Standard/contact precautions	Duration of illness	Body fluids and sites contaminated with MRSA	Gloves; personal protective equipment including gown/mask if in contact with site of infection
Tuberculosis (TB) (pulmonary)	Standard/airborne precautions	Until three sputum smears are negative or TB is ruled out	Airborne respiratory droplet nuclei	Special particulate mask; client wears surgical mask when transported outside of negative-airflow room
Vancomycin-resistant enterococci (VRE) (infection or colonization)	Standard/contact precautions	Until three negative cultures from infectious site (1 week apart)	Stool, body sites from which VRE is isolated	Hand hygiene and gloves; gowns if in contact with contaminated material

Health Promotion and Disease Prevention

Nurses contribute greatly to the health of clients and population groups using health promotion and disease prevention strategies. Nursing care of the client incorporates knowledge of early detection of disease and actions to promote optimal health.

Health Promotion

Includes client education, health risk assessment, wellness assessment, lifestyle and behavior changes, and environmental control programs

Health Promotion and Disease Prevention

Preventive Care	Examples of Prevention Activities
Primary prevention: Focus is on promoting health and preventing disease.	• Immunization programs • Child car seat education • Nutrition and fitness activities • Health education programs
Secondary prevention: Focus is on early identification of illness, providing treatment, and conducting activities geared to prevent a worsening health status.	• Communicable disease screening and case finding • Early detection and treatment of hypertension • Exercise programs for older adults who are frail
Tertiary prevention: Focus is on preventing long-term consequences of chronic illness or disability and supporting optimal functioning.	• Prevention of pressure ulcers as a complication of spinal cord injury • Promoting independence for a client following stroke

Disease Prevention

 A. NURSING INTERVENTIONS

1. Conduct a risk factor assessment.
2. Educate clients to follow standards for recommended screenings.
3. Identify lifestyle risk behaviors requiring modification.
4. Encourage client to continue health-promoting behaviors.
5. Instruct client about preventive immunizations.

Screening Guidelines[*]

Test	Female	Male
Routine physical	Begin age 20 Every 1–3 years Annually at age 40	Begin age 20 Every 5 years Annually at age 40
Dental assessments	Every 6 months	Every 6 months
Blood pressure	Begin age 20 Minimum every 2 years	Begin age 20 Minimum every 2 years
Body mass index (BMI)	Begin age 20 Each health care visit	Begin age 20 Each health care visit
Blood cholesterol	Begin age 20 Minimum every 5 years	Begin age 20 Minimum every 5 years
Blood glucose	Begin age 45 Minimum every 3 years	Begin age 45 Minimum every 3 years
Colorectal screening	Fecal occult blood annually begin age 50 **AND** Flexible sigmoidoscopy every 5 years[*], or • Colonoscopy every 10 years, or • Double-contrast barium enema every 5 years[*], or • CT colonography (virtual colonoscopy) every 5 years **NOTE: Frequency may increase based upon results.**	Fecal occult blood annually begin age 50 **AND** Flexible sigmoidoscopy every 5 years[*], or • Colonoscopy every 10 years, or • Double-contrast barium enema every 5 years[*], or • CT colonography (virtual colonoscopy) every 5 years **NOTE: Frequency may increase based upon results.**
Pap test	Annually, start age 21 (earlier if sexually active) Every 1–2 years	
Clinical breast exam	Begin age 20, every 3 years Begin age 40, yearly	
Mammogram	Begin age 40, yearly	
Prostate-specific antigen test and digital rectal exam		Begin age 50 or as indicated by provider

[*]American Diabetes Association, American Heart Association and American Cancer Society

UNIT THREE

Adult Medical-Surgical Nursing

SECTION 1

Review of Fluids and Electrolytes

Fluids and Electrolytes

Nurses should review the client's health history and laboratory data and perform clinical assessment. Many health problems can cause changes in balance of fluids and electrolytes. The nurse is prepared to manage the client with imbalances.

A. Body Fluids

1. Adults
    a. Women: 50 to 55% body weight is water
    b. Men: 60 to 70% body weight is water
    c. Older adults: 47% body weight is water
2. Infants: 75 to 80% body weight is water
3. Intracellular: 80% of total body water
4. Extracellular: 20% of total body water

NOTE: 1 kilogram (2.2 lb) of body weight is approximate to 1 liter of fluid.

Fluid Imbalance

A. Fluid Volume Deficit (FVD)

1. Definition: Includes hypovolemia-isotonic (loss of H_2O and electrolytes from ECF) and dehydration-osmolar (loss of H_2O, no electrolyte loss)
2. Contributing Factors
    a. Excess GI loss
    b. Diaphoresis
    c. Fever
    d. Excess renal loss
    e. Hemorrhage
    f. Insufficient intake
    g. Age-related changes
3. Manifestations
    a. Weight loss/poor skin turgor
    b. Dry mucus membranes
    c. Increased heart rate and respirations
    d. Hyperthermia
    e. Capillary refill > 3 sec
    f. Weakness, fatigue
    g. LATE SIGNS: Oliguria, decreased CVP, flattened neck veins
    h. Laboratory data (due to hemoconcentration)
        1) Elevated Hct
        2) Elevated urine specific gravity and osmolarity
4. Diagnostic Procedures
    a. Serum: electrolytes, BUN, creatinine, Hct
    b. Urine: specific gravity and osmolarity

5. Collaborative Care

NURSING INTERVENTIONS

   a. Assess vital signs.
   b. Assess skin turgor.
   c. Maintain strict I&O.
   d. Weigh client daily.
   e. Assess laboratory data.
   f. Replace fluids orally.
   g. Initiate and maintain IV therapy as ordered.
   h. Correct underlying cause.

B. Medications

1. Electrolyte replacement
2. Intravenous fluids

Intravenous Fluids

Isotonic	Hypotonic	Hypertonic
Indication: treatment of vascular system fluid deficit	**Indication**: treatment of intracellular dehydration	**Indication**: used only when serum osmolality is critically low
Characteristics: • Concentration equal to plasma • Prevent fluid shift between compartments	**Characteristics:** • Lower osmolality than the ECF • Shift fluid from ECF to ICF	**Characteristics:** • Osmolality higher than the ECF • Shift fluid from ICF to ECF
Isotonic Solutions: • Normal saline (0.9% NS) • Ringer's lactate solution (RL) • 5% dextrose in water (D_5W)	**Hypotonic Solutions:** • 0.45% normal saline (0.45% NS) • 2.5% dextrose in 0.45% saline ($D_{2.5}$ 45% NS)	**Hypertonic Solutions:** • 10% dextrose in water ($D_{10}W$) • 50% dextrose in water ($D_{50}W$) • 5% dextrose in 0.9% saline (D_5NS) • 5% dextrose in 0.45% saline (D_5W in 0.45% NaCL) • 5% dextrose in Ringer's lactate (D_5LR)

C. Fluid Volume Excess (FVE)

1. **Definition:** Includes hypervolemia-isotonic (water and sodium retained in abnormally high proportions) and overhydration-osmolar (more water gained than electrolytes)
2. Contributing Factors
    a. Abnormal renal function
    b. Heart failure
    c. Hepatic failure
    d. Interstitial to plasma fluid shifts (hypertonic fluids, burns)

e. Excessive sodium intake

f. Age-related changes

g. Water replacement without electrolyte replacement

h. Excess intake of hypotonic fluid

3. Manifestations

a. Cough, dyspnea, crackles

b. Increased blood pressure, pulse rate/amplitude, and respirations

c. Headache

d. Weight gain (1 L of water = 1 kg of weight)

e. Hemodilution of Hct and electrolytes

f. LATE signs: JVD, tachycardia, pitting edema, increased CVP

4. Diagnostic Procedures

a. Serum: electrolytes, BUN, creatinine, Hct

b. Urine: specific gravity and osmolarity

c. Chest x-ray if respiratory complications present

5. Collaborative Care

a. Assess respiratory rate, symmetry, and effort.

b. Assess breath sounds.

c. Assess for edema.

d. Assess for ascites, and measure abdominal girth.

e. Monitor I&O and vitals signs.

f. Weigh the client daily.

g. Administer diuretics (osmotic, loop) as prescribed.

h. Limit fluid intake.

i. Provide frequent skin care.

j. Use semi-Fowler's position; reposition every 2 hours.

Electrolyte Imbalances

A. Electrolytes

1. Extracellular

a. Na^+ 135 to 145 mEq/L

b. Ca^{++} 8.5 to 10 mg/dL

c. Cl^- 85 to 115 mEq/L

d. HCO_3^- 22 to 26 mEq/L

2. Intracellular

a. K^+ 3.5 to 5.0 mEq/L

b. PO_4 2.5 to 4.5 mg/dL

c. Mg^+ 1.8 to 3.0 mEq/L

B. Function

1. Maintain homeostasis

2. Promote neuromuscular excitability

3. Maintain fluid volume

4. Distribute water between fluid compartments

5. Maintain cardiac stability

6. Regulate acid-base balance

Major Electrolytes: Imbalance/Interventions

Electrolyte/Imbalance	Manifestations	Interventions
Potassium (K⁺)		
Hypokalemia **Risk factors:** • GI loss • Diuretics • Aminoglycosides • ↓ intake	**K⁺ < 3.5 mEq/L** • Muscle weakness, fatigue • Nausea and vomiting • Dysrhythmias • Flat T waves (ECG)	• ECG monitor • Administer K⁺ • Teach dietary sources of K⁺ **NOTE: NEVER give K⁺ IV bolus; MUST dilute.** **NOTE: "No P = No K."**
Hyperkalemia **Risk factors:** • Tissue injury • K⁺-sparing diuretics • Renal failure • Adrenal insufficiency • ↑ intake	**K⁺ > 5.0 mEq/L** • Muscle cramps, weakness, paralysis • Bradycardia • Dysrhythmias • Tall T waves (ECG)	• ECG monitor • Kayexalate • 50% glucose with insulin • Calcium gluconate • Loop diuretics • Dialysis **NOTE: BS assessment with Kayexalate**

(continues)

Major Electrolytes: Imbalance/Interventions (continued)

Electrolyte/Imbalance	Manifestations	Interventions
Sodium (Na⁺)		

Hyponatremia **Risk factors:**
• GI loss
• SIADH
• Adrenal insufficiency
• Diuretics
• Water intoxication
• ↓ intake
	Na⁺ < 135 mEq/L
	• Weakness
	• Lethargy
	• Confusion
	• Seizures
	• Coma
		• Daily weight
		• Assess CNS changes
		• I&O
		• Administer IVF:
		  – hypertonic (acute)
		  – isotonic (restore volume)
		• Seizure precautions
		• Teach sodium-rich food
		• If etiology is FVE, restrict fluids
		
		NOTE: Risk with hypertonic solutions— cerebral edema

Hypernatremia **Risk factors:** • Water deficit • GI loss • DI • ↑ intake	**Na⁺ > 145 mEq/L** • Thirst, dry mucous membranes • Restless, weak • Orthostatic hypotension • Muscle irritability, seizures • Coma	• Daily weight • Assess CNS changes • I&O • Administer IVF: – isotonic (restore volume) • Seizure precautions • Teach food sources
Calcium (Ca⁺⁺)		
Hypocalcemia **Risk factors:** • Hypoparathyroidism • Hypomagnesemia • Renal failure • Vitamin D deficiency • Loop diuretics • Phenytoin	**Ca⁺⁺ < 8.5 mg/dL** • Tetany, cramps • Paresthesias • Dysrhythmias • Trousseau's sign • Chvostek's sign • Seizures	• Seizure precautions • IV calcium replacement • Daily calcium supplements **NOTE: Calcium has inverse relationship with phosphorus**
Hypercalcemia **Risk factors:** • Hyperparathyroidism • Malignant disease • Prolonged immobilization • Vitamin D excess • Thiazide diuretics • Lithium	**Ca⁺⁺ > 8.5 mg/dL** • Muscle weakness • Decreased DTRs • Hypercalciuria/renal stones • Dysrhythmias • Confusion • Anxiety • Lethargy/coma	• Increase mobility • Isotonic IVF • Furosemide • Calcitonin • Glucocorticoids • Biosphosphonates **NOTE: Increase risk of fractures**
Magnesium (Mg⁺⁺)		
Hypomagnesemia **Risk factors:** • GI loss • Alcoholism • Diuretics • Pancreatitis • Hypocalcemia • Hypokalemia • Insulin resistance • DKA	**Magnesium < 1.8 mEq/L** • Tetany, cramps • Increased DTRs • Paresthesias • Dysrhythmias • Trousseau's sign • Chvostek's sign • Agitation, confusion	• Seizure precautions • Assess for difficulty swallowing • Correct underlying cause • IV magnesium • Teach food sources **NOTE: Monitor for signs of magnesium toxicity with IV replacement and treat with calcium.**

Major Electrolytes: Imbalance/Interventions (continued)

Electrolyte/Imbalance	Manifestations	Interventions
Hypermagnesemia **Risk factors:** • Renal failure • Excessive Mg++ therapy • Adrenal insufficiency • Laxative abuse	**Magnesium > 3.0 mEq/L** • Hypotension • Drowsiness • Decreased DTRs • Bradycardia • Bradypnea • Coma • Cardiac arrest	• Decrease intake • IV calcium gluconate • Mechanical ventilation • Temporary pacemaker
Phosphorus		
Hypophosphatemia **Risk factors:** • Alcoholism • Chronic diarrhea • Starvation • Vitamin D deficiency	**Phosphorus < 2.5 mg/dL** • Muscle weakness • Decreased DTRs • Hypercalciuria/renal stones • Dysrhythmias • Confusion • Anxiety • Lethargy/coma	• Correct etiology • Oral phosphate replacement • Vitamin D • Decrease calcium level
Hyperphosphatemia **Risk factors:** • Renal failure • Chemotherapy • High vitamin D • High phosphorus intake • Excessive enema use (Fleet's)	**Phosphorus > 4.5 mg/dL** • Tetany, cramps • Paresthesias • Dysrhythmias • Trousseau's sign • Chvostek's sign • Seizures	• Aluminum hydroxide (with meals) • Decrease dialysis (RF) **NOTE:** Phosphorus has inverse relationship with calcium.

Acid-Base Balance

A. Definition: Acid-base imbalances range from simple to complex. The four basic imbalances include:

Imbalance	pH	PCO₂	HCO₃
Normal value	7.35–7.45	35–45 mm Hg	22–26 mEq/L
Metabolic acidosis	↓	Normal	↓
Metabolic alkalosis	↑	Normal	↑
Respiratory acidosis	↓	↑	Normal
Respiratory alkalosis	↑	↓	Normal

B. ROME: "Respiratory Opposite Metabolic Equal"

C. Regulation of acid-base balance is primarily controlled by:
1. Lungs (regulate carbonic acid through respiration)
2. Kidneys (regulate bicarbonate by retention or excretion)

Acid-Base Imbalances

Imbalance	Manifestations	Interventions
Metabolic acidosis **Risk factors:** • Diarrhea • Fever • Hypoxia • Starvation • Seizure • Overdose: salicylates or ethanol • Renal Failure	• VS: bradycardia, weak pulses, hypotension, tachypnea • Flaccid paralysis • Confusion	• Treat underlying cause • Administer fluids, electrolytes
Metabolic alkalosis **Risk factors:** • Ingestion of antacids • GI suction • Hypokalemia • TPN • Blood transfusion	• Dizziness • Paresthesias • Hypertonic muscles • Decreased respirations	• Treat underlying cause • Administer fluids, electrolytes

(continues)

Acid-Base Imbalances (continued)

Imbalance	Manifestations	Interventions
Respiratory acidosis **Risk factors:** • Respiratory depression • Pneumothorax • Airway obstruction • Inadequate ventilation	• Dizziness • Palpitations • Muscle twitching • Convulsions	• Maintain patent airway • Reversal agents for narcotics • Regulation ventilation therapy • Bronchodilators • Mucolytics
Respiratory alkalosis **Risk factors:** • Hyperventilation • Hypoxemia • Altitude sickness • Asphyxiation • Asthma • Pneumonia	• Tachypnea • Anxiety, tetany • Paresthesias • Palpitations • Chest pain	• Regulate Oxygen therapy • Reduce anxiety • Rebreathing techniques

SECTION 2

Review of Respiratory System Alterations

The respiratory system includes upper airways, lungs, lower airways and alveolar air sacs (base of lungs). The lungs aid the body in oxygenation and tissue perfusion.

Diagnostic Tests for Respiratory Disorders

A. Noninvasive Procedures

1. Chest x-ray (CXR) (Use lead shield for adults of childbearing age.)
2. Pulse oximetry
3. Pulmonary function tests
4. Sputum culture

B. Invasive Procedures

1. Arterial blood gas (ABGs via arterial puncture or arterial line) allows the most accurate method of assessing respiratory function

   a. Perform Allen test if no arterial line.

   b. Sample is drawn into heparinized syringe.

   c. Keep on ice and transport to laboratory immediately.

   d. Document amount and method of oxygen delivered for accurate results.

   e. Apply direct pressure to puncture site 5–10 minutes (longer for clients at risk for bleeding).

2. Bronchoscopy: visualize larynx, trachea, bronchi; obtain tissue biopsy

   a. Informed consent

   b. NPO 8–12 hours

   c. Local anesthetic throat spray

   d. Position upright

   e. Sedation

   f. Observe postprocedure:
      1) Gag reflex
      2) Bleeding
      3) Respiratory status

3. Mantoux test: positive test indicates exposure to tuberculosis. Diagnosis must be confirmed with sputum culture for presence of acid-fast bacillus (AFB).

   a. Administer 0.1 mL of purified protein derivation intradermal to upper ⅓ inner surface of forearm (insert needle bevel up).

   b. Assess for reaction in 48–72 hours; induration if 10 mm or greater is positive test.

4. QuantiFERON®-TB Gold In-Tube test (QFT-GIT) and T-SPOT®.TB: Identify the presence of *Mycobacterium tuberculosis* infection by measuring the immune response to the TB bacteria in whole blood

5. Thoracentesis: Surgical perforation of the pleural space to obtain specimen, or to remove fluid or air

   a. Informed consent

   b. Educate client: remain still, feeling of pressure, positioning

   c. Position upright

   d. Monitor vital signs

   e. Label specimens

   f. Chest tube at bedside

Disorders of the Respiratory System: Airflow Problems

A. **Asthma:** Chronic inflammatory disorder of the airways resulting in intermittent and reversible airflow obstruction of the bronchioles

1. Contributing Factors

   a. Extrinsic: antigen–antibody reaction triggered by food, medications, or inhaled substances

   b. Intrinsic: pathophysiological abnormalities within the respiratory tract

   c. Older clients: beta receptors are less responsive to agonist and trigger bronchospasms

2. Manifestations

   a. Sudden, severe dyspnea with use of accessory muscles

   b. Sitting up, leaning forward

   c. Diaphoresis and anxiety

   d. Wheezing, gasping

   e. Coughing

   f. Cyanosis (late sign)

   g. Barrel chest

3. Diagnostic Procedures

    a. ABGs

    b. Sputum cultures

    c. Pulmonary function tests

4. Collaborative Care

 a. **NURSING INTERVENTIONS**

    1) Remain with the client during the attack.

    2) Position in high Fowler's.

    3) Assess lung sounds and pulse oximetry.

    4) Administer oxygen therapy.

    5) Maintain IV access.

  b. Medications

    1) Bronchodilators

      a) Short-acting inhaled: Proventil, Ventolin for rapid relief

      b) Methylxanthines: theophylline (Theo-Dur); monitor therapeutic range for toxicity

  c. Anti-inflammatory

    a) Corticosteroids: fluticasone (Flovent) and prednisone (Deltasone)

    b) Leukotriene antagonsists: montelukast (Singulair)

    1) Combination agents

      a) Ipratropium and albuterol (Combivent)

      b) Fluticasone and salmeterol (Advair)

NOTE: With inhaled agents, administer bronchodilators BEFORE anti-inflammatory medication.

  d. Therapeutic Measures

    1) Respiratory treatments

    2) Oxygen administration

  e. Client Education and Referral

    1) Avoidance of allergens and triggers

    2) Proper use of inhaler

B. Status Asthmaticus

1. **Definition:** A life-threatening episode of airway obstruction that is often unresponsive to treatment

2. Manifestations

    a. Extreme wheezing

    b. Labored breathing

    c. Use of accessory muscles

    d. Distended neck veins

    e. High risk for cardiac and/or respiratory arrest

 3. **NURSING INTERVENTIONS**

    a. Place in high Fowler's.

    b. Prepare for emergency intubation.

    c. Administer oxygen, epinephrine, and systemic steroid as prescribed.

    d. Provide emotional support.

C. Chronic Obstructive Pulmonary Disease (COPD) encompasses pulmonary emphysema and chronic bronchitis. COPD is not reversible.

1. Pulmonary emphysema

  a. **Definition:** destruction of alveoli, narrowing of bronchioles, and trapping of air resulting in loss of lung elasticity

    1) Contributing Factors

      a) Cigarette smoking (main causative factor)

      b) Advanced age

      c) Exposure to air pollution

      d) Alpha-antitrypsin deficiency (inability to break down pollutants)

    2) Manifestations

      a) Dyspnea with productive cough

      b) Difficult exhalation, use of pursed-lip breathing

      c) Wheezing, crackles

      d) Barrel chest with clubbed fingernails

      e) Shallow, rapid respirations

      f) Respiratory acidosis with hypoxia

      g) Anorexia, weight loss

      h) Weakness

2. Chronic bronchitis

  a. **Definition:** inflammation of the bronchi and bronchioles caused by chronic exposure to irritants

  b. Contributing Factors

    1) Cigarette smoking (main causative factor)

    2) Exposure to air pollution

  c. Manifestations

    1) Productive cough

    2) Thick, tenacious sputum

    3) Hypoxemia

    4) Respiratory acidosis

  d. Diagnostic Procedures for COPD

    1) Chest x-ray shows consolidation

    2) Pulmonary function tests: stale air remains trapped in lungs

    3) Pulse oximetry: often < 90%

    4) ABGs: chronic respiratory acidosis

  e. Collaborative Care

    1) **NURSING INTERVENTIONS**

      a) Assess respiratory effort.

      b) Assess cardiac status for signs of right-sided failure.

      c) Position upright and leaning forward.

      d) Schedule activities to allow for frequent rest periods.

      e) Administer low-flow oxygen therapy (maximum is 3 L).

      f) Use incentive spirometry.

      g) Encourage fluids 3 L per day.

h) Encourage high-calorie diet (increased protein, decreased carbohydrates).

i) Provide emotional support.

2) Medications

a) Bronchodilators

b) Methylxanthines

c) Anti-inflammatory agents

d) Mucolytic agents

3) Therapeutic Measures

a) Chest physiotherapy/pulmonary drainage

b) Lung reduction surgery

4) Client Education and Referral

a) Breathing techniques

b) Portable oxygen therapy

c) Medications

d) Nutrition

e) Promote smoking cessation

f) Avoid crowds

g) Encourage immunizations for pneumonia and influenza

h) Pulmonary rehabilitation

3. Complications of COPD

a. Cor pulmonale: right-sided heart failure caused by pulmonary disease

1) Manifestations

a) Hypoxia and hypoxemia

b) Extreme dyspnea

c) Cyanotic lips

d) JVD

e) Dependent edema

f) Metabolic and respiratory acidosis

g) Pulmonary hypertension

2) Collaborative Care

 a) **NURSING INTERVENTIONS**

(1) Monitor for respiratory distress.

(2) Monitor oxygen therapy and oximetry.

(3) Ensure adequate rest periods.

(4) Encourage low-sodium diet.

b) Medications

(1) Diuretics

(2) Digoxin

c) Therapeutic Measures

(1) Mechanical ventilation

D. Carbon Dioxide Toxicity: Stuporous secondary to increased CO$_2$ retention

1. Contributing Factors

a. Carbon dioxide retention

b. Excessive oxygen delivery

2. Manifestations

a. Drowsiness, irritability

b. Hallucinations

c. Convulsions and coma

d. Tachycardia with dysrhythmias

3. Collaborative Care

a. Monitor pulse oximetry and ABGs.

b. Avoid excessive concentrations of oxygen: below 3 L/min (Cannula 40%, mask 60%, nonrebreather 100%).

c. Administer CPAP or BiPAP.

E. Pneumonia

1. **Definition:** An inflammatory process in the lungs that produces excess fluid and exudate that fill the alveoli; classified as bacterial, viral, fungal, or chemical

2. Contributing Factors

a. Older adult

b. Chronic lung disease

c. Immunocompromised

d. Mechanical ventilation

e. Postoperative

f. Prolonged immobility

g. Tobacco use

3. Manifestations

a. Tachypnea and tachycardia

b. Sudden onset of chills, fever, flushing

c. Productive cough

d. Dyspnea with pleuritic pain

e. Crackles

f. Elevated WBC

g. Decreased O$_2$ saturation

4. Diagnostic Procedures

a. Chest x-ray

b. Pulse oximetry

c. Sputum culture

5. Collaborative Care

 a. **NURSING INTERVENTIONS**

1) Assess respiratory pattern and effort.

2) Administer oxygen.

3) Assess sputum.

4) Monitor vital signs.

5) Encourage fluids to 3 L/day.

6) Provide pulmonary toilet.

7) Encourage mouth care.

b. Medications

1) Anti-infectives

2) Cough suppressants

3) Bronchodilators

4) Anti-inflammatories

c. Client Education

1) Medication administration

2) Preventive measures

3) Pneumonia vaccine

F. Tuberculosis

1. **Definition:** A highly communicable infectious disease caused by *Mycobacterium tuberculosis* and transmitted through aerosolization (airborne route)

2. Contributing Factors

    a. Older and homeless populations

    b. Lower SES

    c. Foreign immigrants

    d. Those in frequent contact with untreated persons

    e. Long-term care facilities

    f. Prisons

3. Manifestations

    a. Cough, hemoptysis

    b. Positive sputum culture for AFB

    c. Fever with night sweats

    d. Anorexia, weight loss

    e. Malaise, fatigue

4. Diagnostic Procedures

    a. Screening test: Mantoux

    b. Sputum culture and smear

    c. Serum analysis, QuantiFERON-TB Gold (QFT-G)

    d. Chest x-ray

5. Collaborative Care

     a. **NURSING INTERVENTIONS**

    1) Initiate airborne isolation precautions.
    2) Obtain sputum sample before administering medications.
    3) Maintain adequate nutritional status.
    4) Teach the client to avoid foods containing tyramine.
    5) The nurse should wear a particulate mask when entering the client's room.
    6) Isolate the client in a negative pressure room.

    b. Medications: Combination drug therapy

    1) Administer medications on an empty stomach at the same time every day.
    2) Medications should be taken for 6 to 12 months, as directed.
    3) Instruct the client to watch for signs and symptoms of hepatotoxicity, and notify a primary care provider of signs of nephrotoxicity, and visual changes.
    4) Medications to treat TB:
        a) Isoniazid (INH)
        b) Rifampin
        c) Pyrazinamide
        d) Streptomycin
        e) Ethambutol

    c. Client Education and Referral

    1) Encourage the client to practice good hand hygiene and to always cover his nose and mouth when sneezing or coughing.
    2) Ensure medication compliance and follow-up care.

6. Cases of diagnosed TB are reported to local or state health department.

    a. Refer all high-risk clients to local health department for testing and prophylactic treatment regimen.

G. Laryngeal Cancer

1. Definition: Malignant cells occurring in the mucosal tissue of the larynx; more common in men between the ages of 55 and 70

2. Contributing Factors

    a. Smoking

    b. Radiation exposure

    c. Chronic laryngitis and/or straining of vocal cords

3. Manifestations

    a. Hoarseness extending longer than 2 weeks

    b. Dysphagia

    c. Dyspnea

    d. Cough

    e. Gray, dark brown or black color of tongue

    f. Hard, immobile lymph nodes in neck

    g. Weight loss, anorexia

4. Diagnostic Procedures

    a. MRI

    b. Direct laryngoscopy with biopsy

    c. X-ray and CT

    d. Bone scan

5. Collaborative Care

     a. **NURSING INTERVENTIONS**

    1) Maintain patent airway
    2) Swallowing precautions
    3) Emotional support
    4) Nutrition
    5) Pain management
    6) Administer medications as elixir when possible

    b. Therapeutic Measures

    1) Partial or total laryngectomy

    c. Client Education and Referral

    1) Communication method
    2) Stoma care
    3) Swallowing

6. Speech therapy

H. Lung Cancer

1. **Definition:** Leading cause of cancer-related deaths for both men and women in the U.S.; primary or metastatic disease; most commonly occurs between the ages of 45 and 70 years

2. Contributing Factors

    a. Smoking (first- and secondhand smoke)

    b. Radiation exposure

    c. Chronic exposure to inhaled irritants

    d. Older adult

3. Manifestations

    a. Chronic cough

    b. Chronic dyspnea

    c. Hemoptysis

    d. Hoarseness

    e. Unilateral wheezing

    f. Fatigue, weight loss, anorexia

    g. Clubbing of fingers

    h. Chest wall pain

4. Diagnostic Procedures

    a. Chest x-ray and computed tomography (CT) scan

    b. Bronchoscopy with biopsy

    c. TNM system for staging

      1) **T**umor

      2) **N**odes

      3) **M**etastasis

5. Collaborative Care

     a. **NURSING INTERVENTIONS**

      1) Maintain patent airway.

      2) Suction PRN.

      3) Monitor vital signs and pulse oximetry.

      4) Monitor nutritional status.

      5) Position high Fowler's.

      6) Provide emotional support.

      7) Assess and treat stomatitis.

      8) Ensure protection for immunocompromised client.

    b. Medications

      1) Chemotherapeutic agents

      2) Opioid narcotics

    c. Therapeutic Measures

      1) Palliative care

        a) Medication

        b) Thoracentesis

      2) Surgical

        a) Tumor excision

        b) Pneumonectomy, lobectomy, wedge resection

    d. Client Education and Referral

      1) Medications

      2) Constipation

3) Mouth care

4) Nutrition

6. Respiratory services

7. Radiology

8. Rehabilitation

9. Nutrition

10. Hospice

Respiratory Emergencies

A. Pulmonary Embolism

1. **Definition:** A life-threatening hypoxic condition caused by a collection of particulate matter (blood clot, air, fat) that enters venous circulation and lodges in the pulmonary vessels causing pulmonary blood flow obstruction

2. Contributing Factors

    a. Chronic atrial fibrillation

    b. Hypercoagulability

    c. Long bone fracture

    d. Long-term immobility

    e. Oral contraceptive or estrogen therapy

    f. Obesity

    g. Postoperative

    h. PVD

    i. Sickle cell anemia

3. Manifestations

    a. Tachypnea

    b. Tachycardia

    c. Diaphoresis

    d. Decreased SaO_2

    e. Pleural effusion

    f. Crackles and cough

    g. Pleurisy

NOTE: Petechial rash is present with fat embolus.

4. Diagnostic Procedures

    a. ABGs

    b. D-dimer

    c. Chest x-ray

    d. V/Q scan

    e. Pulmonary angiography

5. Collaborative Care

     a. **NURSING INTERVENTIONS**

      1) Provide oxygen therapy.

      2) Position in high Fowler's.

      3) Initiate IV access.

      4) Provide emotional support.

    b. Medications

      1) Thrombolytics

      2) Anticoagulants

c. Therapeutic Measures
  1) Embolectomy
  2) Vena cava filter
d. Client Education and Referral
  1) Preventive measures
  2) Dietary precautions with vitamin K
  3) Follow-up for PT or INR
  4) Bleeding precautions
6. Cardiology and pulmonary services
  a. Respiratory care

B. Respiratory Emergencies

1. Pneumothorax
  a. **Definition:** A collection of air or gas in the chest or pleural space that causes part or all of a lung to collapse due to a loss of negative pressure
2. Hemothorax
  a. Definition: Accumulation of blood in the pleural cavity
3. Contributing Factors
  a. Blunt chest trauma
  b. COPD
  c. Closed/occluded chest tube
  d. Older adults
  e. Penetrating chest wounds
4. Manifestations
  a. Respiratory distress
  b. Tracheal deviation to unaffected side (tension pneumothorax)
  c. Reduced or absent breath sound (affected side)
  d. Asymmetrical chest wall movement
  e. Hyperresonance on percussion due to trapped air (pneumothorax)
  f. Subcutaneous emphysema
5. Diagnostic Procedures
  a. Chest x-ray
  b. Thoracentesis (hemothorax)
6. Collaborative Care
   a. **NURSING INTERVENTIONS**
  1) Administer oxygen.
  2) Position in high Fowler's.
  3) Monitor chest tube and dressing.
  4) Provide emotional support.
  b. Therapeutic Measures
  1) Chest tube insertion
    a) Chest tube: inserted to pleural space for draining fluid, blood, or air; reestablishes a negative pressure; facilitates lung expansion
    (1) Position supine or semi-Fowler's.
    (2) Verify consent form is signed.

(3) Prepare chest drainage system prior to insertion.
(4) Administer pain and sedation medication as ordered.
(5) Apply dressing to insertion site.
(6) Maintain chest tube system.
(7) Monitor respiratory status and pulse oximetry.
(8) Monitor for complications.

Chest Tube Complication	Nursing Interventions
Air leak (continuous rapid bubbling in the water seal chamber)	1. Start at the chest and move down tubing to locate leak; tighten connection or replace drainage system. 2. Keep connection taped securely.
No tidaling in water seal chamber	1. Assess for kinks in the tubing. 2. Assess breath sounds (lungs re-expanded).
No bubbling in suction control chamber	1. Verify tubing is attached. 2. Verify water is filled to prescribed level. 3. Increase wall suction regulator.
Chest tube is disconnected from system	Insert open end of the chest tube into sterile water until system can be replaced.
Chest tube accidentally pulled from patient	1. Cover insertion site with gauze 4 × 4. **NOTE: Tape 3 sides.** 2. Contact physician. 3. Prepare for reinsertion.

Airway Management

A. Oxygen Therapy is used in many acute and chronic respiratory problems to improve cellular oxygenation and prevent hypoxia or hypoxemia.

  1. Clinical Manifestations (hypoxia and hypoxemia)

Early	Late
Tachypnea	Bradypnea
Tachycardia	Bradycardia
Restlessness	Confusion and stupor
Pale skin and mucous membranes	Cyanotic skin and mucous membranes
Elevated blood pressure	Hypotension
Use of accessory muscles, nasal flaring, adventitious lung sounds	Cardiac dysrhythmias

2. Collaborative Care

Oxygen Delivery Devices

Device	FiO$_2$/Flow Rate
Nasal cannula	24–44% at 1–6 L/min
Simple face mask	24–44% at 1–6 L/min
Partial rebreather mask	60–70% at 6–11 L/min
Non-rebreather mask	80–95% at 10–15 L/min
Venturi mask	24–55% at 2–10L/min
Aerosol mask, face tent	24–100% at least 10 L/min
T-piece	24–100% at least 10 L/min

3. Client Education

    a. Assess for electrical hazards.

    b. Post "oxygen in use sign."

    c. Wear cotton gown.

    d. No smoking.

B. Suctioning

1. **Definition:** Use of a suction machine and catheter to remove secretions from the airway

2. Clinical Manifestations (indicating a need for suctioning)

    a. Restlessness

    b. Tachypnea

    c. Tachycardia

    d. Decreased SaO$_2$

    e. Adventitious breath sounds

    f. Visualization of secretions

    g. Absence of spontaneous cough

3. Collaborative Care

    a. Perform hand hygiene.

    b. Don required PPE.

    c. Position patient to semi or high Fowler's.

    d. Obtain baseline breath sounds, VS, and SaO$_2$.

    e. Use medical aseptic technique (oral suction).

    f. Use surgical aseptic technique for all other types.

    g. Hyperoxygenate patient.

    h. Suction 10–15 seconds (rotating motion); limit to 2–3 attempts.

    i. Allow recovery between attempts (20–30 seconds).

C. Tracheostomy Care

1. **Definition:** Care of a tracheostomy to maintain a patent airway and optimal ventilation

2. Collaborative Care

    a. Explain the procedure.

    b. Position patient in semi or high Fowler's.

    c. At all times, keep two extra tracheostomy tubes (one size is the client's size and one is a smaller size) at the bedside in the event of accidental decannulation.

    d. Suction client only as clinically indicated (never on routine schedule).

    e. Assess for respiratory distress.

    f. Provide tracheostomy care every 8 hours.

    g. Change tracheostomy tubes every 6 to 8 weeks or per protocol.

3. Client Education and Referral

    a. Tracheostomy care

    b. Prevention of respiratory infections

    c. Nutrition

4. Home health care agency

5. Community support group

SECTION 3

Review of Perioperative Care

A. Preoperative Phase: Procedures or teaching completed prior to a surgical procedure to reduce potential complications, reduce postoperative discomfort, relieve client anxiety, and increase client participation.

1. **Definition of preoperative:** Care of the client before surgery

2. Collaborative Care

    a. **NURSING INTERVENTIONS**

        1) Take patient history.

        2) Identify risk factors.

        3) Check for informed consent (a nurse may witness only).

        4) Perform baseline assessment.

        5) Assess for latex allergy.

        6) Verify NPO status.

    b. Medications

        1) Anesthesia

           a) Inhalation

           b) Intravenous

           c) Regional

           d) Topical

        2) Antibiotics

        3) Anticholinergics

        4) Narcotics

        5) Sedatives

c. Therapeutic Measures
  1) Laboratory profile
  2) Chest x-ray
  3) ECG

d. Client Education
  1) Fears and anxiety
  2) Medications
  3) Invasive procedures
  4) Incentive spirometry
  5) Turn, position, and perform early ambulation, including leg exercises
  6) Analgesics and pain control methods
  7) Routine and expected postoperative care
  8) Pre-, intra-, and postoperative routines (frequent VS, monitoring, setting)

B. Intraoperative Phase: Begins when client enters the surgical suite and ends with transfer to post-anesthesia recovery area. Nursing focus is on safety, patient advocacy, and health team collaboration.

1. Collaborative Care

  a. Perioperative Nursing Staff
    1) Holding area
    2) Circulator
    3) Scrub
    4) Specialty

 b. **NURSING INTERVENTIONS**
    1) Implement role according to established standards.
    2) Maintain safe environment.
    3) Ensure strict asepsis.
    4) Apply grounding devices.
    5) Ensure correct sponge, needle, and instrument count.
    6) Position patient.
    7) Remain alert to complications.
    8) Communicate with surgical team.

  c. Therapeutic Measures
    1) Blood transfusion
    2) Radiology
    3) Biopsy
    4) Laboratory profiles

C. Postoperative Phase: Begins when client enters the post-anesthesia recovery area and continues until discharge from the health care facility

1. Collaborative Care

 a. **NURSING INTERVENTIONS**: Immediate recovery period
    1) Ongoing assessment
      a) Pulmonary
        (1) Verify airway and check gag reflex.
        (2) Check for bilateral breath sounds.
        (3) Encourage coughing and deep breathing.
      b) Circulatory
        (1) Compare vital signs to baseline.
        (2) Assess tissue perfusion.
      c) Neurological
        (1) Evaluate the level of consciousness.
        (2) Assess reflexes and movement.
      d) Genitourinary
        (1) Monitor I&O.
        (2) Assess urinary output (color, clarity, and amount).
      e) Gastrointestinal
        (1) Assess for bowel sounds.
        (2) Assess for abdominal distention.
      f) Integument
        (1) Assess color.
        (2) Assess wound.
        (3) Assess drainage insertion sites.
      g) Equipment
        (1) Verify IV fluid type, rate, and site.
        (2) Check dressings for type and amount of drainage.
        (3) Identify drainage tubes and amount and color of drainage.
        (4) If NG tube, determine type and amount of suction ordered.
        (5) Position to facilitate maximum oxygenation.
        (6) Ensure thermoregulation.
        (7) Provide pain management.
        (8) Maintain NPO until the client is alert and a gag reflex returns.
        (9) Prevent complications (see table).
        (10) Transfer or discharge patient.

Common Postoperative Complications

Complication	Occurrence	Manifestations	Interventions
Atelectasis	First 48 hr	Tachycardia Tachypnea Shallow respirations	Incentive spirometer T,C,DB q 2 hr Early ambulation Hydration
Hypostatic pneumonia	After 48 hr	Febrile Tachycardia Tachypnea Crackles, rhonchi	Incentive spirometer T,C,DB q 2 hours Early ambulation Hydration Mucolytics
Respiratory depression	Immediate to 48 hr	Bradypnea Shallow respirations Decreased LOC	Monitor client Regulate narcotics Oxygen therapy Narcotic antagonist
Hypoxia	Immediate to 48 hr	Confusion Increased BP, P Tachypnea	Monitor client Oxygen therapy Resolve underlying problem
Nausea	Immediate to 48 hr	Nausea	Comfort measures Relaxation Mouth care Antiemetic NGT to decompress
Shock	Immediate to 48 hr	Decreased BP, pulse, UOP Cold, clammy, pale skin Lethargy Stupor	Monitor VS Replace fluids I&O
Urinary retention/hesitancy	Immediate to 3 days	Inability to void Bladder distention Restlessness Increased BP	Privacy Bladder scan Offer bedpan I&O
Decreased peristalsis	2–4 days	Hypoactive/absent bowel sounds No flatus	NG to decompress Limit narcotics Ambulation
Wound hemorrhage	Immediate to discharge	Bleeding from drainage tubes or surgical site Signs of shock	Assess site Identify early signs Monitor drainage device, keep patent Avoid tension at surgical site
Thrombophlebitis	7–14 days	Redness, warmth, calf tenderness/pain, edema at site	Early ambulation Apply antiembolus stockings or sequential compression devices as prescribed Avoid actions that decrease venous flow Anticoagulant prophylaxis
Delayed wound healing	5–6 days	Edema, redness, pallor, separation at edges, absence of granulation tissue	Splint incision as needed Use incision support devices (abdominal binder) Promote high-protein diet
Wound infection	3–5 days	Signs of delayed healing with purulent/dis-colored drainage, pain in incisional area	Actions for delayed healing Wound care Antibiotics as prescribed
Wound dehiscence/evisceration	4–15 days	Open wound revealing underlying tissue (dehiscence) or organs (evisceration)	Position client to decrease tension at suture line Apply sterile saline-soaked gauze Notify surgeon
Urinary tract infection	5–8 days	Frequency, urgency, dysuria Malodorous, cloudy urine	Limit use of indwelling catheters Encourage voiding Increase fluids 3 L/day Cranberry juice Antibiotics Uroanalgesics

Gastrointestinal, Hepatic, and Pancreatic Disorders

A. Definition: Impaired function of the GI tract, pancreas, and liver resulting from structural, mechanical, motility, infection, or cancerous conditions

B. Contributing Factors

1. Alcohol
2. Autoimmune
3. Diet history
4. Genetics
5. NSAIDs
6. Older adult
7. Obesity
8. Smoking
9. Sedentary lifestyle
10. Stress

Diagnostic Procedures

A. Laboratory Profiles: Gastric Aspirate

1. Hydrochloric acid and pepsin (evaluate Zollinger-Ellison syndrome)
   a. NPO 12 hours
   b. Must avoid alcohol, tobacco, medications changing gastric pH for 24 hours
   c. Insert NG tube
   d. Aspirate gastric contents
   e. pH (normal is 1.5–2.5)

B. Laboratory Profiles: Hepatic or Pancreatic Disease (normal ranges are provided)

1. Albumin (3.5–5.0 g/dL)
2. Ammonia: liver's ability to break down protein by-products (normal ammonia level is 15–110 mg/dL)
3. Bilirubin: measured directly in the blood
   a. Total 0–1.0 mg/dL
   b. Unconjugated (indirect) bilirubin (0.2–0.8 mg/dL)
   c. Conjugated (direct) bilirubin (0.1–1.0 mg/dL)
4. Cholesterol
   a. Total < 200 mg/dL LDL ("bad") < 100 mg/dL
   b. HDL ("good") > 40 mg/dL
   c. Triglycerides < 150 mg/dL
5. Liver enzymes (AST, ALT, ALP)
   a. ALT/SGPT (8–20 units/L)
   b. AST/SGOT (5–40 units/L)
   c. ALP (42–128 units/L)

6. Pancreatic enzymes (amylase, lipase)
   a. Amylase (56–90 IU/L)
   b. Lipase (0–110 units/L)
   c. Prothrombin time (0.8–1.2 seconds)

C. Laboratory Profiles: GI Parasites, Bacteria, or Bleeding

1. Stool samples (C&S, O&P)
   a. Approved specimen container
   b. No urine or toilet paper
2. Fecal occult blood
   a. Instruct client
   b. 3 samples needed

NOTE: Anticoagulants, iron therapy, and consumption of red meat may result in positive test.

D. Endoscopy: Allows direct visualization of tissues, cavities, and organs using a flexible fiber-optic tube

1. Colonoscopy: exam of the entire large intestine
   a. Bowel prep to clear fecal contents (1–3 day prep)
   b. Clear liquid diet 12–24 hours before procedure
   c. NPO except water 6–8 hours before procedure
   d. IV sedation
   e. Monitor postprocedure for excessive bleeding or severe pain
2. Virtual colonoscopy
   a. Bowel prep as for traditional colonoscopy
   b. Performed using MRI or CT
   c. Small tube is placed in the rectum
   d. Images viewed on screen
3. Sigmoidoscopy: exam of rectum and sigmoid colon
   a. Clear liquid diet 24 hours before procedure
   b. Laxative the evening before the procedure
   c. Enema the morning of the procedure
   d. Sedation is not required
   e. Tissue biopsy may be performed
   f. Report excessive bleeding
4. Small bowel capsule endoscopy: video exam of small bowel, including distal ileum
   a. Only water is allowed 8–10 hours before test.
   b. NPO 2 hours before test.
   c. Client's abdomen is marked for location of placement for sensors.
   d. Client wears abdominal belt housing data recorder.
   e. Administer video capsule with full glass of water.
   f. Resume normal diet 4 hours after swallowing pill.
   g. Return to the facility with capsule equipment for download of data.
   h. Procedure takes approximately 8 hours.
   i. Capsule will be excreted via stool (may or may not be seen); no action needed.

5. Esophagogastroduodenoscopy (EGD): exam of esophagus, stomach, and duodenum (identify bleeding, Crohn's disease, colitis)

   a. NPO 6–8 hours before procedure.

   b. Avoid anticoagulants, aspirin, or NSAIDs for several days before test.

   c. IV sedation.

   d. Atropine to dry secretions.

   e. Local anesthetic is sprayed to inactivate gag reflex.

   f. Prevent aspiration.

   g. Monitor for signs of perforation, pain, bleeding, or fever.

   h. Comfort measures for hoarseness or sore throat (several days).

6. Endoscopic retrograde cholangiopancreatography (ERCP): exam of liver, gallbladder, bile ducts, and pancreas

   a. NPO 6–8 hours before procedure.

   b. Avoid anticoagulants, aspirin, or NSAIDs for several days before test.

   c. Assess for allergies to x-ray dye.

   d. IV sedation.

   e. May have colicky abdominal discomfort.

   f. Monitor for severe pain, fever, nausea, or vomiting (indicates perforation).

E. Radiographic Studies (with or without contrast)

1. Barium series: x-ray visualization from the mouth to the duodenojejunal junction; may include a small bowel follow-through

   a. NPO 8 hours before procedure.

   b. Avoid opioid analgesics and anticholinergic medications for 24 hours before the test.

   c. Have client drink 16 ounces of barium liquid.

   d. Client will assume multiple positions during the x-ray exam.

   e. Teach client to include additional fiber and fluids to promote barium elimination.

   f. Visualize stool for barium contents next 24–72 hours (will be chalky white).

   g. Brown stool should return when barium is evacuated.

   h. Mild laxative or stool softener as needed to promote bowel elimination.

F. Liver Biopsy: Needle inserted through abdominal wall to obtain sample for biopsy or tissue examination; performed under fluoroscopy

1. Preparation

   a. Obtain informed consent.

   b. Assess coagulation studies (PT. aPTT, INR, platelet count).

   c. NPO 8–10 hours before procedure.

   d. Position on affected side to promote hemostasis.

   e. Monitor for bleeding complications.

G. Paracentesis: Needle inserted through abdominal wall into peritoneal cavity, withdrawing fluid accumulated due to ascites

1. Have client void.

2. Obtain baseline vital signs.

3. Position upright.

4. Administer mild sedation.

5. Administer prescribed IV fluids or albumin to restore fluid balance (as much as 4 L of fluid is slowly drained from the abdomen).

6. Monitor vital signs.

7. Record weight pre- and postprocedure.

8. Measure abdominal girth pre- and postprocedure.

9. Assess laboratory profile pre and post procedure: albumin, amylase, protein, BUN, creatinine.

Gastrointestinal Therapeutic Procedures

Gastrointestinal Tubes

Tube	Purpose	🩺 Nursing Interventions
Nasogastric Levin: single lumen **Salem sump:** double lumen— (1) suction, aspiration, (2) vent	Decompress stomach (ileus, gastric atony, or intestinal obstruction) Obtain specimens for analysis (pH of gastric fluid and the presence of blood)	Elevate head of bed Verify placement Frequent mouth care Maintain NPO
Miller-Abbott: double lumen— (1) aspiration, (2) inflate balloon at tip	Small bowel suction	Reposition q 1 hour Do NOT tape tube to nose Monitor advancement of tube Assess color of gastric contents
Sengstaken-Blakemore: triple lumen—(1) esophageal balloon, (2) gastric balloon, (3) suction, irrigation	For treatment of esophageal varices; can cause potential trauma and complications for the client, such as rebleeding, pneumonia, and respiratory obstructions	Monitor for respiratory distress (most clients have ETT) Keep scissors at bedside Monitor signs of shock

A. Enteral Feeding Tubes

1. Definition: delivery of a nutritionally complete feeding directly into the stomach, duodenum, or jejunum

2. Small-bore nasogastric feeding tubes

   a. Obtain x-ray to determine placement.

   b. Assess gastric pH before each feeding; every 4 hours for continuous feeding.

   c. Maintain a semi-Fowler's position while feeding is infusing.

   d. Assess residual in the stomach and refeed the residual (unless the amount exceeds 100 mL).

   e. Provide nose and mouth care.

   f. Tube is replaced every 4 weeks.

3. Small-bore nasointestinal/jejunostomy tubes: inserted through the skin and occasionally sutured in place for long-term feeding

   a. Obtain x-ray to determine placement (prior to initial feeding).

   b. Assess length of exposed tubing (tube migration).

   c. Assess placement prior to feeding using gastric pH

   d. Monitor for dumping syndrome.

   e. Maintain a semi-Fowler's position.

   f. Assess residual (should be < 100 mL; greater volume indicates upward migration).

4. Percutaneous endoscopic gastrostomy (PEG)

   a. Assess skin integrity.

   b. Assess residual volume.

   c. Allow feeding to infuse slowly (raise/lower syringe).

   d. Flush with 30 mL warm water before and after feeding.

   e. Maintain semi-Fowler's position 1–2 hours after feeding.

B. Total Parenteral Nutrition

1. Definition: IV administration of a hypertonic intravenous solution made up of glucose, insulin, minerals, lipids, electrolytes, and other essential nutrients. Total parenteral nutrition (TPN) must be administered through a central venous line. Used to correct severe nutritional deficiencies and minimize adverse effects of malnourishment.

2. Contributing Factors

   a. Gastrointestinal mobility disorders

   b. Inability to achieve or maintain adequate nutrition for body requirements

   c. Short bowel syndrome

   d. Chronic pancreatitis

   e. Severe burns

3. Collaborative Care

 a. **NURSING INTERVENTIONS**

   1) Confirm placement by chest x-ray.

   2) Monitor central line insertion site for local infection.

   3) Maintain strict surgical asepsis for dressing change (every 72 hours).

   4) Change tubing and remaining TPN every 24 hours.

   5) Monitor for signs of systemic infection.

   6) Monitor client's glucose, electrolytes, and fluid balance.

   7) Prevent air embolism.

   8) Use infusion pump.

   9) Keep 10% dextrose/water available.

Gastrointestinal Disorders

A. Gastroesophageal Reflux Disease

1. Definition: A condition in which the lower esophageal sphincter does not close properly allowing stomach contents to back up into the esophagus.

B. Hiatal Hernia

1. Definition: a portion of the stomach protrudes through the esophageal hiatus of the diaphragm into the chest

2. Contributing Factors

   a. High-fat diet

   b. Caffeinated beverages

   c. Tobacco products

   d. Medications: Ca^{++} channel blockers, anticholinergics, nitrates

3. Manifestations

   a. Regurgitation

   b. Persistent heartburn and dysphagia

   c. Flatulence and belching

   d. Epigastric pain

   e. Hoarseness in the morning, dry cough

   f. Hypersalivation

4. Collaborative Care

 a. **NURSING INTERVENTIONS**

   1) Manage client care for diagnostic tests.

   2) Assess diet history.

   3) Encourage small frequent meals.

   4) Avoid eating 3 hours prior to bedtime.

   5) Sit upright 1–2 hours after meals.

   6) Elevate head of bed.

   7) Sleep in right side-lying position.

   8) Encourage weight reduction for client's with BMI >25.

9) Monitor for complications:
   a) Bleeding or esophageal ulcers
   b) Barrett's esophagus
   c) Aggravation of asthma, chronic cough, and pulmonary fibrosis

b. Medications
1) Antacids
2) Histamine receptor antagonists
3) Prokinetic agents
4) Proton pump inhibitors

c. Client Education
1) Dietary medication regimen
2) Precautions to prevent aspiration

d. Therapeutic Measures
1) Hiatal hernia—fundoplication if other measures ineffective

C. Peptic Ulcer Disease (PUD)

1. Definition: ulcerations in the stomach or duodenum as a result of mucosal tissue destruction; high risk of perforation and bleeding

2. Contributing Factors
a. NSAIDs
b. Corticosteroids
c. *H. pylori* infection
d. Uncontrolled stress
e. Smoking

3. Manifestations
a. Dyspepsia
b. Upper epigastric pain 1–2 hours after meals
c. Symptoms worsen with empty stomach
d. Relief noted with antacids
e. Belching
f. Bloating

4. Collaborative Care
a. **NURSING INTERVENTIONS**
1) Monitor stools and emesis for signs of bleeding.
2) Encourage small frequent meals.
3) Avoid bedtime snacks.

b. Medications
1) Mucosal healing agents
2) Stool softeners
3) Antacids
4) Histamine receptor antagonists
5) Prokinetic agents
6) Proton pump inhibitors

c. Therapeutic Measures
1) EGD
2) Chest and abdominal x-ray
3) Hematocrit and hemoglobin
4) Stool specimen

d. Client Education
1) Symptom management
2) Medication therapy
3) Nutrition therapy
4) Stress reduction

D. Irritable Bowel Syndrome (IBS)

1. Definition: chronic disorder with recurrent diarrhea, constipation, and/or abdominal pain and bloating (most common digestive disorder seen in clinical practice)

2. Contributing Factors
a. Diverticular disease
b. Smoking
c. Caffeine
d. NSAIDs
e. Milk allergy
f. Stress
g. Mental or behavioral illness

3. Manifestations
a. Weight loss
b. Fatigue and malaise
c. Erratic bowel patterns
d. Abdominal pain relieved by defecation
e. Abdominal distention
f. Mucus with passage of stool
g. Colicky abdomen with diffuse tenderness

4. Collaborative Care
a. **NURSING INTERVENTIONS**
1) Monitor for signs of complication
2) Client education
3) Administer medications

b. Medications
1) Antibiotics
2) Mucosal healing agents
3) Stool softeners
4) Antacids
5) Histamine receptor antagonists
6) Prokinetic agents
7) Proton pump inhibitors

c. Therapeutic Measures
1) Endoscopy
2) Chest and abdominal x-ray
3) Test for *H. pylori*

d. Client Education
1) Keeping diary to identify triggers
2) Avoidance of causative agents
3) Symptom management
4) Medication therapy
5) Nutrition therapy
6) Stress reduction

E. **Inflammatory Bowel Disease is a group of conditions of the large intestine (and in some cases the small intestine).** Do not confuse it with irritable bowel syndrome, which is less severe. Included in this group are Crohn's disease and ulcerative colitis.

1. Crohn's Disease

    a. Definition: chronic inflammatory disease affecting the entire intestinal mucosa (cobblestone appearance); most common site is terminal ileum

    b. Contributing Factors

       1) Family history

       2) Jewish ancestry

       3) Bacterial infection

       4) Smoking

       5) Adolescents or young adults (ages 15 to 40)

    c. Manifestations

       1) Abdominal pain (RLQ); does not resolve with defecation

       2) Low-grade fever

       3) Diarrhea, steatorrhea

       4) Weight loss (may become emaciated)

       5) Formation of fistulas (abnormal tracts between bowel and skin/bladder or vagina)

 Point to Remember: Bleeding is rare with Crohn's disease.

    d. Collaborative Care

    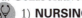 1) **NURSING INTERVENTIONS**

       a) Promote adequate rest periods.

       b) Record color, volume, frequency, and consistency of stools.

       c) Monitor and prevent fluid deficit.

       d) Nutrition therapy includes high calorie, protein, low fiber, no dairy.

       e) Manage fistula (F&E, prevent infection).

       f) Provide supportive care.

      2) Medications

       a) Steroids

       b) Antifungals

       c) Aminosalicylates (5-ASAs)

       d) Immune modulators: infliximab (Remicade), adalimumab (Humira), certolizumab (Cimzia), and natalizumab (Tysabri)

       e) TPN

      3) Therapeutic Measures

       a) Bowel resection (possible ileostomy)

       b) Stricturoplasty

       c) Laboratory profiles: Hct, hemoglobin, C-reactive protein, WBC, ESR

       d) Abdominal x-ray

      4) Client Education

       a) Refer to support group

       b) Dietary

       c) Health promotion and relaxation

2. Ulcerative Colitis

    a. Definition: widespread inflammation of the rectum and rectosigmoid colon (can extend to entire colon)

    b. Contributing Factors

       1) Family history

       2) Jewish ancestry

       3) Isotretinoin (Accutane) use

       4) Young and middle-age adults (15–25 years; 55–65 years)

    c. Manifestations

       1) Liquid, bloody stool (10–20 per day)

       2) Low-grade fever

       3) Abdominal distention along the colon

       4) Rebound tenderness indicates perforation/peritonitis

NOTE: Bleeding is common with ulcerative colitis.

    d. Collaborative Care

    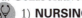 1) **NURSING INTERVENTIONS**

       a) Promote adequate rest periods.

       b) Record color, volume, frequency, and consistency of stools.

       c) Maintain NPO status during acute phase.

       d) Monitor and prevent fluid deficit.

       e) Nutrition therapy includes high calorie, protein, low fiber, no dairy.

       f) Manage pain.

       g) Provide supportive care.

      2) Medications

       a) Antidiarrheals (monitor for megacolon)

       b) Aminosalicylates (5-ASAs)

       c) Immune modulators: infliximab (Remicade), adalimumab (Humira), certolizumab (Cimzia), and natalizumab (Tysabri)

       d) TPN

      3) Therapeutic Measures

       a) Surgical management is indicated for bowel perforation, toxic megacolon, hemorrhage, and colon cancer.

         (1) Colectomy and ileostomy

         (2) Total proctocolectomy with permanent ileostomy

         (3) Laboratory profiles: Hct, hemoglobin, C-reactive protein, WBC, ESR

         (4) Abdominal x-ray

      4) Client Education

       a) Refer to support group

       b) Dietary

       c) Health promotion and relaxation

F. Diverticular Disease

1. Definition: includes three conditions that involve numerous small sacs or pockets in the wall of the colon, including any of the following:

   a. Diverticulosis: the presence of pouchlike herniations (diverticula) along the wall of the intestines

   b. Diverticular bleeding: results from injury of small vessels near the diverticula

   c. Diverticulitis: inflammation of one or more diverticula

2. Contributing Factors

   a. Older adult

   b. Constipation

   c. Low dietary fiber and high-fat diet

   d. Diet risk: low fiber, high fat, and red meat

   e. Connective tissue disorders causing weakness in the colon wall

3. Manifestations (Diverticulitis)

   a. Alternating diarrhea with constipation

   b. Painful cramps or tenderness in the lower abdomen (LLQ)

   c. Chills or fever

4. Collaborative Care

    a. **NURSING INTERVENTIONS**

      1) Provide high-fiber diet to prevent diverticulitis.

      2) Provide low-fiber diet during inflammation (diverticulitis).

      3) Avoid foods such as popcorn, nuts, and any food with seeds.

      4) Increase fluids to 3 L/day.

      5) Manage pain.

      6) Avoid laxatives.

      7) Monitor bowel elimination patterns.

      8) Monitor for complications (obstruction, hemorrhage, infection).

   b. Medications

      1) Bulk laxatives (preventive)

      2) Metronidazole (Flagyl)

      3) Trimethoprim/sulfamethoxazole (Bactrim, Septra)

      4) Ciprofloxacin (Cipro)

   c. Therapeutic Measures

      1) Emergency colon resection for peritonitis, bowel obstruction, or abscess

   d. Client Teaching

      1) High-fiber versus low-fiber diet

      2) Collaborate with nutritionist

      3) Preventive measures

G. Abdominal Hernia

1. Definition: protrusion of bowel through the muscle wall of abdominal cavity (umbilical, ventral, inguinal). **May become strangulated if blood supply to the herniated segment is cut off.**

2. Contributing Factors

   a. Older age

   b. Male

   c. Obesity

   d. Heavy lifting or straining

   e. Abdominal surgery

3. Manifestations

   a. Client reports "lump" felt at the involved site

   b. Pain in groin when bending, coughing, or lifting

   c. Absent bowel sounds (strangulated)

   d. Palpation of mass

4. Collaborative Care

   a. **NURSING INTERVENTIONS**

      1) Wear abdominal binder for support of herniated tissue

      2) Prevent constipation

   b. Therapeutic Procedures

      1) Herniorrhaphy laparoscopic repair

   c. Client Education

      1) Avoid lifting 4–6 weeks after surgery

      2) Measures to prevent constipation

H. Intestinal Obstruction

1. Definition: partial or complete blockage of intestinal contents

2. Etiologies: mechanical (adhesions, tumors, volvulus), neurogenic (paralytic ileus), or vascular (mesenteric artery occlusion)

3. Contributing Factors

   a. Crohn's disease

   b. Radiation therapy

   c. Fecal impaction

   d. Carcinomas

   e. Surgical procedures

   f. Narcotics

   g. Hypokalemia

   h. Diverticulitis

4. Manifestations

   a. Inability to pass flatus or stool for > 8 hours

   b. Abdominal distention

   c. Hyperactive bowel sound above site of obstruction

   d. Hypoactive or active bowel sounds below site of obstruction

Comparison of Intestinal Obstruction Manifestations

Small Bowel	Large Intestine
Sporadic, colicky pain	Diffuse and constant pain
Visible peristaltic waves	Significant abdominal distention
Profuse, projective vomitus with fecal odor (vomiting relieves pain)	Infrequent vomiting, leakage of fecal fluid around impaction

5. Collaborative Care

 a. **NURSING INTERVENTIONS**

   1) NPO
   2) Assess bowel sounds
   3) IV fluids
   4) Preoperative care
   5) NGT for decompression
   6) Prevent fluid and electrolyte deficit

b. Therapeutic Measures

   1) Abdominal x-rays
   2) Endoscopy
   3) CT scan
   4) Surgical intervention (remove obstruction, resection)

c. Client Teaching

   1) Preventive measures based on etiology
   2) Diet

Gastric Surgical Procedures

A. **Bariatric Surgery:** Used as a treatment for morbid obesity when other weight control methods have failed

1. Contributing Factors

   a. Long history of morbid obesity

2. Manifestations

   a. BMI > 40
   b. BMI > 35 with other diseases

3. Collaborative Care

 a. **NURSING INTERVENTIONS**

   1) Assess psychosocial issues related to weight loss.
   2) Provide perioperative care.
   3) Monitor bowel sounds.
   4) Ambulate as soon as possible.
   5) Prevent dumping syndrome.
   6) Provide diet therapy, liquids, and pureed foods 1st 6 weeks, then progress.

b. Medications

   1) Vitamin and mineral supplements

c. Client Education

   1) Consume 4–6 meals per day
   2) Consume 2 servings of protein per day
   3) Limit meal size to 1 cup
   4) Walk 30 minutes each day
   5) Supplements
   6) Symptoms and measures to prevent dumping syndrome

4. Referral and Follow-up

   a. Dietician
   b. Support groups

B. **Colostomy:** A surgical procedure that brings the end of the colon through the abdominal wall, creating an opening for the evacuation of fecal material. May be temporary or permanent

1. Contributing Factors

   a. Cancer or tumors
   b. Obstructive bowel disease
   c. Colectomy
   d. Severe diverticulitis or Crohn's disease
   e. Trauma

2. Collaborative Care

 a. **NURSING INTERVENTIONS**

   1) Assess ostomy site.
   2) Assess output from stoma (the higher an ostomy is placed in the small intestine the more liquid and acidic the output will be).
   3) Empty ostomy bag when ¼ to ½ full.
   4) Fit appliance to prevent leakage.
   5) Monitor for complications related to blood supply.
   6) Offer emotional support.

b. Client Education

   1) Avoid foods that cause excessive gas formation and odor
   2) Stoma care and irrigations as prescribed
   3) How to burp the flange to remove gas and prevent the bag from dislodging

NOTE: Clients with ileostomy have no control over stool evacuation and must always wear an ostomy bag.

Hepatic Disorders

A. **Cirrhosis**

1. Definition: scarring of the liver and poor liver function as a result of chronic liver disease

2. Contributing Factors

   a. Alcohol induced (Laennec's)
   b. Postnecrotic (hepatitis, chemicals)
   c. Biliary disease
   d. Severe right-sided heart failure

3. Manifestations

   a. Early stage

      1) Enlarged liver
      2) Jaundice
      3) Gastrointestinal disturbances
      4) Weight loss

   b. Late stage

      1) Liver becomes smaller and nodular
      2) Splenomegaly

3) Ascites, distended abdominal veins; increased pressure in the portal system

4) Bleeding tendencies; decreased vitamin K and prothrombin, anemia

5) Esophageal varices, internal hemorrhoids; increased pressure in the portal area

6) Dyspnea from ascites and anemia

7) Pruritus from dry skin

8) Clay-colored stools; no bile in stool

9) Tea-colored urine; bile in urine

c. End stage

1) Prodromal: slurred speech, vacant stare, restlessness, neuro deterioration

2) Impending: asterixis (flapping tremors), apraxia, lethargy, confusion

3) Stuporous: marked mental confusion, somnolence

4) Coma: unarousable, fetor hepaticus, seizures, high mortality rate

4. Collaborative Care

 a. **NURSING INTERVENTIONS**

1) Encourage rest.

2) Weigh the client daily and measure abdominal girth.

3) Assess skin integrity frequently.

4) Monitor I&O.

5) Assess for bleeding and hemorrhoids.

6) Avoid hepatotoxic medications.

7) Maintain a high-calorie, low-protein (20–40 g/day), low-fat, low-sodium diet (maintain protein restriction during stages I and II of encephalopathy; no protein allowed during stages III and IV).

8) Limit sodium and fluid intake as prescribed

9) Monitor liver enzymes, bilirubin, hematologic testing: CBC, WBC, and platelets, PT/INR and Ammonia levels

b. Medications

1) Diuretics: spironolactone (Aldactone), Furosemide (Lasix)

2) Neomycin and metronidazole (Flagyl)—reduces intestinal bacteria

3) Lactulose (Chronulac)—decreases ammonia levels.

4) Provide supplemental vitamins (B_1 and B complex, A, C, and K; folic acid; and thiamine) as prescribed.

5) Fat-soluble vitamin supplements and folic acid may need to be given IV.

6) Proton pump inhibitors and H_2 receptor antagonist

7) Albumin IV to decrease ascites

c. Therapeutic Measures

1) Liver biopsy

2) EGD

3) Paracentesis

4) Transjugular Intrahepatic Portosystemic Shunt (TIPS)

d. Client Education

1) Alcohol abstinence

2) Dietary guidelines

3) Bleeding risk and precautions

5. Referral and Follow-up

a. Alcohol recovery program

b. Nutrition

c. Social services

B. Hepatitis

1. Definition: inflammation of the liver caused by infectious organisms, chemicals, or toxins. Cases must be reported to the local health department.

Hepatitis

Characteristics	Type A (HAV)	Type B (HBV)	Type C (HCV)
Mode of transmission	• Fecal-oral route • Person to person • Food contamination	• Unprotected sex • Sharing needles • Needlesticks • Blood products; organ transplant before 1992	• Blood to blood • Illicit IV drug sharing • Blood products, organ transplant before 1992
Manifestations	• Mild course • "Flu-like" • Advanced age and chronic disease increase severity	• May be asymptomatic • RUQ pain • Anorexia, N/V • Fatigue • Febrile • Dark urine • Light-colored stool • Jaundice	• Most are asymptomatic • Diagnosis with blood testing • Chronic inflammation progresses to cirrhosis
Prevention	• Hand washing • Vaccine for ages 2 and older • 2 doses 6–18 months apart	• Vaccine infants and high-risk populations • 3 doses over 6-month period	Avoid high-risk behaviors
Treatment	• Symptom specific • May have change in medication regimen to "rest liver"	• Antiviral drugs • PEG-Intron • Monitor renal function	Same as Type B

C. Nonviral Hepatitis

1. Definition: liver injury and inflammation caused by ingestion of drugs and chemicals (industrial toxins, alcohol, drugs)
2. Contributing Factors
   a. Inhalation of hepatotoxic agents
   b. Drug toxicity
   c. Alcohol
   d. Secondary infection may occur with Epstein-Barr, herpes simplex, varicella-zoster, and cytomegalovirus
3. Manifestations
   a. Jaundice
   b. Liver enlargement
   c. Liver necrosis
4. Collaborative Care
   a. Monitor signs of liver impairment
   b. Monitor client for RUQ pain
   c. Monitor weight
   d. Treatment is specific to symptoms and causative factors

D. Gallbladder Disease

1. Definitions
   a. Cholecystitis: inflammation of the gallbladder
   b. Cholelithiasis: presence of stones in the gallbladder
2. Contributing Factors
   a. Female
   b. Fertile
   c. Over age forty
   d. Overweight
3. Manifestations
   a. Right upper quadrant, epigastric, or shoulder pain
   b. Nausea and vomiting
   c. Dietary fat intolerance
   d. Murphy's sign
   e. Jaundice (indicates obstruction)
4. Diagnostic Procedures
   a. Ultrasound
   b. Hepatobiliary scan
   c. ERCP
   d. Cholangiography
5. Collaborative Care
   a. **NURSING INTERVENTIONS**
      1) Administer analgesics as prescribed.
      2) Prevent F&E imbalances.
      3) Maintain low-fat diet.
      4) Provide postoperative care.
      5) Cholecystectomy client may have T-tube:
         a) Monitor drainage; keep below level of GB.
         b) Empty collection bag every 8 hours.
         c) Report drainage amounts > 1,000 mL/day.
         d) Never irrigate without physician order.
      6) Observe color of stool.
      7) Monitor for signs of postcholecystectomy syndrome (symptoms of cholecystitis after surgery) and report to physician.
   b. Medications
      1) Meperidine (Demerol) or hydromorphone (Dilaudid): AVOID morphine to prevent biliary spasms
      2) Antiemetics
      3) Anticholinergics
   c. Therapeutic Measures
      1) Sphincterotomy with stone removal may be done with ERCP
      2) Extracorporeal shock wave lithotripsy (ESWL) to break up stones (only for small cholesterol stones)
      3) Cholecystecomy
   d. Client Education
      1) Resume regular low-fat diet
      2) Prevent dumping syndrome
      3) Care of T-tube at home

Pancreatic Disorders

A. Acute Pancreatitis

1. Definition: serious life-threatening inflammatory process of the pancreas

B. Chronic Pancreatitis

1. Definition: progressive disease of the pancreas characterized by remissions and exacerbations resulting in diminished function
2. Contributing Factors
   a. Alcoholism
   b. Gallstones
   c. Drug use
   d. Infection
   e. Blunt abdominal trauma
   f. Operative manipulation and trauma
3. Manifestations
   a. Severe mid-epigastric or left upper quadrant pain
   b. Pain intensifies after meals and when lying down
   c. Nausea and vomiting
   d. Abdominal tenderness
   e. Elevated amylase and lipase
   f. Steatorrhea
   g. Turner's sign
   h. Cullen's sign

4. Diagnostic Procedures

    a. Laboratory profiles: liver enzymes, bilirubin, pancreatic enzymes

    b. CT scan with contrast

5. Collaborative Care

    a. **NURSING INTERVENTIONS**

        1) NPO

        2) NGT for decompression of stomach

        3) Pain management

        4) Position for comfort (fetal, sitting up, leaning forward)

        5) Prevent F&E imbalances

    b. Medications

        1) Antibiotics

        2) Opioid analgesics

        3) Anticholinergics

        4) Pancreatic enzymes

    c. Therapeutic Measures

        1) TPN

        2) ERCP to create an opening in sphincter of Oddi if cause is gallstones

        3) Cholecystectomy

        4) Pancreaticojejunostomy (Roux-en-Y) to "reroute" pancreatic secretions to the jejunum

    d. Client Education for Chronic Pancreatitis

        1) Take enzymes before meals and snacks

        2) Follow up with all scheduled laboratory testing

        3) Nutrition: high caloric needs

        4) Alcohol abstinence

        5) Avoid high fat intake

6. Referral and Follow-up

    a. Alcohol recovery program Nutritionist

    b. Home health for clients requiring long-term TPN

C. Pancreatric Cancer

Carcinoma has vague symptoms and is usually diagnosed in late stages after liver or gallbladder involvement

1. Contributing Factors

    a. Older age; tobacco use

    b. Chronic pancreatitis

    c. Diabetes mellitus

    d. Cirrhosis

    e. High intake of red meat, processed meat

    f. Obesity

    g. Small number have an inherited risk

2. Manifestations

    a. Fatigue, anorexia, flatulence

    b. Pruritis

    c. Weight loss, palpable abdominal mass, abdominal pain that may radiate to the back

    d. Hepatomegaly, jaundice (late sign when cancer blocks the bile duct)

    e. Ascites

    f. Clay colred stools, dark urine, ascites

    g. Glucose intolerance

3. Diagnostic Procedures

    a. Carcinoembryonic antigen (CEA) elevated: Nonsmoker 2.5-5 ng/ml; Smoker up to 5 ng/ml

    b. Elevated serum amylase and lipase

    c. Elevated alkaline phosphatase and bilirubin

    d. ERCP

    e. Ultrasound, CT scan

4. Collaborative Care

    a. Nursing Interventions

        1) palliative care measures

        2) Pain management

        3) Monitor blood glucose levels

        4) Provide nutritional support (enteral supplements and TPN)

    b. Medications

        1) Opioid analgesics

    c. Therapeutic Measures

        1) Chemotherapy may be used to shrink the tumor size. The nurse monitors for myelosuppression and pancytopenia

        2) Radiation Therapy

        3) Partial pancreatectomy done for small tumors

        4) Whipple procedure: Pancreatoduodenectomy is the most common operation to remove (resect) pancreatic cancers. Procedure done when cancer is located in the head of the pancreas. Involves removing the head of the pancreas, duodenum, parts of the jejunum and stomach, gallbladder and possibly the spleen. The pancreatic duct is reconnected to the common bile duct and the stomach is connected to the jejunum. May be done laparoscopically.

        a) Nursing interventions

           (1) Provide routine postop care

           (2) Monitor NG output. Observe for bloody or bile tinged drainage which can indicate anastomotic disruption.

           (3) Maintain a semi-fowler's position to prevent stress on suture line

           (4) Facilitate coughing and deep breathing and use of incentive spirometer

           (5) Monitor blood glucose and administer insulin as needed.

           (6) Provide analgesia

    d. Client Education

        1) Encourage client to seek palliative care at home, cancer support group and available community resources.

        2) Support measures for pain, anorexia and weight loss

Diagnostic Tests for Musculoskeletal Disorders

A. Bone Scan: Radioactive medium is injected for viewing entire skeleton, primarily to detect tumors, arthritis, osteomyelitis, osteoporosis, vertebral compression fractures, and unexplained bone pain.

1. Technician or physician administers the isotope 4 to 6 hours prior to testing.
2. Client must lie still for 30–60 minutes as imaging is performed.
3. Increase fluids post procedures.

B. Dual-Energy X-ray Absorptiometry (DEXA) Scan: Most common screening tool for measuring bone mineral density for diagnosis of osteopenia and osteoporosis

1. Baseline for women in their 40s.
2. Client should wear loose clothing without zippers or metal
3. Client must remove jewelry.
4. Instruct client to stop vitamin D and calcium supplementation 48 hours prior to scan.

C. Electromyography (EMG) and Nerve Conduction Studies: Used to evaluate muscle weakness by emission of low-frequency electrical stimulation

1. Client will be asked to perform activities for measurement of muscle activity.
2. Observe needle insertion sites for hematoma.
3. Support client with anxiety related to testing.

D. Magnetic Resonance Imaging (MRI): Imaging produced through interaction of magnetic fields, radio waves, and atomic nuclei to diagnose muscle, tissue, and bone disorders

1. Client must remove all metal objects (inquire about surgical implanted devices, nonvisible piercings). Canes, crutches, and walkers generally must be left outside of the MRI room; assist client as necessary to stretcher.
2. Contraindicated for clients with pacemakers, stents, and surgical clips.
3. Clients with titanium joint replacements may have MRI.
4. Assess client for claustrophobia if closed scanner is used.
5. Assess client for ability to lie still in supine position for 45–60 minutes.

Arthritis

Definition: Inflammation of one or more joints, which results in pain, swelling, stiffness, and limited movement

A. Osteoarthritis: Progressive deterioration and loss of cartilage in one or more joints

1. Contributing Factors
   a. Older adult
   b. Female
   c. Metabolic disease
   d. Obesity
   e. Repetitive use or abuse of joints
   f. Smoking
2. Manifestations
   a. Chronic joint pain and stiffness
   b. Pain diminished after rest and worsens after activity
   c. Crepitus
   d. Limited movement
   e. Heberden nodes (closest to the end of the fingers and toes)
   f. Bouchard's nodes (middle joints of fingers or toes)
   g. Excess joint fluid (especially with knee involvement)
   h. Skeletal muscle atrophy from disuse
3. Diagnostic Procedures
   a. X-rays
   b. MRI
   c. Erythrocyte sedimentation rate (ESR) and serum C-reactive protein (CRP) show slight elevation
4. Collaborative Care
    a. **NURSING INTERVENTIONS**
      1) Assess and manage pain.
      2) Instruct client to use ice or heat for comfort.
      3) Encourage client to perform range of motion and isometric exercises.
      4) Encourage adequate rest and sleep as need to relieve pain.
      5) Involve physical therapy as appropriate.
      6) Utilize assistive devices to help increase independence and completion of activities of daily living.
   b. Medications
      1) NSAIDs
      2) Corticosteroids
      3) Topical analgesics
   c. Therapeutic Measures
      1) Total joint arthroplasty
      2) Total joint replacement

d. Client Education
1) Use of mobility devices and safety
2) Prevention of complications
3) Perform exercises per treatment plan

5. Referral and Follow-up
a. Physical therapy
b. Rehabilitation therapy

B. Rheumatoid Arthritis: Chronic, progressive autoimmune connective tissue disorder primarily affecting synovial joints

1. Contributing Factors
a. Cause is unknown
b. Increased incidence in middle-age females
c. Infection, genes, and hormones may be linked to the disease.

2. Manifestations
a. Morning stiffness and pain
b. Bilateral joint inflammation with decreased range of motion
c. Joint deformity in late stages
d. Warmth, redness, and edema of affected areas
e. Dry eyes and mouth (Sjögren syndrome)
f. Numbness, tingling, or burning in the hands and feet

3. Diagnostic Procedures
a. X-ray
b. MRI
c. Positive rheumatoid factor
d. Synovial fluid analysis

4. Collaborative Care
a. **NURSING INTERVENTIONS**
1) Assess and manage pain.
2) Instruct client to use ice or heat for comfort.
3) Encourage physical activity to maintain joint mobility (within client's capacity).
4) Monitor client for signs of fatigue.
5) Monitor for signs of complications related to therapy (secondary osteoporosis, vasculitis).

b. Medications
1) NSAIDs
2) Corticosteroids
3) DMARDs

c. Therapeutic Measures
1) Plasmapheresis for severe, life-threatening exacerbation
2) Synovectomy
3) Total joint arthroplasty if unresponsive to medication

d. Client Education
1) Use of mobility devices and safety
2) Prevention of complications
3) Perform exercises per treatment plan

5. Referral and Follow-up
a. Occupational/physical therapy
b. Rehabilitation therapy
c. Arthritis support group

C. Gouty Arthritis: Systemic inflammatory disease caused by (1) problems with purine metabolism (primary gout) or (2) hyperuricemia (secondary gout)

1. Contributing Factors
a. Family history
b. Excessive alcohol intake
c. High intake of foods with purines (organ meats, yeast, sardines, spinach)
d. Obesity
e. Comorbid conditions of DM and/or renal disease

2. Manifestations
a. Excruciating pain and inflammation in one or more small joints (great toe is most common joint; appears warm and red)
b. Appearance of tophi (deposits of sodium urate crystals; generally appear after years of gouty arthritis)
c. Progressive joint damage and deformity
d. Increased incidence of uric acid renal stone

3. Diagnostic Procedures
a. Serum uric acid > 7 mg/dL
b. ESR
c. Synovial fluid analysis (will show uric acid crystals)

4. Collaborative Care
a. **NURSING INTERVENTIONS**
1) Maintain bed rest during acute attacks.
2) Use bed cradle to keep linen elevated above affected joint.
3) Promote fluid intake 3 L daily.
4) Limit foods high in purine.

b. Medications
1) Acute phase: Colchicine
2) Chronic treatment: Allopurinol
3) NSAIDs
4) Corticosteroids
5) Injection of corticosteroid into affected joint may be performed by provider

c. Client Education
1) Foods to avoid (high in purine)
2) Instruct client to keep diary of triggering factors
3) Avoid alcohol
4) Lose weight slowly (rapid weight loss may precipitate a flare-up or increase the incidence of uric acid renal stones)

Fractures

Definition: A break or disruption in the continuity of bone tissue

A. Types of Fractures

1. Closed
2. Comminuted (fragmented)
3. Compression
4. Displaced
5. Greenstick
6. Impacted
7. Oblique
8. Open (compound)
9. Pathologic (tumors, infection, bone disease)
10. Spiral
11. Stress (small crack in bone)

B. Collaborative Care

1. Assess client's neurovascular status (6 Ps) noting bilateral comparisons.
   a. Pain, Pressure, Paralysis, Pallor, Pulselessness, Paresthesia
2. Monitor for changes in skin temperature.
3. Monitor for complications of fat embolism (most common with long bone fractures):
   a. Confusion, anxiety
   b. Tachycardia
   c. Tachypnea
   d. Hemoptysis
   e. Petechiae over neck, upper arms, chest, abdomen (late sign)
4. Monitor for complications of compartment syndrome (irreversible if compromise persists beyond 4–6 hours):
   a. Pain unrelieved by positioning or medication
   b. Cyanosis
   c. Tingling
   d. Paralysis
5. Maintain correct body alignment.
6. Provide nursing care specific to therapeutic measures of fracture reduction.

C. Therapeutic Measures

1. Cast: application of plaster or fiberglass to immobilize and maintain alignment of the bone
   a. Collaborative Care
      1) Assess neurovascular status.
      2) Allow plaster cast to air dry and handle cast with palms while drying.
      3) Elevate affected extremity.
      4) Monitor for complications.
      5) Client may "petal" plaster cast if irritation around edges develops.
      6) Remind client to place NO objects down cast to help reduce risk of infection.

2. Traction
   a. Skin traction: provides a mechanical pulling force to overcome muscle spasms, to immobilize or relieve pain
      1) Buck's
      2) Bryant's
      3) Cervical halter
      4) Pelvic
   b. Skeletal traction: applied directly to a bone to reduce a fracture or maintain surgically manipulated bone alignment
      1) Pins or wires inserted through skin and soft tissue into the bone
      2) Balanced suspension using splints, slings, weights

D. External Fixation Device: Rigid metal frames with attached percutaneous pins or wires used to align and immobilize

1. Collaborative Care
   a. Assess pulses and vascular status.
   b. Maintain proper body alignment.
   c. Verify weights are free hanging.
   d. Monitor skin for pressure points or breakdown.
   e. Promote strengthening exercises for uninjured areas.
   f. Consult with physical therapy.

Osteoporosis

Definition: Chronic disease in which bone loss causes decreased density and possible fracture. Osteopenia is the precursor of osteoporosis.

A. Contributing Factors

1. Primary Osteoporosis
   a. Women age 65 and older
   b. Men age 75 and older
   c. Asian and Caucasian ethnicity
   d. Family history
   e. Estrogen or androgen deficiency
   f. Protein deficiency
   g. Sedentary lifestyle
   h. Smoking and alcohol intake
2. Secondary Osteoporosis
   a. Bone cancer
   b. Cushing's syndrome
   c. Diabetes mellitus
   d. Medications: corticosteroids, phenytoin, cytotoxic agents, immunosuppressants, loop diuretics
   e. Paget's disease
   f. Prolonged immobilization
   g. Rheumatoid arthritis
   h. Manifestations
3. Shortened height
4. History of fractures
5. Thoracic kyphosis
6. Decreased bone mass

B. Collaborative Care

 1. **NURSING INTERVENTIONS**

    a. Encourage safe weight-bearing exercises.

    b. Administer medications as prescribed.

    c. Instruct client to increase foods rich in calcium and vitamin D.

    d. Promote safety.

  2. Medications

    a. Biophosphonates

    b. Calcium supplements

    c. Vitamin D supplements

  3. Client Education

    a. Instruct client to continue health screenings and diagnostic evaluations.

    b. Instruct client to avoid activities with increased risk of falls (ice, slippery surfaces).

    c. Instruct client to take medications as prescribed.

Osteomyelitis

Definition: An acute or chronic bone infection

A. Contributing Factors

  1. Diabetes

  2. Hemodialysis

  3. Injection drug use

  4. Poor blood supply

  5. Recent trauma

B. Manifestations

  1. Bone pain

  2. Fever

  3. General discomfort, uneasiness, or ill feeling (malaise)

  4. Local swelling, redness, and warmth

  5. Other symptoms that may occur with this disease:

    a. Chills

    b. Excessive sweating

    c. Low back pain

    d. Swelling of the ankles, feet, and legs

C. Diagnostic Procedures

  1. Bone biopsy (which is then cultured)

  2. Bone scan

  3. Bone x-ray

  4. Complete blood count (CBC)

  5. CRP

  6. ESR

  7. MRI of the bone

  8. Needle aspiration of the area around affected bones

D. Collaborative Care

 1. **NURSING INTERVENTIONS**

    a. Obtain blood cultures as ordered prior to administering antibiotics.

    b. Administer antibiotic therapy as scheduled.

    c. Administer pain medication as needed.

  2. Medications

    a. Antibiotics

    b. Analgesics

  3. Therapeutic Measures

    a. Surgical excision of dead and infected bone may be needed.

    b. Bone grafting may be performed in large impacted areas.

Total Joint Arthroplasty (Replacement)

Definition: Surgical procedure performed to replace a joint with a prosthetic system. Arthroplasty may be performed for ankle, finger, elbow, shoulder, toe, and wrist. The hip and knee arthroplasties are the most commonly performed procedures.

A. Contributing Factors

  1. Impaired mobility and uncontrolled pain related to osteoarthritis

  2. Congenital anomalies

  3. Trauma

  4. Osteonecrosis

B. Collaborative Care

 1. **NURSING INTERVENTIONS**

    a. Position client correctly, maintaining alignment:

      1) Hip arthroplasty: keep abductor pillow in place while in bed, do not flex hip more than 90 degrees

      2) Knee arthroplasty: maintain continue passive motion (CPM) machine to promote joint mobility

    b. Assess for pain, rotation, and extremity shortening.

    c. Assess neurovascular status.

    d. Use aseptic technique for wound care and emptying of drains.

    e. Monitor for signs of infection.

    f. Prevent venous thromboembolism.

    g. Use toilet seat extender.

  2. Medications

    a. Anticoagulants

    b. NSAIDs

    c. Opioid narcotics

  3. Client Education

    a. Instruct client to participate in exercise regimen.

    b. Instruct client in use of ambulatory devices.

C. Referral and Follow-up

1. Physical therapy for ambulation, transfer, and joint movement

2. Occupational therapy to meet goals of independence and self-care

Amputations

Definition: Removal of a part of the body; may be elective or traumatic

A. Types of Amputations

1. Above the knee

2. Below the knee

3. Mid-foot

4. Toe

B. Contributing Factors

1. Peripheral vascular disease

2. Severe crushing of tissues or significant vessels

3. Malignant tumors

4. Osteomyelitis

C. Collaborative Care

 1. **NURSING INTERVENTIONS**

a. Assess neurovascular status.

b. Assess psychosocial status.

c. Assess client's willingness and motivation to withstand prolonged rehabilitation.

d. Manage phantom limb and residual limb pain.

e. Monitor for signs of wound healing.

f. Monitor for complications:
   1) Hemorrhage
   2) Infection
   3) Phantom limb pain
   4) Flexion contractures

g. Promote mobility and range of motion.

h. Promote independence.

i. Maintain aseptic technique with dressing changes.

2. Medications

a. Opioids for residual limb pain

b. Calcitonin to reduce phantom limb pain

c. Antispasmodics for muscle spasms

d. Beta blockers for constant, dull, burning pain

e. Antiepileptic drugs for knifelike or sharp burning pain

3. Client Education

a. Types of pain and management regimen

b. Measures to prevent contractures

c. Use of ambulatory devices or prosthetics

D. Referral and Follow-up

1. Rehabilitation therapy

2. Support group

Endocrine System Functions and Disorders

Overview of the endocrine system: The endocrine system is made up of glands, organs, and hormones. The endocrine system works with the nervous system to regulate body function and maintain homeostasis through feedback loops. Endocrine glands include the hypothalamus, pituitary gland, adrenal glands, thyroid gland, parathyroid glands, islet cells of the pancreas, and gonads.

Pituitary Gland

The anterior lobe of the pituitary gland promotes growth of body tissue, is responsible for the secretory activity of the adrenal cortex, and controls the activity of thyroid hormone secretion. The anterior lobe is the major producer of thyrotropic hormone (TSH), adrenocorticotropic hormone (ACTH), luteinizing hormone (LH), follicle-stimulating hormone (FSH), and gonadotropic hormones. The posterior pituitary, controlled mainly by the hypothalamus (known as the master gland), directly affects the function of the other endocrine glands.

Disorders of the Anterior Pituitary Gland

A. Acromegaly: Hypersecretion of growth hormone (GH) that occurs after puberty; commonly associated with benign pituitary tumors. Occurs in approximately 6 out of every 100,000 people

1. Manifestations

a. Enlargement of skeletal extremities; sudden increase in adult height

b. Protrusion of the jaw and orbital ridges

c. Headache, visual problems, and blindness

d. Hyperglycemia, insulin resistance, skin tags, and acanthosis nigricans

e. Hypercalcemia

f. Body odor and excessive perspiration

g. Carpal tunnel syndrome; decreased muscle strength and fatigue; and joint pain and limited range of motion in joints

h. Hoarseness

i. Widely spaced toes and teeth

j. In females: male pattern or excessive hair growth/ menstrual irregularities

k. In males: erectile dysfunction

l. Unintentional weight gain

m. Sleep apnea

2. Diagnostic Procedures

a. Serum studies, showing:
   1) Elevated GH levels
   2) High insulin-like growth factor levels

---

3) Elevated fasting plasma glucose

4) Abnormal glucose tolerance test

b. CT and MRI

1) Pituitary MRI may show a pituitary tumor

c. Spinal x-rays show abnormal bone growth

d. Echocardiogram

1) May show an enlarged heart, leaky mitral or aortic valve

3. Collaborative Care

 a. **NURSING INTERVENTIONS**

1) Provide emotional support.

2) Provide symptomatic care.

3) Prepare client as necessary for surgery if pituitary tumor is to be removed.

4) Prepare client as necessary for pituitary radiation if radiation therapy is warranted.

b. Key Assessment Findings

1) Backache and arthralgias (arthralgias are commonly caused from overgrowth of bone and cartilage, leading to arthritis symptoms)

2) Changes in hat, glove, ring, or shoe size

3) Complaints of excessive perspiration and/or body odor

4) Changes in facial symmetry and size

c. Medications

1) Ocreotide (Sandostatin)—a somatostatin analog (SSA)

a) First line of medication therapy to lower GH levels; can be administered IM or SQ monthly; may cause GI upset and gallstones; generally improves insulin uptake and reduces insulin needs in clients with acromegaly

2) Pegvisomant (Somavert)—GH receptor antagonists

a) Second line of medication therapy to block the effects of excessive GH; does not normalize GH levels; administered SQ once a day

b) Overuse will cause severe fatigue and cardiovascular collapse; educate clients that extra doses will not make the disease go away "faster"

3) Bromocriptine mesylate (Parlodel) or pergolide (Permax)—dopamine agonists

a) Third line of therapy; not as effective as other therapies; generally used in conjunction with SSAs; side effects include headache, nausea, and lightheadedness

d. Therapeutic Measures

1) Surgical removal of pituitary gland (transsphenoidal hypophysectomy); surgery is generally the first treatment option. If surgery is successful, facial appearance and symmetry improve within 3–4 days.

2) Surgery may impact ADH secretion from the pituitary gland; RN should assess for SIADH postoperatively.

3) Irradiation of pituitary gland generally only performed if tumor remains after surgery; irradiation done in conjunction with medications generally requires supplementation of other pituitary hormones.

4. Client Education and Referral

a. Medication adherence

b. Continued compliance with follow-up appointments with all providers

B. Gigantism: Hypersecretion of GH that occurs in childhood prior to closure of the growth plates

1. Manifestations

a. Proportional overgrowth in all body tissue

b. Overgrowth of long bones: height during childhood may reach 8 or 9 ft

1) Generally diagnosed during routine well child visits

2) Parents will report that the child "shot up"

2. Diagnostic procedures and Collaborative Care same as acromegaly

C. Dwarfism: Hyposecretion of GH during fetal development or childhood that results in an adult height of < 4 ft. 10 inches; higher incidence in children with cleft lip and cleft palate. May be congenital or result from damage to the pituitary gland.

1. Manifestations

a. Head and extremities are disproportionate to torso

1) Face may appear younger than peers'

b. Short stature; slow or flat growth rate

1) Slowing in growth rate generally is not recognized until child is between 2–3 years of age.

2) The child will be much shorter than children of the same gender and age.

3) Child may appear "chubby" due to increased body fat to muscle percentage.

c. Progressive bowed legs and lordosis

d. Delayed adolescence or puberty

2. Diagnostic Procedures

a. Comparison of height/weight against growth charts; slowed growth rate will be noted

b. Serum growth hormone level; most providers will also evaluate other hormonal levels to ensure that no secondary deficiencies exist

c. DEXA scans or hand x-rays to determine bone age

d. MRI of the head (to assess pituitary gland)

3. Collaborative Care

 a. **NURSING INTERVENTIONS**

   1) Teach child and family adaptive measures available for ADLs.

   2) Teach child and family how to administer supplemental growth hormone.

      a) Growth hormone will generally increase stature 3–4 inches in years 1 through 3.

      b) The earlier the therapy is initiated, the better the prognosis.

      c) GH therapy does not work in all children.

   3) Provide positive feedback to child to help boost self-esteem.

b. Medications

   1) Human growth hormone injections; generally administered SQ once a day or three times a week; monitor for fluid retention, muscle and joint aches

c. Therapeutic Measures

   1) Limb-lengthening surgery (rarely performed anymore; GH injections are very effective)

Disorders of the Posterior Pituitary Gland

A. **Diabetes Insipidus (DI):** A deficiency of antidiuretic hormone (ADH or vasopressin) that results in the inability of the kidneys to conserve water appropriately. DI is considered central (caused from an injury to the hypothalamus or pituitary gland due to head injury, infection, surgery, or tumors), nephrogenic (congenital is most common; also PKD or hypercalcemia), or drug-induced (lithium, demeclocycline, or amphotericin B). The underlying cause of DI should be identified and treated.

1. Manifestations

   a. Urine chemistry (dilute)

      1) Decreased urine specific gravity

      2) Decreased urine osmolarity (< 300 mmol)

   b. Serum chemistry (concentrated)

      1) Hypernatremia

      2) Increased serum osmolality

      3) Hypokalemia

   c. Polyuria and polydipsia

      1) Urinary output can exceed 50 mL/kg/day

      2) Clients may crave ice water

   d. Dehydration, weight loss, and dry skin

   e. Hemoconcentration

   f. Enuresis/nocturia/urinary frequency

2. Diagnostic Procedures

   a. Water (fluid) deprivation test

      1) Nurse measures body weight and urine volume hourly.

      2) Urine and serum chemistries will become concentrated in cases of DI.

   b. Vasopressin test

      1) Performed only if fluid deprivation test is inconclusive

      2) IV vasopressin is administered

      3) Client urine and serum chemistries will improve

   c. MRI of hypothalamus and pituitary

   d. 24-hour urine

3. Collaborative Care

 a. **NURSING INTERVENTIONS**

   1) Weigh client daily.

   2) Monitor urine specific gravity.

   3) Assess the client's blood pressure and heart rate.

   4) Maintain fluid and electrolyte balance.

b. Medications

   1) Desmopressin acetate (DDAVP)

   2) Vasopressin (Pitressin)

   3) If DI is nephrogenic in origin, thiazide diuretics will be prescribed

      a) Thiazides stimulate ADH production and retain sodium.

c. Client Education and Referral

   1) Lifetime vasopressin replacement therapy

   2) Report weight gain, polyuria, or polydipsia to the health care provider

   3) Monitor fluid intake

   4) Avoid foods with diuretic action

B. **Syndrome of Inappropriate Secretion of Antidiuretic Hormone (SIADH):** The inappropriate, excessive release of antidiuretic hormone resulting in water intoxication; caused by neoplastic tumors, head injury, meningitis, respiratory disorders, and drugs (lithium, phenytoin, NSAIDs, and alcohol).

1. Manifestations

   a. Urine chemistry (concentrated)

      1) Increased urine sodium (> 30 mEq/L)

      2) Increased urine osmolality (> 200 mOsm/kg)

   b. Serum chemistry (dilute)

      1) Decreased serum sodium

      2) Decreased serum osmolality

   c. Mental confusion, irritability, lethargy, and seizures

   d. Increased vasopressin levels

   e. Weight gain

   f. Weakness, anorexia, nausea, and vomiting

   g. *Clinical caution: If the client has edema plus hyponatremia, SIADH is generally not the culprit!* Notify provider promptly if edema is noted.

2. Collaborative Care

 a. **NURSING INTERVENTIONS**

    1) Restrict oral fluids to 500–1,000 mL/day (amount of fluids should be equal to urinary output plus 500 mL/day). Monitor I&O very closely.

    2) Weigh client daily.

    3) Monitor mental status frequently; initiate seizure precautions.

b. Medications

    1) Sodium infusions if profoundly hyponatremic

    2) Loop diuretics; used to treat hypervolemic hyponatremia

    3) Osmotic diuretics; allows free water excretion

    4) Vasopressin receptor antagonists (initiated if serum sodium is less than 125 mEq)

      a) Conivaptan (Vaprisol)

      b) Tolvaptan (Samsca)

c. Therapeutic Measures

    1) Treat the underlying cause with surgery, chemotherapy, and/or radiation.

Adrenal Gland

The adrenal cortex produces glucocorticoids (cortisol) and mineralocorticoids (aldosterone), which regulate glucose metabolism and electrolyte balance. The adrenal cortex also produces androgens and estrogens. The adrenal medulla produces epinephrine and norepinephrine.

Disorders of the Adrenal Cortex

A. Addison's Disease: The hyposecretion of adrenal cortex hormones from insufficiency of cortisol, aldosterone, and androgens caused by autoimmune disease, TB, tumors, HIV; can be induced by abrupt cessation of steroid medications

Memory hint: With Addison's you need to ADD cortisol.

1. Manifestations

    a. Fatigue, muscle pain and weakness, and joint pain

    b. Anorexia, chronic diarrhea, nausea, vomiting, and weight loss

    c. Hyperpigmentation/patchy skin color

    d. Hypotension and syncope; increased heart rate

    e. Hypoglycemia, hyponatremia, hyperkalemia, hypercalcemia

    f. Craving salty foods

    g. Irritability and depression

    h. Diminished libido

2. Diagnostic Procedures

    a. ACTH stimulation test

    b. Electrolyte panels

    c. Abdominal/renal CT scan

3. Collaborative Care

 a. **NURSING INTERVENTIONS**

    1) Assess blood pressure and heart rhythm.

    2) Monitor fluid and electrolyte balance.

    3) Monitor and treat hypoglycemia.

    4) Monitor for Addisonian crisis (also known as adrenal crisis): sudden extreme weakness; severe abdominal, back, and leg pain; hyperpyrexia; coma; death. It occurs secondary to infection, trauma, surgery, pregnancy, or stress. The client will require IV steroids and may require respiratory support.

    5) Monitor for side effects of hormone replacement therapy, which are the same symptoms as hypersecretion of the adrenal cortex.

b. Medications

    1) Hydrocortisone (Cortef)

    2) Prednisone (Deltasone)

    3) Cortisone (Cortisone Acetate)

    4) Fludrocortisone (Florinef)

      a) Most clients are treated with a combination of glucocorticoids and mineralocorticoids.

c. Client Education and Referral

    1) Provide emotional support to the client and provide instruction on lifelong disease management (medications, prompt treatment of infection and illness, and stress management).

    2) Educate about lifelong medication replacement, including the potential need for increased steroid therapy during times of stress or illness.

      a) The client should be educated to promptly notify the provider in cases of infection, injury, and stress. Doses of hormones will need to be individually adjusted during these times.

    3) Teach the client signs and symptoms of Addisonian crisis.

    4) Teach the client to avoid using caffeine and alcohol.

    5) Teach the client to have appropriate medical identification with them at all times in case of emergency.

    6) Advise the client to eat a high-protein and high-carbohydrate diet.

B. Cushing's Disease and Cushing's Syndrome: The hypersecretion of the glucocorticoids from an adenoma of the pituitary gland that stimulates an overproduction of ACTH or a carcinoma of the adrenal gland that stimulates an overproduction of cortisol. Cushing's syndrome is caused by exogenous use of steroid medications.

1. Manifestations

    a. Upper body obesity and thin extremities; moon face, buffalo hump, and neck fat

    b. Skin fragility with purple striae

    c. Osteoporosis

d. Hyperglycemia, hypernatremia, hypokalemia

e. Hirsutism

f. Amenorrhea

g. Elevated triglycerides and hypertension

h. Sexual dysfunction; ED in men

i. Immunosuppression

j. Peptic ulcer disease

k. In children: slower growth rate

l. Backache, bone pain, or tenderness

m. Increased thirst and urination

n. CVA tenderness/flank pain/kidney stones

2. Collaborative Care

 a. **NURSING INTERVENTIONS**

1) Monitor the client for infection.

2) Protect the client from accidents and falls.

3) Monitor and treat hyperglycemia.

4) Assess blood pressure and heart rhythm.

b. Medications

1) Bromocriptine (Parlodel), mitotane (Lysodren), or aminoglutethimide (Cytadren)

c. Therapeutic Measures

1) For a pituitary adenoma, the client may need a transsphenoidal adenomectomy.

2) For an adrenal carcinoma, the client may need a unilateral or bilateral adrenalectomy.

d. Client Education and Referral

1) For clients prescribed exogenous steroid therapy, educate the client concerning long-term self-administration of hormone suppression therapy in Cushing's disease and the need for tapering steroid doses in Cushing's syndrome.

2) Advise the client to eat foods high in protein, low in carbohydrates, and low in sodium, with potassium supplementation.

C. **Hyperaldosteronism (Conn's Syndrome):** The hypersecretion of aldosterone from the adrenal cortex (usually due to a tumor). Primary hyperaldosteronism is fairly rare (generally occurs between 30 and 50 years old); secondary hyperaldosteronism may be caused from cirrhosis, heart failure, or nephrotic syndrome.

1. Manifestations

a. Hypokalemia and hypernatremia

b. Hypertension from hypernatremia

c. Muscle weakness, numbness, and cardiac problems

d. Fatigue

e. Headache

2. Diagnostic Procedures

a. Abdominal CT

b. EKG

c. Serum aldosterone/renin and potassium

d. Urine aldosterone

3. Collaborative Care

 a. **NURSING INTERVENTIONS**

1) Provide the client with a quiet environment.

2) Assess the client's blood pressure and cardiac activity.

3) Monitor the client's potassium level and be prepared to replace potassium.

4) Closely monitor I&O, as acute renal failure has been known to develop from hyperaldosteronism.

b. Medications

1) Antihypertensive medications: spironolactone (Aldactone)

2) Eplerenone (Inspra): blocks action of aldosterone

c. Therapeutic Measures

1) Surgical removal of tumor/adrenal gland if primary cause

Disorders of the Adrenal Medulla

A. **Pheochromocytoma:** A rare, usually benign tumor of the adrenal medulla that causes hypersecretion of epinephrine and norepinephrine; generally seen in young men and women

1. Manifestations

a. Generally sudden onset

b. Hypertensive crisis

c. Tachycardia/palpitations

d. Diaphoresis

e. Apprehension

f. Nausea, vomiting

g. Orthostatic hypotension

h. Headache

i. Pallor

j. Fight-or-flight symptoms

k. Hyperglycemia

l. Tremors

m. Insomnia

2. Diagnostic Procedures

a. 24-hour urine to determine levels of the hormones adrenaline (epinephrine) and noradrenaline (norepinephrine) and their breakdown products (metanephrines)

b. CT, MRI, or PET scan

c. Adrenal biopsy

3. Collaborative Care

 a. **NURSING INTERVENTIONS**

1) Carefully assess vital signs.

2) Provide a high-calorie, nutritious diet and avoid caffeine.

3) Encourage frequent rest periods.

4) Provide a quiet environment.

5) Assess for hypertension to prevent stroke secondary to hypertensive crisis

6) Do not palpate or assess for CVA tenderness, as this can cause rupture of the tumor.

b. Medications

1) Alpha and beta-blocker medication to diminish the effect of norepinephrine prior to surgery

c. Therapeutic Measures

1) Surgical removal of tumor

Thyroid Gland

The thyroid gland has a rich blood supply and produces throxine (T_4), triiodothyronine (T_3), and calcitonin. T_4 and T_3 regulate metabolism, and calcitonin helps regulate serum calcium levels.

Disorders of the thyroid gland

A. Hypothyroidism: A malfunction of the thyroid gland in which there is a slow, but progressive decrease in secretion of thyrocalcitonin and hyposecretion of thyroxine (T_4) and triiodothyronine (T_3); more commonly seen in women, peaking between the ages of 50 and 60.

1. Manifestations

a. Fatigue and weakness

b. Increased sensitivity to cold

c. Constipation

d. Dry skin, brittle hair and nails

e. Weight gain

f. Deepened, hoarse voice

g. Joint pain and stiffness

h. Hyperlipidemia and anemia

i. Depression

j. Heavy menstrual cycle

k. Facial edema/goiter

l. Puffy appearance (non-pitting edema)

2. Diagnostic Procedures/Findings

a. Low serum T_4 and T_3

b. Elevated TSH (seen in primary hypothyroidism)

c. A goiter may be seen due to increased gland activity initiated by elevated TSH levels

3. Myxedema coma is a rare and serious condition seen in untreated or uncontrolled hypothyroidism. The severely decreased metabolism causes the heart muscle to become flabby, resulting in decreased cardiac output and organ failure. High mortality rate.

4. Collaborative Care

 a. **NURSING INTERVENTIONS**

1) Provide the client with a warm environment.

2) Provide a low-calorie, low-cholesterol, and low-fat diet.

3) Increase roughage and fluids.

4) Avoid sedatives.

5) Plan rest periods for the client.

6) Weigh the client daily.

7) Observe for manifestations of overdose of thyroid preparations (palpitations, insomnia, increased appetite, and tremors).

b. Medications

1) Levothyroxine (Synthroid)

c. Client Education and Referral

1) Educate the client regarding lifelong medication therapy

2) Continued follow-up with provider

3) Take medication on an empty stomach each morning

4) Know signs and symptoms of medication toxicity

5) Eat a diet high in fiber

6) Monitor need for sleep

B. Hyperthyroidism: The hypersecretion of thyroxine; typically from the immune system (Grave's disease); more common in women older than 20.

1. Manifestations

a. Anxiety and irritability

b. Insomnia and fatigue

c. Tachycardia

d. Tremors

e. Diaphoresis

f. Intolerance of heat

g. Weight loss (despite food intake)

h. Exophthalmos and photosensitivity

i. Diarrhea

j. Light or absent menstrual cycle

2. Diagnostic Procedures/Findings

a. Elevated T_4 and T_3

b. Elevated thyrotropin receptor antibodies (seen in Grave's disease)

3. Thyroid storm is a rare and life-threatening condition seen in untreated or uncontrolled hyperthyroidisms. Hyperpyrexia, tachycardia, and systolic hypertension are classic symptoms.

4. Collaborative Care

a. **NURSING INTERVENTIONS**

1) Assess VS.

2) Promote comfort.

3) Encourage the client to get adequate rest in a cool, quiet environment.

4) Provide a high-caloric (4,000 to 5,000 cal/day), high-protein, and high-carbohydrate diet without stimulants or extra fluids.

5) Weigh the client daily.

6) Provide the client emotional support.

7) Provide eye protection for the client by giving ophthalmic medicine, taping the client's eyes at night, and decreasing sodium and water.

8) Elevate the head of the client's bed.

b. Medications

1) Beta-blocker medications are needed to manage tachycardia, anxiety, and tremors.

a) Nadolol (Corgard), propranolol (Inderal), atenolol (Tenormin), metoprolol (Lopressor)

2) Propylthiouracil (Propyl-Thyracil or PTU): blocks thyroid hormone production.

3) Methimazole (Tapazole): short-term use to block production of thyroxine; usually used no more than 8 weeks. Monitor CBC frequently for occurrence of agranulocytosis.

4) Iodides decrease vascularity and inhibit the release of thyroid hormones.

a) Lugol's solution (use is decreasing)

b) Saturated solution of potassium iodide (SSKI); used prior to thyroidectomy

5) A radioactive iodine treatment shrinks the thyroid gland prior to surgery.

a) Sodium iodide 131

c. Therapeutic Measures

1) Thyroidectomy: the removal of all or part of the thyroid gland. Requires a lifelong intake of levothyroxine (Synthroid) and calcium

a) Preoperative goal: decrease thyroid function toward normal range (euthyroid) using saturated solution of potassium iodide (SSKI) and antithyroid medication

b) Postoperative interventions

(1) Place the client in the semi-Fowler's position.

(2) Assess the client's dressing, especially the back of the neck.

(3) Observe for respiratory distress. Keep a tracheostomy tray, oxygen, and suction apparatus at the client's bedside.

(4) Assess for signs of hemorrhage.

(5) Note any hoarseness, which is indicative of laryngeal nerve injury; limit talking.

(6) Observe for signs of tetany (Chvostek's and Trousseau's sign), which may indicate damage or accidental removal of parathyroid glands and subsequent hypocalcemia.

(7) Keep calcium gluconate IV at the client's bedside.

(8) Observe for thyroid storm caused by an increased release of the thyroid hormone due to manipulation of the thyroid gland.

(9) Gradually increase the range of motion to the neck and support the client when sitting up.

Parathyroid Gland

The parathyroid gland maintains calcium and phosphate balance

Disorders of the Parathyroid Gland

A. Hypoparathyroidism: The hyposecretion of PTH, resulting in hypocalcemia and hyperphosphatemia

1. Manifestations

a. Paresthesia

b. Muscle cramps and tetany

c. Chvostek's sign: tapping the side of the cheek causes muscle spasms and twitching around the mouth, throat, and cheeks

d. Trousseau's sign: pressure from the blood pressure cuff induces muscle spasms in the distal extremity

e. Alopecia

f. Dry skin, brittle hair and nails

g. Painful menstruation

h. Poor development of tooth enamel

i. Lethargic, low energy

j. Thin hair and brittle nails

k. Mental retardation

l. Circumoral paraesthesia with numbness and tingling of the fingers

2. Collaborative Care

a. **NURSING INTERVENTIONS**

1) Place the client in a quiet room with no stimuli.

2) Assess the client for signs of neuromuscular irritability.

3) Provide a high-calcium, low-phosphorous diet.

4) Institute seizure precautions.

b. Medications

1) Acute: IV calcium gluconate

2) Chronic:

a) Oral calcium salts (generally calcium carbonate)

b) Vitamin D

B. Hyperparathyroidism: A hypersecretion of PTH (caused by tumor or renal disease) that leads to the loss of calcium from the bones into the serum, resulting in hypercalcemia and hypophosphatemia

1. Manifestations

a. Kidney stones and hyperuricemia

b. Osteoporosis/renal osteodystrophy

c. Hypercalcemia and hypophosphatemia

d. Abdominal pain, nausea, and vomiting

e. Muscle weakness and fatigue

f. Polyuria and polydipsia

g. Hypertension

2. Collaborative Care

 a. **NURSING INTERVENTIONS**

1) Force fluids.

2) Provide the client a low-calcium, low-vitamin D diet.

3) Prevent constipation and fecal impaction.

4) Strain all of the client's urine.

5) Instruct the client about safety measures to prevent fractures.

b. Medications

1) Plicamycin (Mithracin) or gallium nitrate (Ganite)

2) Calcitonin decreases the release of skeletal calcium and increases the kidney excretion of calcium; enhanced if given along with glucocorticoids.

3) Hydration and diuretics: furosemide (Lasix); promotes excretion of excess calcium.

c. Therapeutic Measures

1) Subtotal surgical resection of the parathyroid gland

Pancreas

The pancreas is a gland that produces insulin designed to decrease blood glucose by stimulating active transport of glucose into muscle and adipose tissue, stimulating protein synthesis, and promoting the conversion of glucose to glycogen for storage; also produces glucagon, which converts glycogen back to glucose when needed.

Disorders of the pancreas

A. Diabetes mellitus: A chronic disorder of carbohydrate metabolism, characterized by an imbalance between insulin supply and demand; either a subnormal amount of insulin is produced or the body requires abnormally high amounts.

1. Type 1: insulin-dependent diabetes mellitus; usually juvenile onset. The body does not make insulin.

2. Type 2: Noninsulin-dependent diabetes mellitus:

a. Of the over 25 million Americans with diabetes mellitus, approximately 90% have type 2.

b. Diabetes mellitus is caused by the dual defects of insulin resistance and beta-cell secretory dysfunction. The pancreas does not make enough insulin or the body does not respond to the insulin.

c. Insulin resistance is the classic symptom of type 2 DM.

d. More common in people of color and those who are obese or have a sedentary lifestyle.

3. Glycemic Control

a. Maintaining tight glycemic control substantially reduces the risk for the onset or progression of the complications of diabetes mellitus.

b. Glucose control is monitored on a day-to-day basis by capillary blood glucose levels.

1) Normal preprandial (fasting) blood glucose is 70–99 mg/dL.

2) Normal postprandial blood glucose is 70–140 mg/dL.

c. Glucose control is monitored on a long-term basis by HbA1c (glycosylated hemoglobin).

1) Normal (nondiabetic) HbA1c level is less than 6%.

2) The goal of the American Diabetes Association is a HbA1c level of less than 7% in diabetics.

4. Manifestations: "3 Polys"

a. Polyuria

b. Polydipsia

c. Polyphagia

5. Long-Term Complications

a. Diabetic neuropathy: Causes pain in the legs, decreased sensation, and impotence in men

b. Renal: Affects microcirculation of the kidneys; results in renal failure

c. Cardiovascular: Clients with diabetes mellitus are four times more likely to have acute coronary syndromes; DM also increases the occurrence of hypertension and decreased peripheral circulation

d. Eyes: DM is the number one cause of blindness and cataracts

e. Infections: Increased glucose in body fluids makes for an ideal medium for growth of micro-organisms, urinary tract infections, and cellulitis

6. Collaborative Care

 a. **NURSING INTERVENTIONS**

1) Balance the client's diet with insulin and exercise.

2) Administer insulin therapy as prescribed.

a) Insulin is necessary to open the door for glucose to enter the cell and be used for energy.

b) Rotate areas of insulin injection to avoid lipodystrophy (indurated areas of subcutaneous tissue secondary to injecting cold insulin or not rotating sites).

3) Provide the client with adequate nutrients for proper cell growth and function.

4) Teach the client proper foot care.

a) Cleanse feet daily in warm, soapy water; rinse and dry carefully; don't break blisters; trim nails to follow natural curve of the toe; always wear breathable shoes such as leather; no crossing of the legs; no cream between toes; inspect each foot daily.

5) Instruct the client about the importance of weight management.

6) Encourage the client not to smoke.

7) Teach stress-reduction techniques.

8) Assist the client in developing lifestyle changes that support the maintenance of dietary insulin and blood glucose control. Referral to a diabetic educator is appropriate.

9) Monitor all systems for complications.

a) Hypoglycemia occurs when the blood glucose level falls below 60 mg/dL.

(1) Causes: decreased dietary intake, excess insulin, and increased exercise

(2) Manifestations

(a) Tachycardia

(b) Diaphoresis

(c) Weakness, fatigue

(d) Irritability, anxiety

(e) Confusion

 (3) **NURSING INTERVENTIONS**

(a) Give the client 15 g of a fast-acting simple carbohydrates (hard candy, 4 tsp of sugar, one Tbsp of honey, ½ cup fruit juice)

(b) Pure glucose may be the preferred treatment, but any form of carbohydrate that contains glucose will raise blood glucose. Adding protein to carbohydrate does not affect the glycemic response and does not prevent subsequent hypoglycemia. Adding fat may retard and then prolong the acute glycemic response.

(c) For severe hypoglycemia (blood glucose of less than 20 mg/dL), the client may not be able to swallow. If he is unconscious or seizing, administer 1 mg of glucagon IM or subcutaneous.

(d) Follow the 15/15/15 rule:

1. Administer 15 g of simple carbohydrates.

2. Wait 15 minutes and recheck serum glucose.

3. Administer 15 more grams of carbohydrates.

b. Medications (see Pharmacology Content)

1) Insulin pump: An external device that provides a basal dose of rapid-acting or regular insulin with a bolus dose before meals; does not read blood glucose

a) Needles are inserted into subcutaneous abdominal tissue (change site every 24 to 48 hr)

b) Complications are secondary to continuous administration of insulin

c) Allows for liberalization of diet and a sense of normalcy

c. Client Education

1) Maintain diet therapy.

2) Maintain a balance between the amount of glucose in the body and the amount of insulin present to use the glucose.

3) The provider may advise the client to follow food exchanges or carb counting from the American Diabetes Association's diet.

B. **Diabetic Ketoacidosis:** Complication of diabetes mellitus due to deficient insulin production; exacerbated hyperglycemia causes production of ketones resulting from fat used for energy; the most common is type 1 diabetes mellitus.

1. Contributing Factors

a. Illness, fever, or infection

b. Surgery

c. Fever

d. Substance abuse

e. Noncompliance with insulin therapy

2. Manifestations

a. Exacerbated polyuria, polydipsia, polyphagia

b. Anorexia, nausea, and vomiting

c. Metabolic acidosis with ketonuria

d. Kussmaul's respirations

e. Fruity, scented breath

f. Monitor for level of consciousness changes (coma can result)

3. Collaborative Care

 a. **NURSING INTERVENTIONS**

1) Provide vascular support.

2) Administer fluid and electrolyte replacements as prescribed by the provider.

3) Administer regular insulin IV therapy.

a) In any hyperglycemic emergency, the goal of therapy is to return the client to a normal blood glucose level. However, too rapid of a drop in serum blood glucose levels will precipitate a hypoglycemic response. The goal of therapy is to reduce blood glucose by 25% over the first 4 hours and to return to baseline during the next 24 hours.

C. **Hyperglycemic–Hyperosmolar State (HHS)**

1. Manifestations

a. Extremely high glucose levels cause dehydration

1) The glucose level in HHS is higher than in DKA

b. Generally not seen with ketosis

c. elevated BUN

2. Collaborative Care

a. **NURSING INTERVENTIONS**

1) Replace fluids as prescribed.

2) Administer insulin and electrolytes as prescribed.

D. Transient Hyperglycemia: An elevated blood glucose level greater than 140 mg/dL; generally treated with sliding scale insulin to return serum blood glucose to normal range

1. Prompt treatment is necessary to avoid hyperglycemic emergencies.

a. Treated with regular insulin

b. Gold standard in sliding scale insulin is blood glucose 100/30

1) 100 is used as "normal" blood glucose

2) Divisor is 30 as one unit of regular insulin will decrease BG by 30 mg/dL

a) Example: client's BG is 220 mg/dL

$$(220 - 100)/30 = 120/30 = 4$$

Administer 4 units of regular insulin as the sliding scale dose.

SECTION 7

Blood Disorders

A. Anemia: A deficiency of RBCs characterized by a decreased RBC count, Hgb, or Hct. Anemia is a clinical sign that results in decreased oxygen delivery to the cells.

1. Contributing Factors

a. Acute or chronic blood loss (gastrointestinal bleeding)

b. Greater than normal destruction of RBCs (spleen diseases)

c. Abnormal bone marrow function (chemotherapy)

d. Decreased erythropoietin (renal failure)

e. Inadequate maturation of RBCs (cancer)

f. Nutritional deficiencies (iron, B_{12}, folic acid, intrinsic factor)

2. Manifestations

a. Fatigue, dizziness, and weakness

b. Pallor: first seen in conjunctival area (Caucasian) and oral area (dark-skinned population), as well as the nail beds, the palmar creases, and around the mouth

c. Tachycardia, murmurs and gallops, and orthostatic hypotension

d. Decreased activity tolerance

e. Decreased Hgb, Hct, and RBC levels

f. Shortness of breath and dyspnea; decreased oxygen saturation levels

g. Increased fatigue and headache

3. Collaborative Care

a. **NURSING INTERVENTIONS**

1) Monitor labs (RBC, Hgb, and Hct).

2) Encourage activity as tolerated by the client with frequent rest periods.

3) Monitor skin integrity and implement measures to prevent breakdown.

4) Provide oxygen therapy to the client as needed.

5) Administer blood products and medications as prescribed. (see individual anemias)

B. Types of Anemia

1. Anemia secondary to renal disease: Anemia due to lack of erythropoietin

a. Medications

1) Erythropoietin (Procrit, Epogen)

2. Iron deficiency anemia: Anemia resulting from low iron levels; the iron stores are depleted first, followed by hemoglobin stores

a. Contributing Factors

1) Chronic blood loss (bleeding ulcer)

2) Nutritional deficiency

3) Common in infants, young adult women, and older adults

b. Manifestations

1) Microcytic red blood cells

2) Weakness and pallor

3) Low serum ferritin levels:
   Male: 12-300 ng/mL; *Female*: 12-150 ng/mL

c. Collaborative Care

 1) **NURSING INTERVENTIONS**

a) Monitor for symptoms of bleeding

b) Monitor labs

2) Medications

a) Administer iron preparations

3) Therapeutic Measures

a) Follow provider prescriptions for ulcer treatment

3. Aplastic anemia: Bone marrow suppression of new stem cell production resulting in a deficiency of circulating WBCs, platelets, and/or RBCs. Can be due to medications, viruses, toxins, and/or radiation exposure

a. Manifestations

1) Hypoxia, fatigue, and pallor (related to anemia)

2) Increased susceptibility to infection (related to leukopenia)

3) Hemorrhage, ecchymosis/petechiae (related to thrombocytopenia)

4) Pancytopenia (decrease in RBC's, WBC's and Platelets)

b. Collaborative Care

 1) **NURSING INTERVENTIONS**

a) Monitor labs.

b) Provide the client protective isolation.

c) Monitor for manifestations of infection.

d) Provide emotional and psychological support to the client.

e) Implement protective barrier precautions.

2) Medications

a) Immunosuppressive therapy (prednisone, cyclosporine)

b) Chemotherapy drugs (Cytoxan, Procytox)

3) Therapeutic Measures

a) Hematopoietic stem cell transplantation

b) Splenectomy

c) Cautious use of blood transfusions

4. Pernicious anemia: Anemia due to a lack of dietary intake or absorption of vitamin B$_{12}$

a. Contributing Factors

1) Atrophy of the gastric mucosa/hypochlorhydria (underproduction of hydrochloric acid by the stomach)

2) Total gastrectomy (lack of intrinsic factor decreases intestinal vitamin B$_{12}$ absorption)

3) Malnutrition

b. Manifestations

1) Numbness and tingling of extremities; paresthesia

2) Hypoxemia

3) Pallor

4) Jaundice

5) Glossitis

6) Poor balance

c. Diagnostic Procedures

1) Shilling test measures the presence of vitamin B$_{12}$ in the urine after the client is given an oral dose of radioactive vitamin B$_{12}$.

2) CBC: megoblastic RBCs (macrocytic)

d. Collaborative Care

 1) **NURSING INTERVENTIONS**

a) Monitor labs.

b) Promote rest for the client and encourage a balanced dietary intake.

2) Medications

a) Cobalamin (vitamin B$_{12}$); standard dose is 1,000 mcg IM daily for 2 weeks, then weekly until Hct level is therapeutic, then monthly for life. Nascobal intranasally maintains vitamin B$_{12}$ levels.

5. Folic acid deficiency anemia: Anemia due to folic acid deficiency. Symptoms similar to vitamin B$_{12}$ deficiency, but nervous system functions remain normal.

a. Contributing Factors

1) Poor nutrition

2) Malabsorption (secondary to Crohn's disease)

3) Drugs (chronic alcohol abuse, anticonvulsants, and oral contraceptives)

b. Collaborative Care

1) **NURSING INTERVENTIONS**

a) Identify high-risk clients: alcoholics, elderly, debilitated clients

2) Medications

a) Folic acid replacement

6. Hemolytic anemia: A group of anemias that occur when the bone marrow is unable to increase production to make up for the premature destruction of red blood cells. Sickle cell and Thalassemia are hemolytic anemias.

a. Contributing Factors

1) Trauma; crushing injuries

2) Lead poisoning

3) Tuberculosis

4) Infections

5) Transfusion reactions

6) Toxic agents

b. Manifestations

1) Chills

2) Dark urine

3) Enlarged spleen

4) Pallor

5) Rapid heart rate

6) Shortness of breath

7) Jaundice

c. Collaborative Care

1) **NURSING INTERVENTIONS**

a) Treat the underlying cause.

b) Hydrate the client.

c) Blood transfusion when kidney function is normal.

2) Medications

a) In severe immune-related hemolytic anemia, steroid therapy is sometimes necessary.

7. Sickle cell anemia: A genetic defect found in clients of African American or Mediterranean origin, in which the Hgb molecule assumes a sickle shape and delivers less oxygen to tissues; the sickle cells become lodged in the blood vessels, especially the brain and the kidneys.

a. Contributing Factors (precipitate crisis by enhancing sickling)

1) Stress

2) Dehydration

3) Hypoxia

4) High altitudes

b. Manifestations

1) Severe pain and swelling

2) Fever

3) Jaundice

4) Susceptibility to infection

5) Hypoxic damage to organs

c. Diagnostic Procedures

   1) Percentage of hemoglobin S (Hbs) seen on electrophoresis. Sickle cell trait has less than 40% Hbs and sickle cell disease may have 80–100% Hbs.

d. Collaborative Care

   1) **NURSING INTERVENTIONS**

     a) Maintain adequate hydration.

     b) Provide oxygen therapy to the client.

     c) Encourage the client to rest.

     d) Teach the client to identify triggers, get immunizations in a timely manner, and refer for genetic counseling.

   2) Medications

     a) Morphine sulfate or hydromorphone (Dilaudid) to manage the client's pain

     b) Hydroxyurea (Droxia) to reduce the amount of sickling and number of painful episodes

8. Thalassemia: Inherited blood disorder in which the body makes an abnormal form of hemoglobin, resulting in excessive destruction of red blood cells, which leads to anemia.

  a. Contributing Factors

   1) Must inherit the defective gene from both parents to develop thalassemia major

   2) Asian, Chinese, Mediterranean, or African American ethnicity

   3) Family history of the disorder.

  b. Manifestations

   1) Develop during the first year of life.

   2) Bone deformities in the face

   3) Fatigue

     a) Growth failure

   4) Shortness of breath

   5) Yellow skin (jaundice)

  c. Diagnostic Procedures

   1) Red blood cells appear small and abnormally shaped.

   2) Complete blood count (CBC) reveals anemia.

   3) Hemoglobin electrophoresis shows the presence of an abnormal form of hemoglobin.

   4) Mutational analysis detects alpha thalassemia that cannot be seen with hemoglobin electrophoresis.

  d. Collaborative Care

   1) **NURSING INTERVENTIONS**

     a) Encourage increase of folate in the diet by including dark green leafy vegetables, dried beans and peas (legumes), and citrus fruits and juices.

     b) Administer blood transfusions.

     c) Encourage rest

     d) Provide genetic counseling

  2) Therapeutic Measures

     a) Treatment often involves regular blood transfusions.

     b) Clients receiving blood transfusions should not take iron supplements as this can cause high iron levels in the blood.

     c) Chelation therapy may be necessary to remove excess iron from the body.

     d) Bone marrow transplant may help treat the disease in some clients, especially children.

  3) Medications

     a) Folic acid

SECTION 8

Cardiovascular System Disorders

A. Cardiovascular Overview

1. Efficiently pumps blood to all parts of the body, indicating healthy working cardiac muscles and system

2. Circulates adequate blood volume to meet the body's needs

3. Adequate blood pressure is maintained by peripheral vascular.

4. Normal heart rate is 60 to 100 per minute.

B. Diagnostic Procedures

1. Laboratory tests

  a. Serum electrolytes

  b. Erythrocyte sedimentation rate (ESR); indicator of inflammation

  c. C-reactive protein

  d. Blood coagulation tests

   1) PTT (16–40 seconds): most significant if the client is on heparin therapy

   2) PT (11–14 seconds): most significant if the client is on warfarin sodium (Coumadin) therapy

   3) INR

     a) Normal INR is 1.

     b) Universal test is not affected by variations in laboratory norms.

     c) If the client requires anticoagulation, the desired value is increased to approximately 2 to 3.

     d) BUN and creatinine: reflect renal function and perfusion; levels may increase in MI, CHF, and cardiomyopathy

     e) Total serum cholesterol desirable: less than 200 mg/dL; risk for cardiac or stroke event with levels greater than 200

       (1) Low-density lipids: desirable less than 100 mg/dL

       (2) High-density lipids: desirable greater than 40 mg/dL for men, 50 mg/dL for women

(3) Triglycerides: desirable less than 150 mg/dL

(4) B-type natriuretic peptide (BNP): indicator for diagnosing heart failure; normal is less than 50 pg/mL

f) Enzymes (test indicates death of myocardial muscles; heart attack)

(1) Creatinine phosphokinase MB (CPK–MB) isoenzyme is an enzyme that increases within 4 to 6 hr following an MI and remains elevated from 24 to 72 hr. Normal value is 30 to 170 units/L.

(2) Troponin is a protein that is considered the gold standard in diagnosing MI. A series of three tests completed over 12 hr can remain elevated for 1 to 2 weeks following an event. Normal level < 0.2 ng/dL.

g) Central venous pressure (normal = 5 to 10 cm water)

(1) Provides an indication of pressure in the right atrium

(2) Trends are more important than values

2. ECG: A record depicting the electrical activity of the heart

a. Interpretation

1) P wave: atrial depolarization

2) PR interval: 0.12 to 0.2 seconds

3) QRS complex: ventricular depolarization; 0.08 to 0.1 seconds

4) T wave: ventricular repolarization

b. Sinus dysrhythmias

1) Atrial fibrillation

a) Rapid, irregular quivering of the atria

b) Loss of atrial kick

c) May lead to stroke and/or heart failure

d) Managed with cardioversion, beta-blockers, digoxin, and warfarin (Coumadin)

2) Sinus tachycardia

a) Heart rate exceeds 100/min

b) Occurs with hypoglycemia, hypokalemia, digoxin toxicity, anxiety, fever, hypotension, and stimulants

c) Treated by removing the cause

3) Sinus bradycardia

a) Rate below 60/min

(1) Normal in athletes

(2) Significance related to how it affects cardiac output

(3) Treated by administering anticholinergic medication (Atropine)

4) Atrioventricular (AV) heart block: Cardiac electrical conduction transmission is blocked from sinoatrial node to the AV node causing bradycardia, syncope, and palpitations

a) First degree

(1) Delayed transmission of impulse through the AV node

(2) Prolonged PR interval (greater than 0.2)

(3) No treatment necessary

b) Second degree

(1) Not all impulses pass through the AV node

(2) May progress to more lethal heart block

(3) Pacemaker may be necessary

c) Third degree

(1) No impulses pass through AV node

(2) Atria and ventricles beat independently of each other

(3) Ventricular pacemaker takes over; the ventricles are slow and an unreliable source to generate cardiac heart rate

(4) Indication for a permanent pacemaker

c. Ventricular dysrhythmias

1) Premature ventricular contraction

a) Ventricles contract prematurely, causing palpitations

b) Caused by stress, caffeine, acidosis, alcohol, infection, MI, CHF, anemia, hypokalemia, or hypomagnesemia

c) Side effects: slowing of the heart rate, decreased blood pressure, and tissue perfusion

d) Untreated in clients without underlying disease; eliminate possible causes

e) PVCs in MI may be treated with amiodarone (Cordarone), beta blockers, or lidocaine

2) Ventricular tachycardia

a) Pulse rate above 150/min

b) Decreases cardiac output

c) Treatment: pulse (cardioversion); no pulse (defibrillation)

d) Treat with antiarrhythmic medications

(1) amiodarone (Cordarone)

(2) lidocaine (Xylocaine)

3) Ventricular fibrillation

a) Most serious dysrhythmia

b) Synonymous with cardiac arrest; treat with CPR and defibrillation

3. Cardiac catheterization: A diagnostic or therapeutic procedure introducing a catheter into the right or left side of the heart through either the femoral or brachial artery.

a. Types:

1) **Angiography**: A procedure utilizing the injection of a contrast medium into the vascular system to outline an area of the body

2) **Angioplasty**: Includes a variety of procedures.

b. Purpose

1) Measure oxygen concentration, saturation, tension, and pressure in various chambers of the client's heart

2) Detect coronary shunts

3) Balloon angioplasty

4) Stent placement

5) Obtain blood samples

6) Determine cardiac output and pulmonary blood flow

7) Determine the client's need for cardiac bypass surgery

 c. **NURSING INTERVENTIONS**

1) Prior to catheterization

a) Verify that procedural consent has been obtained.

b) Know approach for shave prep—right (venous) side, or left (arterial) side.

c) NPO for 6 hours prior to the procedure.

d) Mark distal (baseline) pulses.

e) Explain to the client that the procedure may leave a metallic taste, and may feel flushed when the dye is injected.

f) Verify that the client does not have any history of allergy to dye or shellfish.

2) After catheterization

a) Monitor the client's blood pressure and apical pulse every 15 min for 2 to 4 hr.

b) Perform a neurovascular assessment on the client every 15 min, for the first 2 hr; then every 30 min until the client is able to sit up.

c) Monitor for hematoma at catheter insertion site.

d) Apply pressure for a minimum of 15 min to prevent bleeding or hematoma formation.

e) Monitor for vasospasm, dysrhythmia, or rupture of the coronary vessel.

f) Assess the client for chest pain.

g) Keep the extremity extended for 4 to 6 hr.

h) Maintain bed rest; no hip flexion and no sitting up in bed.

i) Increase fluid intake to enhance flushing of dye.

C. Cardiac Disorders

1. Angina (stable, unstable, and variant): A manifestation of myocardial ischemia caused by arterial stenosis or blockage, uncontrolled blood pressure, or cardiomyopathy

   • **Stable angina**. Usually triggered by physical exertion. Factors such as emotional stress, cold temperatures, heavy meals and smoking also can narrow arteries and trigger angina.

   • **Unstable angina**. If fatty deposits in a blood vessel rupture or a blood clot forms, it can quickly block or reduce flow through a narrowed artery, suddenly and severely decreasing blood flow to the heart muscle. Unstable angina can also be caused by conditions such as severe anemia when narrowed coronary arteries are present; is not relieved by rest or medications.

   • **Variant angina**. Also called Prinzmetal's angina, is caused by a spasm in a coronary artery in which the artery temporarily narrows. Accounts for about 2 percent of angina cases.

a. Contributing Factors

1) Coronary artery disease
2) Diabetes; hypertension
3) Obesity; hypercholesterolemia
4) Family history and stress

b. Manifestations

1) Chest pain or discomfort
2) Pain in arms, neck, jaw, shoulder or back accompanying chest pain
3) Nausea
4) Fatigue
5) Shortness of breath
6) Anxiety
7) Sweating
8) Dizziness

c. Diagnostic Procedures

1) ECG, stress test, echocardiogram, chest x-ray
2) Coronary angiography and cardiac enzymes

d. Collaborative Care

1) **NURSING INTERVENTIONS**

a) Assess the client's pain:
   (1) Location: jaw and/or arm, as well as chest
      (a) Character
      (b) Duration: relieved with rest and/or nitroglycerine (Nitro-Bid)
      (c) Precipitating factors (once identified, eliminate or minimize to avoid attacks)

2) Administer oxygen as needed.

3) Provide environment conducive to rest; avoid activities

4) Administer Medications
   a) Aspirin
   b) Nitrates
   c) Beta blockers
   d) Statins
   e) Calcium channel blockers
   f) Angiotensin-converting enzyme (ACE)

5) Client Education
   a) Educate the client regarding lifestyle changes to prevent further episodes of angina:
      (1) Avoid constipation.
      (2) Avoid excessive activity in cold weather.
      (3) Decrease stress.
      (4) Exercise.
      (5) Low-sodium, low-fat diet.
      (6) Maintain healthy weight.
      (7) Rest after meals.
      (8) Stop smoking.
   b) Disease process (peripheral vasodilation decreases myocardial oxygen demand; coronary artery vasodilation increases the supply of oxygen to the myocardium).

c) Provide teaching on the correct use of nitroglycerin:
   (1) Take as needed at onset of chest pain or tightness or in preparation of exertional activity.
   (2) Take nitroglycerin as prescribed, at onset of attack, and every 5 min up to three doses. If pain is not relieved, call 9-1-1.
   (3) Store nitroglycerin in a dark, dry spot, and replace every 6 months.
   (4) Side effects of taking nitroglycerin include headache and hypotension.
   (5) Types of nitroglycerin are tablets, ointment, patch, or spray.
   (6) If the client is given nitroglycerin for prevention, the client must be nitroglycerine free daily for 12 hr to prevent developing a tolerance.
   (7) If the client uses a nitro patch, instruct to apply it in the morning and remove it at bedtime.
   (8) Instruct the client to take nitroglycerine (Nitrostat) while sitting down and stopping all activity.
   (9) Erectile dysfunction therapy is contraindicated with the use of nitrates.

2. Myocardial infarction (MI): The process by which myocardial tissue is destroyed due to reduced coronary blood flow and lack of oxygen; actual necrosis of the heart muscle (myocardium) occurs.
   a. Contributing Factors
      1) Atherosclerotic heart disease
      2) Coronary artery embolism
   b. Manifestations
      1) Severe chest pain
      2) Unrelieved with nitroglycerin or rest
      3) Crushing quality, radiates to jawline, left arm, neck, and/or back
      4) Diabetics and women often report no pain
      5) Diaphoresis, nausea, vomiting, anxiety, fear
      6) Vital sign changes: tachycardia, hypotension, dyspnea, dysrhythmias
   c. Diagnostic Procedures
      1) Laboratory results: elevated troponin and CK-MB enzymes, elevated LDH
      2) ECG changes: ST elevation, T-wave inversion
   d. Collaborative Care
      1) **NURSING INTERVENTIONS** (aimed at resting the myocardium and preserving the heart muscle)
         a) Early
            (1) Administer oxygen.
            (2) Medications:
                (a) Aspirin
                (b) Antidysrhythmics: amiodarone (Cordarone), lidocaine (Xylocaine)
                (c) Analgesics: morphine sulfate
                (d) Anticoagulants: heparin IV
                (e) Thrombolytics within 6 hr of a cardiac event: streptokinase (Streptase), alteplase recombinant (Activase)
                (f) Vasodilators: nitroglycerine
                (g) Beta-blockers: metoprolol (Lopressor)
                (h) Calcium channel blockers: verapamil (Calan), nifedipine (Procardia)
            (3) Frequently monitor vital signs, O_2 saturation, and ECG.
            (4) Provide emotional support to the client.
         b) Later
            (1) Administer stool softeners to prevent straining with bowel movements and/or Valsalva maneuver.
            (2) Provide the client a soft, low-fat, low-cholesterol, low-sodium diet.
            (3) Use a bedside commode, which requires less energy than using a bedpan.
            (4) Promote self-care, but instruct the client to stop at the onset of pain.
            (5) Plan for cardiac rehabilitation.
            (6) Initiate an exercise program, but stop if fatigue or chest pain occurs.
            (7) Teach and encourage the use of stress management techniques.
            (8) Teach the client to modify any risk factors:
                (a) Obesity
                (b) Stress
                (c) Diet
                (d) Hypertension
                (e) Smoking
                (f) Lack of exercise
            (9) Recognize the risk factors that cannot be modified:
                (a) Heredity
                (b) Race
                (c) Age
                (d) Sex
                (e) Type-A personality
            (10) Ensure bleeding precautions with anticoagulant and antiplatelet therapy.
            (11) Initiate long-term medication therapy:
                (a) Anticoagulants/Antiplatelets: heparin, aspirin, warfarin (Coumadin), enoxaparin (Lovenox), clopidogrel (Plavix)
                (b) Antihypertensives: metoprolol (Lopressor), hydrochlorothiazide (Hydrodiuril), and calcium channel blockers diltiazem (Cardizem)
                (c) Vasodilators: nitroglycerin
                (d) Antilipidemics: simvastatin (Zocor), atorvastatin (Lipitor)

(12) Encourage participation in a cardiac rehabilitation program.

3. Heart failure: The inability of the heart to meet tissue requirements for oxygen (not pumping effectively); the body tries to compensate by increasing the rate (tachycardia), increasing the size of the muscle, and increasing the length of the heart fibers.

a. Left-ventricular failure: An inadequate ejection of blood into the systemic circulation usually associated with MI and hypertension

1) Manifestations (primarily respiratory symptoms)

a) Dyspnea and paroxysmal nocturnal dyspnea

b) Moist cough

c) Crackles, wheezing

d) Orthopnea

(1) Pulmonary edema results, causing excessive fluid in pulmonary interstitial spaces evidenced by:

(a) Moist crackles and frothy sputum

(b) Severe anxiety

(c) Marked dyspnea and cyanosis

2) Collaborative Care

 a) **NURSING INTERVENTIONS**

(1) Deliver high-flow oxygen therapy:

(a) Monitor respiratory status and the need for possible intubation.

(b) Monitor labs.

(c) Maintain bed rest in the semi-Fowler's position.

(2) Administer Medications

(a) Administer digitalis (Digoxin) to increase the efficiency of the myocardium as a pump.

(b) Administer morphine sulfate to decrease respiratory rate and increase effective breathing. This will cause a pooling of blood in the peripheral vessels, which will decrease cardiac return and therefore decrease the work of the heart. Administer furosemide (Lasix) as prescribed.

b. Right-ventricular failure: The inability of the right ventricle to empty completely due to left-ventricular failure, right ventricular MI, or pulmonary hypertension

1) Manifestations

a) Dependent peripheral edema

b) Distended neck veins

c) Weight gain (greater than 2 lb in 1 day)

d) Enlarged liver

e) Elevated central venous pressure, wedge pressures

f) Hypotension and tachycardia

2) Collaborative Care

 a) **NURSING INTERVENTIONS**

(1) Provide the client psychological support for the relief of anxiety and stress.

(2) Administer oxygen as prescribed.

(3) Decrease the client's fluid intake to decrease cardiac preload.

(4) Teach the client to assess the radial pulse, report signs of toxicity, keep laboratory appointments, and avoid St. John's wort and licorice because of risk of toxicity.

(5) Encourage a diet low in sodium and high in potassium.

b) Administer Medications

(1) Improve myocardial contraction with digitalis and dobutamine hydrochloride (Dobutrex).

(2) Digitalis therapy: Decreases the heart rate, and improves ventricular filling, stroke volume, coronary artery perfusion, and strength of contraction

 (a) **NURSING INTERVENTIONS**

1. Monitor the client's potassium levels (decreased levels enhance digitalis toxicity).

2. Monitor the client's apical heart rate (verify greater than 60/min before each dose).

3. Monitor the client for digitalis toxicity (normal digitalis level in serum is 0.8 to 2 ng/mL).

4. Manifestations of digoxin toxicity:

a. Early: nausea, vomiting, anorexia, bradycardia, depression

b. Late: frequent premature ventricular complex, green-yellow halos in visual field, photophobia, diplopia

4. Valvular disorders: Result in narrowing of valve that prevents or impedes blood flow (stenosis) or impaired closure that allows backward leakage of blood (regurgitation); affect mitral, aortic, or tricuspid

a. Contributing Factors

1) History of endocarditis and rheumatic fever is frequently the cause.

b. Manifestations

1) Right-sided heart failure (mitral stenosis, mitral regurgitation, tricuspid stenosis)

2) Left-sided heart failure (aortic stenosis, insufficiency)

3) Murmurs

4) Decreased cardiac output

  c. Collaborative Care

  1) **NURSING INTERVENTIONS**
   a) Allow activities as tolerated.
   b) Implement a low-sodium, low-cholesterol diet.
   c) Encourage the client to implement a low-sodium and low-cholesterol diet at home.
  d. Administer Medications
   1) The client must take anticoagulation medication for life.
   2) Instruct the client in lifelong need for antibiotics prior to any invasive procedures and dental work.
  e. Digoxin and diuretic therapy.
   1) Therapeutic Measures
    a) Surgical Management
     (1) Heart valve replacement (click can be heard on auscultation)
     (2) Valvuloplasty
     (3) Mitral commissurotomy (valvulotomy)

5. Aortic aneurysm: Local distention of an artery wall, usually thoracic or abdominal (4 times more common). Monitored until above 5 cm, when the rate of rupture increases and surgery is required.
  a. Contributing factors
   1) Infections
   2) Congenitally acquired
   3) Atherosclerosis or hypertension
  b. Manifestations (frequently asymptomatic)
   1) Thoracic: pain, dyspnea, hoarseness, cough, dysphagia
   2) Abdominal: abdominal pain, persistent or intermittent low back or flank pain; may be asymptomatic; pulsating abdominal mass; shock
  c. Diagnostic Procedures
   1) CT scan, MRI
   2) X-ray, ultrasound
  d. Collaborative Care

  1) **NURSING INTERVENTIONS**
   2) Treatment usually requires surgery:
    a) Preoperative: careful monitoring for possible rupture; prepare the client for abdominal surgery
    b) Postoperative: careful monitoring of peripheral circulation below the level of the aneurysms
    c) Postoperative complications:
     (1) MI or emboli
     (2) Renal failure
     (3) Spinal cord ischemia

6. Hypertension: Persistent blood pressure above 140/systolic and 90/diastolic; is often called the silent killer
  a. Primary hypertension
   1) Most common type (90%)
   2) Hereditary disease; cause unknown
   3) More common among African Americans
   4) Late manifestations: headaches, fatigue, dyspnea, edema, nocturia, blackouts
   5) Usually no signs or symptoms until end-organ involvement occurs
  b. Secondary hypertension
   1) Due to identifiable cause
   2) Pheochromocytoma
   3) Renal pathology
  c. Collaborative Care

  1) **NURSING INTERVENTIONS**
   a) Teach the client weight control methods.
   b) Encourage the client to stop smoking.
   c) Avoid stimulants by decreasing alcohol and caffeine intake. A moderate amount is less than 1 oz of alcohol or 24 oz of beer a day.
   d) Promote a program of regular physical exercise.
   e) Promote a lifestyle with reduced stress.
   f) The client should maintain a sodium-restricted diet.
   g) Teach the client risk factors.
  2) Medications
   a) Loop diuretic-furosemide (Lasix), bumetanide (Bumex)
   b) Thiazide-hydrochlorothiazide (HCTZ), chlorothiazide (Diuril)
    (1) Interventions for Loop and HCTZ diuretics
     (a) Administer potassium supplements to the client as prescribed.
     (b) Teach dietary sources of potassium.
     (c) Possible interaction between low-potassium and digitalis (Digoxin) preparations.
   c) Potassium-sparing diuretics
    (1) Spironolactone (Aldactone)
    (2) Triamterene (Dyrenium)
    (3) Monitor for increased potassium level
   d) Beta-blockers
    (1) Propranolol HCl (Inderal)
    (2) Atenolol (Tenormin)
    (3) Metoprolol (Lopressor)

     (a) **NURSING INTERVENTIONS** for Beta Blockers
     1. Monitor for major side effects of bradycardia.
     2. Monitor the client's pulse daily.
     3. Monitor for manifestations of heart failure.
     4. Noncardioselective beta-blockers may be contraindicated in asthmatics.
     5. Monitor for reflex tachycardia due to decreased cardiac output and hypotension.

e) Central-acting alpha-blockers (sympatholytics)
  (1) Clonidine HCL (Catapres)
     (a) Monitor for side effects
     (b) Constipation
     (c) Sexual dysfunction
     (d) Dry mouth
     (e) Depression
  (2) Guanfacine HCL (Tenex)
     (a) Monitor for side effects
        1. Rebound hypertension
        2. Drowsiness
        3. Bradycardia
  (3) Methyldopa (Aldomet)
     (a) Monitor for side effects
        1. Aplastic anemia
        2. Thrombocytopenia
f) Angiotensin-converting enzyme (ACE inhibitors)
  (1) Captopril (Capoten)
  (2) Enalapril (Vasotec)
  (3) Lisinopril (Zestril)
  (4) Monitor for side effects
     (a) Cough
     (b) Headache
     (c) Angioedema of face and limbs
g) Calcium-channel blockers
  (1) nifedipine (Procardia)
     (a) Monitor for side effects
        1. Headache/dizziness
        2. Bradycardia
        3. Peripheral edema
  (2) verapamil (Calan), diltiazem (Cardizem)
     (a) Monitor for side effect
        1. Flushing
        2. Arrhythmias
        3. Constipation

7. Thrombophlebitis: A venous blood clot associated with inflammation
  a. Contributing Factors
     1) Stasis
     2) Hypercoagulability
     3) Damage to intima of blood vessels/trauma
     4) Pregnancy or estrogen (oral contraceptives)
     5) Malignancy or obesity
  b. Manifestations
     1) Edema of affected limb
     2) Local swelling, bumpy, knotty
     3) Red, tender, local induration
     4) Venous ulcers usually around the ankle; reddened and bluish; edema often present
  c. Diagnostic Procedures
     1) MRI, CT scan, ultrasound

  d. Collaborative Care
     1) **NURSING INTERVENTIONS**
        a) Maintain bed rest.
        b) Elevate the affected extremity and apply moist, warm compresses.
        c) Monitor labs.
        d) Initiate antiembolism stockings/support hose.
        e) Increase fluids.
        f) Encourage deep breathing to enhance oxygenation.
        g) Assist the client with range of motion.
        h) Avoid eating excessive amounts of green, leafy vegetables while on warfarin (Coumadin).
  e. Medications
     1) NSAIDS
     2) Initial treatment with Heparin
     3) Coumadin for long term management
     4) Dabigatran (Pradaxa) is a newer blood-thinning option that is taken orally.
     5) **Thrombolytic**: alteplase (Activase)
  f. Client Education
     1) Avoid foods high in vitamin K, such as leafy green vegetables, when taking Coumadin.

8. Varicose veins
  a. Contributing Factors
     1) Prolonged standing
     2) Pregnancy
     3) Obesity
     4) Heredity
  b. Manifestations
     1) Enlarged, tortuous veins in lower extremities
     2) Pain
     3) Edema (after upright)
  c. Collaborative Care
     1) **NURSING INTERVENTIONS**
        a) Avoid prolonged sitting or standing.
        b) Instruct the client to wear supportive antiembolism stockings, especially during air flights and pregnancy.
        c) Avoid crossing legs, engage in daily exercise, and maintain an ideal body weight.
        d) Elevate the client's lower extremities to reduce edema and promote venous return.
        e) Promote circulation with thigh-high antiembolism stockings, ambulation, and elevation.
  d. Therapeutic Measures
     1) **Sclerotherapy**. Vein injected with a solution that scars and closes the vein.
     2) **Laser surgeries**. Laser surgery works by sending strong bursts of light onto the vein, which makes the vein slowly fade and disappear. No incisions or needles are used.

3) **Catheter-assisted procedures**. Catheter insertred into an enlarged vein and heats the tip of the catheter. As the catheter is pulled out, the heat destroys the vein by causing it to collapse and seal shut. This procedure is usually done for larger varicose veins.

4) **Vein stripping**. Involves removing a long vein through small incisions.

9. Arterial disorders of the peripheral vascular system: Impeded natural blood flow through arterial vessels

a. Manifestations

1) Intermittent claudication—pain/cramping when walking; resolves with rest

2) Calf muscle atrophy

3) Skin appears shiny with hair loss and thickened toenails

4) Poor neurovascular integrity

5) Necrotic ulcers (looks punched-out; no edema present)

6) Tingling and numbness of the toes

7) Cool extremities with poor pulses

b. Collaborative Care

1) **NURSING INTERVENTIONS**

a) Encourage the client to stop smoking.

b) Provide instruction on maintaining a low-fat diet.

c) The client should avoid crossing legs.

c. Administer Medications

1) Administer pentoxifylline (Trental) and cilostazol (Pletal).

d. Therapeutic Measures

1) Surgical treatment

a) Femoral popliteal bypass surgery

b) Angioplasty or stenting

10. Buerger's disease (thromboangiitis obliterans): Recurring inflammation of the arteries and veins of the lower and upper extremities, resulting in thrombus with occlusion (cause unknown)

a. Contributing Factors

1) Factors are unknown. Thought to have a genetic predisposition. Also cigarette smoking and history of gum disease; occurs in men ages 20-40.

b. Manifestations

1) Intermittent pain in the legs, feet, arms and hands. Pain eases when activity is stopped (claudication).

2) Inflammation along a vein below the skin's surface (due to a blood clot in the vein).

3) Fingers and toes that turn pale when exposed to cold (Raynaud's phenomenon).

4) Painful open sores on fingers and toes.

5) Ulcerations and gangrene with amputation are common.

c. Collaborative Care

1) Interventions

a) Cessation of smoking is important; avoid cold or constrictive clothing.

11. Raynaud's syndrome: Vasospastic or obstructive condition of the arteries/arterioles of upper and lower extremities resulting from exposure to cold/stress; more common in women

a. Contributing Factors

1) Factors that cause of Raynaud's attacks are not clearly understood, but blood vessels in the hands and feet appear to overreact to cold temperatures or stress:

b. Manifestations

1) Coldness, pallor, and pain in extremities secondary to vasospasm

2) Occasional ulceration of the fingertips

3) Color changes from white to blue to red (can be bilateral or symmetrical)

c. Diagnostic Procedures

1) Cold-stimulation test: involves placing the hands in cool water or exposing to cold air, to trigger an episode of Raynaud's.

d. Collaborative Care

1) **NURSING INTERVENTIONS**

a) Teach the client to avoid the cold and keep extremities warm; wear warm, but nonconstrictive gloves.

b) Encourage the client to stop smoking and to limit caffeine intake.

2) Medications

a) Administer nifedipine (Procardia).

D. Cardiac Surgery

1. Pacemaker: An electronic device that provides repetitive electrical stimuli to the heart muscle, in order to control the heart rate.

a. Types

1) Permanent pacemakers

a) Ventricular demand: Fires at a preset rate when the client's heart rate drops below a predetermined/preprogrammed rate

b) Ventricular fixed: Fires constantly at a preset/preprogrammed rate, regardless of the client's own heart rate

c) Dual chamber: Stimulates both the atria and the ventricles

d) Atrial demand: Fires as needed when the atria do not originate a rhythm

e) Variable rate: Senses oxygen demands and increases the firing rate to meet the client's needs

2) Temporary pacemakers

a) Transcutaneous (skin): External, for use in emergency pacing situations

(1) Transvenous

b. Collaborative Care

 1) **NURSING INTERVENTIONS**

a) Monitor ECG for dysrhythmias and check the client.s pulse rate.

b) Assess the wound for hematoma or infection.

c) Administer analgesics as necessary.

d) Maintain an electrically safe environment. Instruct the client to avoid large generators, magnets, and magnetic resonance imaging machines.

e) Observe the client for hiccoughs, which indicates that the pacemaker is malpositioned and is pacing the diaphragm.

f) Use aseptic technique at the insertion site when caring for the wound.

g) To prevent accidental dislodging of the electrode, the client should not raise his arms over his head until the site is healed.

h) Observe for pacemaker malfunction (failure to capture, sense, or pace).

2) Client Education

a) Take pulse daily or when symptomatic.

b) Know pacemaker rate and report changes to provider.

c) Carry identification information at all times.

d) Know and report indications of battery failure.

e) Transmit data via telephone from the pacemaker to the health care provider according to provider protocol.

f) Wear loose-fitting clothes.

g) Avoid contact sports.

h) Keep all provider appointments.

2. Coronary artery bypass graft (CABG): A surgical procedure to replace damaged coronary arteries and reestablish perfusion to the heart muscle in areas of myocardium

a. Most procedures require an open chest/heart approach with a bypass machine; however, the latest techniques may not use bypass, resulting in a shorter recovery period for some clients.

b. Collaborative Care

1) Preoperative/general care

a) Provide psychological support as needed.

b) Prepare client for the possibility of continued postoperative intubation

2) Postoperative care

a) Manage bilateral chest tubes.

b) Provide general postoperative care including pain management and care of wound and drains.

c) Client often has an endotracheal tube postoperatively; provide sterile technique when caring for tube and suctioning.

d) Assess all systems affected by decreased cardiac output (vital signs, urine output, circulation in legs, chest pain).

e) Assess for complications such as MI, pleural effusion, dysrhythmia, and stroke.

f) Monitor for dysrhythmias.

E. **Shock:** Abnormal cellular metabolism due to inadequate oxygenation

1. Types

a. Cardiogenic: failure of the heart to pump adequately

b. Hypovolemic: decreased circulating blood volume

c. Distributive (vasogenic)

1) Neurogenic: increased size of vascular bed due to loss of vascular tone

2) Anaphylactic: hypersensitivity reaction

3) Septic: systemic vasodilation due to infection

2. Manifestations (related to decreased tissue perfusion)

a. Tachycardia with hypotension

b. Tachypnea

c. Oliguria

d. Cold, moist skin

e. Color ashen—pallor

f. Metabolic acidosis

g. Decreased level of consciousness

h. Septic shock—initially warm, flushed skin, fever

3. Collaborative Care

 a. **NURSING INTERVENTIONS**

1) Position the client in modified Trendelenburg.

2) Secure a large-bore IV line (16 or 18 g).

3) Administer oxygen.

4) Record the client's vital signs every 5 min.

5) Promote rest and decrease movement.

6) Monitor the client's urine output.

b. Emergency Medications

1) Atropine: increases heart rate

2) Dopamine (Intropin): vasoconstrictor; increases blood pressure, tissue, and renal perfusion

3) Epinephrine HCl (Adrenalin): increases the body's reaction to stress

4) Isoproterenol (Isuprel): increases heart rate and cardiac output

5) Dobutamine (Dobutrex): inotropic; increases the force of myocardial contraction in cardiogenic shock and increases blood pressure

6) Norepinephrine levarterenol (Levophed): vasoconstrictor; increases tissue perfusion

7) Sodium bicarbonate: decreases acidosis

F. **Cardiopulmonary Resuscitation (CPR)**

1. Indications

a. Absence of palpable carotid pulse

b. Absence of breath sounds

2. Purpose

a. Establish effective circulation and respiration

b. Prevent irreversible cerebral anoxic damage

3. Procedure

   a. Follow the American Heart Association 2010 recommendations:

     1) Call 9-1-1.

     2) Send someone for the automated external defibrillator.

     3) Immediately begin CPR if an adult victim is unresponsive and not breathing normally.

     4) The AHA emphasizes the importance of early, uninterrupted chest compressions; therefore, follow the acronym C-A-B (Compressions–Airway–Breathing).

     5) Untrained rescuers should perform hands-only compressions. Push hard and fast on the center of the victim's chest or follow the directions of EMS dispatchers.

     6) Trained rescuers should provide 30 compressions and 2 rescue breaths to improve outcomes, especially for pediatric victims.

     7) Depth: Compress the chest at least 2 inches (5 cm) in adults or ⅓ the depth of chest in children and infants.

     8) Rate: Provide 100 compressions per minute, to the beat of the Bee Gee's song "Stayin' Alive."

     9) Recoil: Allow the chest to recoil fully between compressions.

     10) Minimize interruptions: Do not delay or interrupt chest compressions to check pulse or rhythm.

   b. Complications

     1) Fractured ribs

     2) Punctured lungs

     3) Lacerated liver

     4) Abdominal distension

   c. Stop CPR when:

     1) A health care provider pronounces the client dead

     2) The rescuer is exhausted

     3) Help arrives

     4) The client's heartbeat returns

   d. Automated external defibrillator: A computerized defibrillator that analyzes cardiac rhythm once pads are placed on the client's chest

     1) A mechanical voice tells the rescuer if/when to deliver shock to the client.

     2) AED is frequently found in public locations, since it is easy for nontrained individuals to use.

     3) Do not use an AED on children who are 1 month to 12 months.

   e. Obstructed airway

     1) Conscious

       a) Establish that the client is choking.

       b) Perform the Heimlich maneuver until it is successful or the client becomes unconscious.

     2) Unconscious

       a) If a conscious choking adult becomes unresponsive, look for the foreign object in the pharynx and perform a finger sweep.

       b) Begin CPR. Every time you open the airway to give breaths, look for the object.

       c) Continue CPR.

SECTION 9
Genitourinary System Disorders

A. Assessment of the Kidney and Urinary System

1. Functions of the kidney

   a. Regulates acid-base balance

   b. Regulates fluid and electrolyte balance

   c. Excretes metabolic wastes (creatinine, urea)

   d. Regulates blood pressure: Renin (stimulated by decreased blood pressure or blood volume) stimulates the production of angiotensin I, which is converted to angiotensin II in the lungs; angiotensin II is a strong vasoconstrictor and stimulates aldosterone secretion; vasoconstriction and sodium reabsorption result in increased blood volume and increased blood pressure.

   e. Secretes erythropoietin

   f. Converts vitamin D to its active form for absorption of calcium

   g. Excretes water-soluble medications and medication metabolites

2. Contributing Factors

   a. History of genitourinary disorder

   b. History of hypertension

   c. History of diabetes

   d. Family history of renal disease, such as PKD

   e. Incontinence, BPH, cancer, or kidney stones

   f. Nephrotoxic medications

3. Manifestations

   a. Flank pain radiating to upper thigh, testis, or labium

   b. Changes in voiding: hematuria, proteinuria, dysuria, frequency, urgency, burning, nocturia, incontinence, polyuria, oliguria, anuria

   c. Thirst, fatigue, generalized edema

B. Diagnostic Tests

1. Urinalysis

   a. Specific gravity: range tested 1.010 to 1.030

   b. Color: yellow, amber, or clear

   c. Negative glucose, protein, nitrites, RBCs, and WBCs

   d. pH: 5 to 8

e. First voided morning sample preferred; 15 mL

f. Sent to laboratory immediately or refrigerated

g. If clean catch, get urine for culture prior to starting antibiotics:

    1) Cleanse labia, glans penis.

    2) Obtain midstream sample.

2. Renal function tests (several tests over a period of time are necessary)

  a. BUN: 10 to 20 mg/dL

  b. Creatinine: 0.5 to 1 mg/dL

  c. 24-hr creatinine clearance: 75 to 120 mL/min

    1) Have the client void and discard the first specimen.

    2) Obtain serum creatinine.

    3) Collect all urine from the client for the next 24 hr (refrigerate or keep container on ice).

    4) At the completion of the 24 hr, the test is stopped following the client's last void.

  d. Uric acid (serum): 3.5 to 7.8 mg/dL

  e. Prostate-specific antigen: greater than 10 increases the risk of prostate cancer

3. Radiologic tests

  a. Kidneys, ureters, bladder (x-ray): shows the size, shape, and position of kidneys, ureters, and bladder; no preparation necessary (verify that the client is not pregnant)

  b. IV pyelography (IV bolus): to help in visualization of the urinary tract

    1) Collaborative Care

      a) **NURSING INTERVENTIONS**

        (1) Verify that informed consent has been signed.

        (2) Verify the client's last creatinine level.

        (3) The client should remain NPO for 8 hr; fluids may be permitted.

        (4) Administer laxatives as prescribed.

        (5) Administer an enema or suppository on the morning of the test (as necessary).

        (6) Check for allergies to iodine or shellfish.

        (7) Inform the client of potential sensations during the exam. The client may experience flushing, warmth, nausea, a metallic or salty taste, or incontinence.

        (8) Emergency equipment should be readily available during the test.

        (9) Encourage fluids to help flush out the dye.

4. Renal angiography: Visualization of renal arterial supply; contrast material injected through a catheter

  a. **NURSING INTERVENTIONS** (preprocedure)

    1) Approach is through the femoral or brachial artery.

    2) Locate and mark peripheral pulses.

    3) Have the client void before the procedure.

    4) Explain that the procedure may create the feeling of warmth along the vessel

  b. **NURSING INTERVENTIONS** (postprocedure)

    1) Maintain bed rest for 6 to 8 hr.

    2) Monitor the client's vital signs until stable.

    3) Observe the client for swelling and hematoma.

    4) Palpate peripheral pulses/vascular checks.

    5) Monitor the client's I&O including urinary status.

5. Cystoscopy: An invasive procedure in which a scope is passed to view the interior of the bladder, urethra, or the position of urethral orifices to remove calculi from the urethra, bladder, and ureter; to treat lesions of the bladder, urethra, and prostate.

  a. **NURSING INTERVENTIONS** (preoperative)

    1) Maintain NPO if the client is given general anesthesia.

    2) Administer preoperative cathartics/enemas as ordered.

    3) Teach the client deep breathing exercises to relieve bladder spasms.

    4) Monitor for postural hypotension.

    5) Inform the client that pink-tinged or tea-colored urine is common following the procedure, but bright, red urine or clots should be reported.

    6) Provide nonpharmacological pain management techniques following the procedure.

  b. **NURSING INTERVENTIONS** (postoperative)

    1) Assess for leg cramps due to lithotomy position.

    2) Assess for back pain or abdominal pain.

    3) Offer warm sitz baths for comfort.

    4) Push fluids and provide analgesics.

    5) Monitor the client's I&O.

6. Renal biopsy

  a. **NURSING INTERVENTIONS** (preprocedure)

    1) Obtain bleeding, clotting, and prothrombin times.

    2) Obtain results of prebiopsy x-rays of kidney.

    3) Administer IV fluids.

    4) Maintain NPO status for 6 to 8 hr.

    5) Position the client with a pillow under her abdomen and her shoulders on the bed.

    6) Verify that the informed consent is signed.

    7) Instruct client to remain still during the procedure.

  b. **NURSING INTERVENTIONS** (postprocedure)

    1) Maintain the client in the supine position. The client should remain in bed for 24 hr.

    2) Monitor the client's vital signs every 5 to 15 min for 4 hr.

    3) Maintain pressure to the puncture site for 20 min.

    4) Observe the client for any pain, nausea, vomiting, and blood pressure changes.

    5) Encourage fluid intake.

    6) Assess Hct and Hgb 8 hr after procedure.

    7) Monitor the client's urine output.

    8) Make sure the client avoids strenuous activity, sports, and heavy lifting for at least 2 weeks.

7. Indwelling urinary catheterization: A sterile procedure to empty the contents of the bladder, obtain a sterile specimen, determine residual urine, initiate irrigation of the bladder, or bypass an obstruction.

a. Collaborative Care

 1) **NURSING INTERVENTIONS**

a) Maintain a closed system.

b) Measure the client's output every shift.

c) Provide meticulous pericare.

d) Keep a drainage bag below the level of the client's bladder.

e) Increase daily fluid intake.

f) Prevent dependent loops in the catheter tubing.

g) Discontinue as soon as possible due to increased risk for urinary tract infection.

C. Specific Disorders

1. Cystitis: Inflammation of the urinary bladder

a. Contributing Factors

1) Wiping back to front after toileting, secondary to ascending infection from *Escherichia coli*

2) Prolonged baths with excessive soap (common in females)

3) Benign prostatic hypertrophy (males)

b. Manifestations

1) Frequency and urgency, and only voiding small amounts of urine each time

2) Dysuria with hematuria

3) Suprapubic tenderness; pain in the bladder region or flank pain

4) Fever, malaise, chills

5) Cloudy, foul-smelling urine

c. Collaborative Care

 1) **NURSING INTERVENTIONS**

a) Obtain the client's clean catch urine sample for culture and sensitivity before initiating antibiotic therapy.

b) Maintain acidic urine pH.

c) Force fluids (greater than 3,000 mL/day).

d) Encourage the client to drink cranberry juice.

e) Apply heat to the perineum for comfort.

2) Medications

a) Antimicrobial medications: Sulfonamides are the medications of choice unless the client is allergic (sulfamethoxazole-trimethoprim [Bactrim] and nitrofurantoin macrocrystal [Macrodantin]).

b) Urinary analgesics (phenazopyridine [Pyridium]): Inform the client that the medication will temporarily turn urine orange.

3) Client Education and Referral

a) Follow appropriate perineal care (wiping front to back).

b) Wear cotton underwear.

c) Avoid bubble baths (they can irritate urethra).

d) Maintain an increased fluid intake.

e) Void after sexual intercourse.

f) Drink cranberry juice daily.

2. Glomerulonephritis: An acute renal disease involving the renal glomeruli of both kidneys; thought to be an antigen–antibody reaction that damages the glomeruli of the kidney (usually in children). The prognosis is good if treatment is implemented.

a. Contributing Factors

1) Beta-hemolytic streptococcal

2) Can follow tonsillitis or pharyngitis

b. Manifestations

1) Hematuria (cola or tea-colored urine), with proteinuria

2) Edema (especially facial and periorbital; ascites)

3) Oliguria or anuria

4) Hypertension with headache

5) Increased BUN; elevated BUN is azotemia

6) Flank or abdominal pain

7) Anemia

c. Collaborative Care

 1) **NURSING INTERVENTIONS**

a) Maintain bed rest to protect the kidney.

b) Restrict fluids.

c) Reduce protein and sodium in the client's diet, but increase calories.

d) Monitor daily weight.

2) Medications

a) Penicillin for streptococcal infection (substitute other antibiotics for clients allergic to penicillin)

b) Corticosteroids for inflammatory disease

c) Antihypertensives for increased blood pressure

3. Nephrosis: A clinical disorder associated with protein wasting; secondary to diffuse glomerular damage

a. Contributing Factors

1) May be autoimmune; the glomerular membrane is more permeable, especially to proteins.

b. Manifestations

1) Insidious onset of pitting edema (generalized edema is anasarca)

2) Proteinuria

3) Anemia

4) Hypoalbuminemia

5) Anorexia malaise and nausea

6) Oliguria

7) Ascites

c. Collaborative Care

 1) **NURSING INTERVENTIONS**

    a) Maintain bed rest (during severe edema only) to preserve renal function.

    b) Make sure the client maintains a low-sodium, low-potassium, moderate-protein, high-calorie diet.

    c) Protect the client from infection.

    d) Monitor I&O.

    e) Weigh the client and measure abdominal girth daily.

2) Medication therapy

    a) Loop diuretics: furosemide (Lasix)

    b) Steroids: prednisone (Deltasone)

    c) Immunosuppressive agents: cyclophosphamide (Cytoxan)

4. Urolithiasis (urinary calculi): Stones in the urinary system

a. Contributing Factors

    1) Obstruction and urinary stasis

    2) Uric acid stones (excessive purine intake)

    3) Immobilization

    4) More common in men ages 20 to 40 and tends to reoccur

b. Manifestations (based on location and size of the stone)

    1) Pain: severe renal colic (ureter); dull, aching (kidney); radiates to the groin

    2) Nausea, vomiting, diarrhea, or constipation

    3) Hematuria

    4) Manifestations of a urinary tract infection

c. Collaborative Care (Goals: to eradicate the stone and prevent nephron destruction)

 1) **NURSING INTERVENTIONS**

    a) Force fluids—at least 3,000 mL/day (IV or by mouth)

    b) Strain all urine

    c) Provide pain control

    d) Maintain proper urine pH (depends on type of stone)

2) Medications

    a) Opioids

    b) Administer allopurinol (Zyloprim) for uric acid stones.

3) Therapeutic Measures

    a) Lithotripsy method to crush the stone through sound waves

4) Client Education

    a) Avoid foods high in oxalates if it is a calcium oxalate stone (spinach, black tea, rhubarb, chocolate).

    b) Maintain fluid intake to maintain hydration.

5. Acute renal failure: An abrupt decrease in renal function; may be the result of trauma, allergic reactions, kidney stones, or shock

a. Contributing Factors

    1) Prerenal: disrupted blood flow to the kidneys; hypovolemic shock, dehydration, heart failure, burn injury, and anaphylaxis

    2) Renal: renal tissue damage; trauma, hypokalemia, acute glomerulonephritis, hemolytic uremic syndrome (infection caused by Escherichia coli; common in children), substance abuse

    3) Postrenal: urine flow from the kidney is compromised; kidney stones, prostate hypertrophy, tumors, and strictures

b. Manifestations (three phases)

    1) Oliguric (8 to 15 days): sudden onset, less than 400 mL in 24 hr, edema, elevated BUN, creatinine and potassium; increased specific gravity; acidosis; heart failure; dysrhythmias

    2) Diuretic: urine output increases followed by diuresis of up to 4,000 to 5,000 mL/day, indicating recovery of damaged nephrons; decreased specific gravity; hypotension and fluid and electrolyte imbalances are a concern

    3) Recovery: may take up to 1 year until renal function returns to normal (baseline); older adults are at increased risk for residual impairment

c. Collaborative Care

1) **NURSING INTERVENTIONS**

    a) Eliminate or prevent cause.

    b) Correct metabolic acidosis, hyperkalemia, hyperphosphatemia, and hypocalcemia:

      (1) Kayexalate (an ion exchange resin given orally or by enema to treat hyperkalemia)

      (2) IV glucose and insulin (causes potassium to enter cells)

      (3) Calcium IV or sodium bicarbonate to stabilize cell membrane

    c) Implement diet:

      (1) For oliguric phase, low-protein, high-carbohydrate diet and restricted potassium intake

      (2) For diuresis phase, low-protein, high-calorie diet and restricted fluids as indicated

        (a) Encourage bed rest in the oliguric phase.

        (b) Monitor daily weights.

        (c) Monitor I&O.

        (d) Implement dialysis (as ordered) until renal function returns.

        (e) Assess for pericarditis (friction rubs).

2) Medications

    a) Phosphate binders to lower phosphorus while replacing calcium (Phos-Lo, calcium acetate)

    b) Epogen (Procrit) to treat anemia

6. Chronic renal failure: Progressive failure of kidney function that results in death unless hemodialysis or transplant is performed; is irreversible

a. Stages of renal failure
1) Diminished renal reserve (creatinine 1.6 to 2)
2) Renal insufficiency (creatinine 2.1 to 5)
3) Renal failure (creatinine > 8)
4) End state renal failure (EDRD) (creatinine > 12)

b. Contributing Factors
1) Diabetes mellitus (leading cause)
2) Uncontrolled hypertension (second cause)
3) Chronic glomerulonephritis
4) Pyelonephritis
5) Congenital kidney disease, such as PKD

c. Manifestations (progressively worsen)
1) Fatigue secondary to anemia
2) Headache and hypertension
3) Nausea, vomiting, diarrhea
4) Irritability
5) Convulsions, coma
6) Edema
7) Hypocalcemia, hyperkalemia
8) Pruritus, uremic frost
9) Pallid, gray-yellow complexion
10) Metabolic acidosis; elevated BUN and creatinine; decreased glomerular filtration rate

d. Collaborative Care
 1) **NURSING INTERVENTIONS**
a) Maintain bed rest.
b) Implement a renal diet for the client—low-protein, low-potassium, high-carbohydrate, vitamins and calcium supplements, low-sodium, and low-phosphate.
c) Monitor for and treat hypertension as prescribed.
d) Strict I&O; fluid replacement—500 to 600 mL more than previous 24-hr urine output.
e) Monitor the client's electrolytes, especially potassium.
f) Do not administer antacids with magnesium or enemas with phosphorous.
g) Maintain dialysis.
h) Administer diuretics in early stages.
i) Provide meticulous skin care.
j) Provide emotional support to the client and the client's family.
k) Assess for bleeding tendencies.

2) Medications
a) Phosphate binders
b) Epoetin alfa/erythropoietin (Epogen, Procrit) for anemia to stimulate RBC formation and transfuse as necessary

7. Dialysis
a. Goals
1) Remove end products of metabolism (urea and creatinine) from the client's blood
2) Maintain safe concentration of serum electrolytes
3) Correct acidosis
4) Remove excess fluid from the client's blood

b. Hemodialysis: The process of cleansing the blood of accumulated waste products and fluids; used for end-stage renal failure or clients who are acutely ill and require short-term treatment
1) Collaborative Care
a) **NURSING INTERVENTIONS**
(1) Weigh the client before and after the procedure.
(2) Monitor the client's blood pressure continuously during the procedure.
(3) Provide care to the access site to prevent clotting and infection.
(4) Assess for presence of thrill and bruit.
(5) Provide adequate nutrition as prescribed.
(6) Post a sign above the client's bed that warns of no blood pressure readings or blood work on the side of the fistula.
(7) Maintain fluid restrictions.
(8) Withhold regular morning medications prior to dialysis.

c. Peritoneal dialysis: An alternative method using the peritoneum to remove fluids, electrolytes, and waste products from the blood. Dialysis is accomplished via a catheter surgically placed into the abdominal cavity.
1) Collaborative Care
a) **NURSING INTERVENTIONS**
(1) Assist the client to void prior to the procedure.
(2) Weigh the client daily.
(3) Monitor the client's vital signs and baseline electrolytes.
(4) Maintain asepsis.
(5) Sterile dressing changes per facility policy.
(6) Keep an accurate record of the client's fluid balance.
(7) Procedure:
(a) Warm dialysate (1 to 2 L of 1.5, 2.5, or 4.25% glucose solution).
(b) Allow to flow in by gravity.
(c) 5 to 10 min inflow time; close clamp immediately.
(d) 30 min of equilibration (dwell time).
(e) 10 to 30 min of drainage (should be clear and pale yellow)
(f) Monitor for complications (peritonitis, bleeding, respiratory difficulty, abdominal pain, and bowel or bladder perforation).

d. Continuous ambulatory peritoneal dialysis (CAPD): Peritoneal dialysis performed by the client without the use of a machine (cycler)

   1) Procedure (differs from acute peritoneal dialysis)

     a) Permanent indwelling catheter inserted into peritoneum

     b) Fluid infused by gravity (1.5 to 3 L)

     c) Dwell time: 4 to 10 hr

     d) Dialysate drains by gravity: 20 to 40 min

     e) Four to five exchanges daily, 7 days/week (some clients may elect to do at night with automatic cycling machines; 10 to 14 hr, 3 times/week)

   2) Collaborative Care

     a) **NURSING INTERVENTIONS**

       (1) Monitor the client for complications.

       (2) Monitor the client for peritonitis (rebound tenderness, fever, cloudy outflow).

       (3) Monitor for bladder perforation (yellow outflow).

       (4) Monitor for hypotension.

       (5) Monitor for bowel perforation (brown outflow).

     b) Advantages to CAPD

       (1) More independence

       (2) Free dietary intake and better nutrition

       (3) Satisfactory control of uremia

       (4) Least expensive dialysis

       (5) Decreased likelihood of future transplant rejection

       (6) More closely approximates normal renal function

8. Renal and urinary tract surgery

  a. Kidney transplantation

    1) For individuals with end-stage renal disease

    2) Requires a well-matched donor

     a) Living donors (most desirable)

     b) Cadaver donors

    3) Preoperative management

     a) Interventions are prescribed to correct the client's metabolic status.

     b) Administer immunosuppressive therapy.

     c) Perform hemodialysis within 24 hr.

     d) Provide the client with emotional support.

    4) **NURSING INTERVENTIONS** (postoperative management)

     a) Monitor labs (CBC, electrolytes, BUN/creatinine).

     b) Administer immunosuppressive medications to the client such as azathioprine (Imuran), cyclosporine (Sandimmune), or steroids.

     c) Monitor the client for rejection. This could include oliguria, edema, fever, tenderness over graft site, fluid and electrolyte imbalance, hypertension, elevated BUN, creatinine, and elevated WBCs.

     d) Monitor the client for infection and maintain protective isolation.

     e) Provide emotional support and monitor for depression.

9. Urinary diversion: Removal of the bladder and surrounding structures to reroute urinary flow through a pouch and abdominal stoma

  a. Collaborative Care

    1) **NURSING INTERVENTIONS**

     a) Monitor the client's vital signs (hemorrhage and shock are frequent complications).

     b) Monitor stoma.

     c) Provide the client with pain control.

     d) Observe for manifestations of paralytic ileus, which are very common.

     e) Provide adequate fluid replacement.

     f) Weigh the client daily.

     g) Maintain function and patency of the drainage tubes:

       (1) Indwelling urinary catheter (dependent position, tape tubing to the thigh)

       (2) Nephrostomy tube

         (a) Never clamp.

         (b) Irrigate only with prescription for 10 mL of 0.9% sodium chloride.

         (c) Assess for leakage of urine.

       (3) Ureteral catheters

         (a) Each catheter drains ½ of the urinary system.

         (b) Bloody drainage is expected after surgery, but should clear within 24 to 48 hr.

         (c) Never irrigate the surgical implant.

         (d) Aseptic technique is required.

10. Benign prostatic hyperplasia: Enlargement of the prostate that may accompany the aging process in males; exact cause is unknown

  a. Manifestations

    1) Difficulty starting stream/dribbling

    2) Decrease in force of the urinary stream

    3) Frequent urinary tract infections

    4) Nocturia

    5) Hematuria

  b. Diagnosis

    1) Digital rectal exam or cystoscopy

    2) Prostate-specific antigen (PSA) for diagnosis

  c. Treatments

    1) Urinary antibiotics

    2) Alpha-blocker medications to promote urinary flow: terazosin (Hytrin), tamsulosin (Flomax), alfuzosin (Uroxatral), and doxazosin (Cardura)

    3) Enzyme inhibitors to decrease the size of the prostate gland: dutasteride (Avodart) and finasteride (Proscar)

4) Transurethral resection of prostate (TURP)

 a) **NURSING INTERVENTIONS** (preoperative)

(1) Insert indwelling urinary catheter.

(2) Administer antibiotics as prescribed.

b) **NURSING INTERVENTIONS** (postoperative)

(1) Monitor the client for shock and hemorrhage.

(2) Teach the client to avoid heavy lifting, prolonged sitting, constipation, or straining (which could cause a rebleed).

(3) Monitor for continuous bladder irrigation (expect bloody drainage; monitor I&O carefully).

(4) Encourage fluid intake (at least 3,000 mL/day).

(5) Assess for TURP syndrome: a cluster of manifestations resulting from absorption of irrigating fluids through prostate tissue (hyponatremia, confusion, bradycardia, hypo/hypertension, nausea, vomiting, and visual changes).

(6) Medicate for pain control: the client may need medication and narcotics to decrease bladder spasm.

(7) Keep the catheter taped tightly to the client's leg (for hemostasis at the surgical site by catheter balloon).

(8) Teach the client Kegel exercises (there may be temporary or permanent loss of sexual function or urinary control).

11. Prostate cancer: A slow-growing cancer of the prostate gland

a. Contributing Factors

1) Men age 50 and older

2) African American

3) Family history

4) Elevated testosterone levels

5) High-fat diet

b. Manifestations

1) Asymptomatic in early stages

2) Hematuria

3) Prostate-specific antigen (PSA) greater than 10

4) Rectal exam: hard, pea-sized nodule

c. Treatment

1) Radical prostatectomy

2) External radiation therapy

3) Internal radioactive seeds

4) Hormone therapy

12. Incontinence

a. Types

1) Urge: Cannot hold urine when stimulus to void occurs

2) Functional: Cannot physically get to the bathroom or is not aware of the stimulus to void

3) Stress: Pressure such as coughing, straining, lifting, bearing down, or laughing causes incontinence; very common in middle-age women

b. Collaborative Care

1) **NURSING INTERVENTIONS**

a) Use adult incontinency devices.

b) Decrease the client's fluid intake after 6 pm.

c) Maintain a regular toilet schedule.

d) Perform the Credé maneuver as needed.

e) Monitor the client for signs of cystitis.

f) Teach the client Kegel exercises to strengthen the sphincter.

g) Assure that the physical environment enhances the ability to get to the bathroom.

2) Medications

a) Urge incontinence

(1) Anticholinergics: tolterodine (Detrol) and oxybutynin (Ditropan)

b) Stress incontinence

(1) Tricyclic antidepressant: imipramine (Tofranil)

13. Urine retention: Caused by a physical obstruction of the urethra from acute or chronic causes (edema, BPH, tumor, inflammation or inability of the bladder to work; postanesthesia, stroke); at risk for hydronephrosis

a. Collaborative Care

1) **NURSING INTERVENTIONS**

a) Stimulate relaxation of the urethral sphincter by providing the client privacy, placing the client's hands in warm water (or just turning on the water), and encouraging guided imagery.

b) Administer bethanechol chloride (Urecholine).

c) Position the client upright.

d) Ensure adequate fluid intake.

SECTION 10

Neurosensory Disorders

A. Neurological Assessment

1. History of present illness

2. Mental status

a. Level of consciousness (alert, lethargic, obtunded, stupor, coma)

b. Orientation (person, place, time)

c. Affect

d. Mood

e. Speech (clarity, consistency, word-finding ability)

f. Cognition (judgment and abstraction ability)

3. Cranial nerves (I through XII)

    a. CN I, olfactory: sensory; smell

    b. CN II, optic: sensory; vision

    c. CN III, oculomotor: motor; eye

    d. CN IV, trochlear: motor; eye

    e. CN V, trigeminal: sensory face; motor chewing

    f. CN VI, abducens: motor; eye

    g. CN VII, facial: sensory; face and hands

    h. CN VIII, acoustic: sensory; hearing and balance

    i. CN IX, glossopharyngeal: sensory; posterior taste

    j. CN X, vagus: sensory; throat, motor; swallow, speech. Cardiac innervation (slows down)

    k. CN XI, accessory: motor; throat, neck muscles, and upper back

    l. CN XII, hypoglossal: motor tongue

4. Motor function

    a. Muscles

        1) Size

        2) Symmetry

        3) Tone

        4) Strength

    b. Coordination

    c. Movement

        1) Voluntary control/involuntary movements

        2) Tremors

        3) Twitches

        4) Balance and gait

    d. Posturing

        1) Decorticate: An abnormal posturing indicated by rigidity, flexion of the arms to the chest, clenched fists, and extended legs; indicative of damage to the corticospinal tract (the pathway between the brain and the spinal cord)

        2) Decerebrate: An abnormal body posturing indicated by rigid extension of the arms and legs, downward pointing of the toes, and backward arching of the head; indicative of deterioration of structures of the nervous system, particularly the upper brain stem

5. Reflexes

    a. Deep tendon reflexes (DTRs)

        1) Biceps, triceps, brachioradial, quadriceps

    b. Superficial reflex

        1) Plantar, abdominal, Babinski

    c. Reflex activity

        1) Absent, no response = 0

        2) Weaker than normal = 1+

        3) Normal = 2+

        4) Stronger/more brisk = 3+

        5) Hyperactive = 4+

        6) Glascow coma scale: neuro assessment tool

    d. Rating: Normal is 8 to 15; 3 or less indicates deep unconsciousness

        1) Eye opening response

            a) Spontaneously = 4

            b) To sound = 3

            c) To pain = 2

            d) No response = 1

        2) Motor response

            a) Obeys verbal command = 6

            b) Localizes pain = 5

            c) Normal flexion: withdrawal to pain = 4

            d) Abnormal flexion: abnormal (decorticate) = 3

            e) Extension: abnormal (decerebrate) = 2

            f) No response to pain on any limb = 1

        3) Verbal response

            a) Oriented × 3 = 5

            b) Conversation (confused) = 4

            c) Speech: inappropriate = 3

            d) Sounds: incomprehensible = 2

            e) No response = 1

6. Pupil check—PERRLA

    a. **P**upils **E**qual in size, **R**ound and regular in shape, **R**eactive to **L**ight and **A**ccommodation

7. Vital signs

    a. Blood pressure or pulse changes may indicate increased intracranial pressure

B. Diagnostic Procedures

1. Lumbar puncture: Procedure that inserts a needle into the subarachnoid space to measure pressure, obtain CSF for analysis, and inject contrast, anesthetics, and certain drugs

     a. **NURSING INTERVENTIONS**

        1) Verify that informed consent has been signed.

        2) Have the client empty his bladder and bowel.

        3) Position the client on his side with his knees pulled toward his chest and his chin tucked downward.

        4) Insert the spinal needle between the third and fourth lumbar vertebrae.

        5) Assist care providers with measuring pressure and collection of fluid.

        6) Postprocedure:

            a) Encourage fluid intake.

            b) Check puncture site for redness, swelling, and clear drainage.

            c) Assess movement of the client's extremities.

2. Computed tomography (CT) scan

   a. Head CT: A computerized tomography image (with or without dye) used to evaluate cranial-facial trauma, subarachnoid or intracranial hemorrhage, and headaches; also used to diagnose a stroke or determine abnormal development of the head and neck

     1) **NURSING INTERVENTIONS** (preprocedure; if dye is used)

       a) Verify that informed consent has been signed.

       b) Check for any allergies to iodine, contrast dyes, or shellfish.

       c) Instruct the client to lie still and flat.

     2) **NURSING INTERVENTIONS** (postprocedure; if dye is used)

       a) Increase fluids to clear dye from the client's system.

       b) Assess dye injection site and monitor the client's distal pulses.

3. Cerebral arteriography: Injection of dye via the femoral artery to allow visualization of the cerebral arteries and assess for brain lesions

   a. **NURSING INTERVENTIONS** (preprocedure)

     1) Verify that informed consent has been signed.

     2) Check for any allergies to iodine, contrast dyes, or shellfish.

     3) Keep client NPO 4 to 6 hr before the procedure.

     4) Mark distal peripheral pulses.

     5) Instruct the client that her face may feel warm during the procedure.

   b. **NURSING INTERVENTIONS** (postprocedure)

     1) Monitor the client for an altered level of consciousness and sensory or motor deficits.

     2) Check for hematoma at the insertion site. Keep the client's leg straight and remain in bed 4–6 hours with sandbag at insertion site.

     3) Check the client's peripheral pulses, color, and temperature of extremities.

4. Electroencephalogram (EEG): Detects problems in the electrical activity of the brain. Electrodes are placed over multiple areas of the scalp to detect and record patterns of electrical activity, and they also check for abnormalities such as seizure disorders, evaluation of head injuries, tumors, infections, degenerative diseases, metabolic disturbances, or to confirm brain death.

   a. **NURSING INTERVENTIONS** (preprocedure)

     1) Verify that informed consent has been signed.

     2) Verify which medications should be administered before the EEG.

     3) Instruct the client to avoid caffeine 8 hr before the test.

     4) Advise the client to wash hair the night before the test, because it must be free of oils, sprays, and conditioners.

     5) Verify if the test is to be done awake, asleep, or sleep-deprived.

5. Magnetic resonance imaging (MRI): A noninvasive procedure that uses magnets and radio waves to construct clear, detailed pictures of the brain and nerve tissues without obstruction

   a. **NURSING INTERVENTIONS**

     1) Verify that informed consent has been signed.

     2) Assess the client for claustrophobia.

     3) Remove all metal objects such as body piercings, jewelry, credit cards, and watch.

     4) No special test, diet, or medications are required.

C. Disorders

1. Increased intracranial pressure: A rise in pressure within the skull that can result from or cause a brain injury

   a. Contributing Factors

     1) Head injury with subdural or epidural hematoma

     2) Cerebrovascular accident or cerebral edema

     3) Brain tumor

     4) Hydrocephalus

     5) Ruptured aneurysm and subarachnoid hemorrhage

     6) Meningitis, encephalitis

   b. Manifestations (vary depending on cause and location; will affect the client's level of consciousness)

     1) Lethargic, drowsy, stupor; motor and sensory changes

     2) Headache, irritability, restlessness

     3) Nausea and vomiting, often projectile

     4) Pupil changes: dilated, unequal, nonreactive

     5) Diplopia

     6) Changes in vital signs

       a) Cushing's triad: severe hypertension, widening pulse pressure, bradycardia

       b) Irregular or decreasing respirations (Cheyne-Stokes respirations)

       c) Elevated temperature

   c. Collaborative Care

     1) **NURSING INTERVENTIONS**

       a) Monitor the client's vital signs and neurological function.

       b) Keep head of bed elevated 30° to 45°.

       c) Keep the client's head in a neutral position to enhance drainage.

       d) Avoid coughing, sneezing, straining, and suctioning.

       e) Maintain maximum respiratory exchange. (Hyperventilation causes CO_2 to decrease, leading to vasoconstriction. This causes a decrease in the intracranial pressure.)

       f) Administer oxygen to increase the supply to the client's brain.

       g) Monitor fluid I&O and restrict fluids to prevent increased cerebral edema.

h) Administer medications as prescribed.

i) Give antihypertensive or anticonvulsant medications if necessary.

j) Use hypothermia as ordered to decrease intracranial pressure.

k) Decrease environmental stimuli.

l) Intensive care is required when monitoring intracranial pressure (ventriculostomy).

2) Medications

a) Avoid opiates and sedatives (contraindicated).

b) Barbiturates (pentobarbital [Nembutal]) may be prescribed for uncontrolled, increased intracranial pressure to place the client into a therapeutic coma with ventilator support and close monitoring of cardiac status.

c) Acetaminophen (Tylenol) may be used for fever.

d) Osmotic diuretics (mannitol [Osmitrol]) and steroids (dexamethasone [Decadron]) may be used to decrease cerebral swelling.

2. Hyperthermia: Body temperature above 40.5° C (105° F). Temperature regulation is controlled by the hypothalamus.

a. Contributing Factors

1) Infections

2) Cerebral edema

3) Environmental heat

b. Manifestations

1) Nausea, vomiting, shivering

2) Hypoxia

c. Collaborative Care

 1) **NURSING INTERVENTIONS**

a) Assess neuro status every hour.

b) Use a cooling blanket as ordered, or place ice packs to axilla, groin, and back of the neck.

c) Monitor the client for tachycardia and dysrhythmias.

d) Monitor for manifestations of dehydration by checking I&O and weighing the client daily.

e) Initiate seizure precautions.

f) Prevent shivering.

(1) Decreases risk of increased intracranial pressure and oxygen consumption

(2) Chlorpromazine hydrochloride (Thorazine)

(3) Meperidine hydrochloride (Demerol)

3. Seizure disorders: Abnormal, sudden, uncontrolled, excessive discharge of electrical activity within the brain

a. Contributing Factors

1) Genetics

2) Trauma

3) Brain tumors

4) Toxicity or infection

b. Classifications

1) Generalized seizures (four types)

a) Tonic-clonic (formerly grand-mal)

b) Absence (formerly petit-mal)

c) Myoclonic

d) Atonic or akinetic (drop attacks)

2) Partial seizures (two types)

a) Complex (loss of consciousness)

b) Simple (no loss of consciousness)

c. Collaborative Care

1) **NURSING INTERVENTIONS**

a) Maintain patent airway (turn to side after tonic phase).

b) Monitor the client for respiratory difficulty.

c) Protect the client from injury.

d) Do not restrain the client.

e) Do not put anything in the client's mouth.

f) Turn client's head to the side to prevent aspiration.

g) Document the length of seizure (most important).

h) Watch for prodromal signs such as irritability, mood change, and insomnia preceding the aura (a sensory warning that the seizure is about to occur).

i) Document how long the client remains unconsciousness.

j) Identify precipitating factors (if any).

k) Monitor and document the client's behavior during the postictal phase (period of lethargy and limpness following seizure).

l) Initiate seizure precautions for clients who are prone to multiple seizures and/or are in poor control.

(1) Bed rest should include padded side rails.

(2) Ensure that immediate access is available for oxygen administration and suction.

m) Determine if there is any incontinence.

2) Medications

a) Phenytoin (Dilantin): gum hypertrophy (must visit the dentist routinely), ataxia, and diplopia; monitor medication levels

b) Carbamazepine (Tegretol): nystagmus, ataxia, blood dyscrasias; monitor CBC, liver function tests, and medication levels

c) Valproic acid (Depakene) and divalproex sodium (Depakote): nausea, bleeding problems, and liver damage; monitor liver function tests and medication levels

d) phenobarbital (Luminal): side effects include drowsiness; monitor liver function test and medication levels

3) Client Education

a) Take medications consistently and never stop abruptly.

b) Get adequate rest and exercise.

c) Avoid alcohol.

d) Wear medic alert tag.

e) Follow state laws regarding operating vehicles and machinery.

f) Keep all follow up appointments.

4. Status epilepticus: A life-threatening condition characterized by prolonged or clustered seizures that develop into continuous seizures for 30 min or more; may be caused by a sudden withdrawal of anticonvulsant medications; can lead to brain damage or death

   a. Collaborative Care

    1) **NURSING INTERVENTIONS**

   a) Initiate seizure precautions.

   2) Medications

   a) Lorazepam (Ativan) is the medication of choice at a loading dose of 4 mg IV every 2 min, up to a maximum of 8 mg.

   b) Diazepam (Valium) may also be used in status epilepticus beginning with a loading dose of 5 to 10 mg IV every 10 min up to a maximum of 30 mg.

   c) Phenytoin (Dilantin) 500 to 1,000 mg IV slowly administering no more than 50 mg/min:

   (1) Do not mix with glucose; administer in 0.9% sodium chloride only.

   (2) Monitor for bradycardia and heart block.

5. Transient ischemic attack (TIA): Temporary episode of neurological dysfunction lasting seconds or minutes secondary to decreased blood flow to the brain; may be a warning sign of an impending stroke, especially in the first 4 weeks after TIA.

   a. Contributing Factors

   1) Atherosclerosis

   2) Microemboli from atherosclerotic plaque

   3) Cerebral artery spasm

   b. Manifestations

   1) Sudden change in visual function

   2) Sudden loss of sensory or motor functions

   c. Diagnostic Procedures

   1) Carotid Doppler studies

   2) CT scan and/or MRI

   3) Arteriography

   d. Collaborative Care

   1) **NURSING INTERVENTIONS**

   a) Encourage the client to stop smoking and limit alcohol intake.

   b) Maintain a diet low in cholesterol and sodium.

   c) Stress the importance of maintaining ideal body weight with regular exercise.

2) Medications

   a) Antiplatelet medications

   (1) Clopidogrel (Plavix)

   (2) Dipyridamole (Aggrenox)

   (3) Ticlopidine (Ticlid)

   b) Anticoagulant medications

   (1) Warfarin (Coumadin)

3) Therapeutic Measures

   a) Angioplasty

   b) Carotid endarterectomy (removal of plaque from one or both carotid arteries)

6. Cerebrovascular accident (CVA): Commonly referred to as a stroke; the sudden loss of brain function resulting from a disruption of blood supply to the involved part of the brain; causes temporary or permanent neurological deficits.

   a. Contributing Factors

   1) Hypertension and obesity

   2) Smoking or cocaine use

   3) Hypercholesterolemia

   4) Diabetes mellitus or peripheral vascular disease

   5) Aneurysm or cranial hemorrhage

   b. Manifestations: The severity of the neurological deficit is determined by location and the extent of tissue ischemia; symptoms manifest on the side opposite of damage to the brain, due to a crossover effect.

   1) Loss of motor balance or function, coordination

   2) Slurred speech, aphasia, and dysphagia

   3) Hemiparesis, hemiplegia

   4) Visual disturbance

   5) Cranial nerve disturbance

   c. Collaborative Care

    1) **NURSING INTERVENTIONS**

   a) Maintain an adequate airway.

   b) Monitor the client's neurological function and vital signs routinely.

   c) Establish level of function and Glasgow coma scale.

   d) Maintain fluid and electrolyte balance.

   e) Monitor for aspiration due to risk of dysphagia; feed the client slowly, placing food in the back of his mouth and to the unaffected side.

   f) Provide psychological support to the client and family.

   g) Establish means of communication with a client who is experiencing aphasia (expressive, receptive, global).

   h) Encourage slow deliberate speech.

i) Range of motion: To prevent flexion contractures, keep extremities in a position of extension or neutrality:
    (1) Hemiparesis, hemiplegia: Will cause safety issues in the client.
    (2) Hemianopsia: Place articles within client's visual range.
j) Help the client to achieve bowel and bladder control.

2) Client Education and Referral
    a) Rehabilitation
    b) Occupational and physical therapy

7. Spinal cord injury: Partial or complete disruption of nerve tracts and neurons; resulting in paralysis, sensory loss, altered activity, and autonomic nervous system dysfunction.
    a. Contributing Factors
        1) Men ages 16 to 25
        2) High-risk activities
            a) Driving while intoxicated
            b) Not wearing a seat belt
            c) No protective sports gear
            d) Firearm use
            e) Diving accidents
    b. Types
        1) Contusion
        2) Laceration
        3) Compression of the cord
        4) Complete transection
    c. Manifestations (determined by the level of injury)
        1) Cervical: causes quadriplegia
            a) Respiratory dysfunction (the client may be ventilator dependent)
            b) Paralysis of all four extremities
            c) Loss of bladder and bowel control
            d) Injury above C3 usually fatal
        2) Thoracic injury: causes paraplegia
            a) Loss of bladder and bowel control
            b) Paralysis of lower extremities and major control of body trunk
            c) Potential complication of autonomic dysreflexia—injury above T6
        3) Lumbar
            a) Paralysis of lower extremities (remain flaccid)
            b) Loss of bladder and bowel control
    d. Collaborative Care
         1) **NURSING INTERVENTIONS**
            a) Immobilize the client as ordered:
                (1) Spinal board
                (2) Halo traction
                (3) Gardner-Wells traction or Crutchfield tongs
            b) Provide care for spinal shock/neurogenic shock (flaccid paralysis below level of injury resulting in spastic reflexes).
            c) Maintain and monitor respiratory function.
            d) Consult with occupational or physical therapy regarding rehabilitation issues (self-care deficits).
            e) Monitor for autonomic hyperreflexia (or dysreflexia), which is a life-threatening syndrome with sudden, severe hypertension triggered by noxious stimuli below damage of cord. May be caused by impaction, bladder distension, pressure points or ulcers, or pain.
                (1) Manifestations
                    (a) Hypertension (250 to 300/100) with bradycardia
                    (b) Headache, flushing, nausea
                    (c) Blurred vision and restlessness
                 (2) **NURSING INTERVENTIONS**
                    (a) Place the client in the high Fowler's position to help decrease blood pressure.
                    (b) Determine stimuli and correct.
                    (c) Teach the client bowel and bladder management.
                    (d) Administer dexamethasone (Decadron) to reduce edema.

8. Head injury: Any trauma that leads to injury of the scalp, skull, or brain, ranging from concussion to skull fracture; classified as either closed or penetrating
    a. Closed-head injury
        1) Head sustains blunt force trauma caused by striking against an object
        2) Concussion
        3) Contusion
        4) Fracture
    b. Basilar skull fracture
        1) Manifestations
            a) Bleeding from the nose and ears
            b) Otorrhea, rhinorrhea: cerebrospinal fluid from the ears or nose; must differentiate between cerebrospinal fluid and mucus by assessing the glucose content of the drainage
            c) Raccoon eyes (periorbital edema and ecchymosis)
            d) Battle's sign (postauricular ecchymosis) noted on mastoid bone
    c. Hematomas
        1) Epidural hematoma: bleeding into the space between the skull and the dura
            a) Commonly involves the middle meningeal artery

b) Typical presentation: client sustains the injury, followed by a brief loss of consciousness; this is followed by a lucid interval, then rapid deterioration

c) Emergency management: burr holes to relieve increasing intracranial pressure

2) Subdural hematoma: bleeding below the dura

a) Usually venous

b) May be acute, subacute, or chronic

c) Management: craniotomy

d) Penetrating head injury—An object penetrates the skull and enters the brain

 3) **NURSING INTERVENTIONS**

a) Assess the client frequently for signs of increased intracranial pressure.

b) Same interventions as head trauma

9. Multiple sclerosis (MS): Chronic, progressive disease of the CNS, characterized by patches of demyelination in the brain and spinal cord (exact cause unknown, probable autoimmune basis)

a. Manifestations

1) Occurs in young adults 20 to 40 years of age

2) Nystagmus, blurred vision, diplopia

3) Slurred hesitant speech and fatigue

4) Spastic weakness of extremities, paresthesia, and difficulty with balance

5) Emotional lability, depression

6) Intention tremors

7) Spastic bladder

8) MRI shows sclerotic patches through the brain and spinal cord

b. Management

1) There is no cure or specific treatment, only symptomatic relief. MS is characterized by long periods of remissions and exacerbations.

2) During exacerbation, administer corticosteroids as prescribed.

3) Stress management techniques may be helpful to prevent exacerbations.

c. Collaborative Care

 1) **NURSING INTERVENTIONS**

a) As much as possible, encourage the client to maintain an active and normal life style.

b) Teach the client self-catheterization techniques.

c) Promote daily exercise with fall precautions.

d) Instruct the client to avoid stressors that exacerbate the condition (infections)

e) Teach the client self-injection technique for beta interferon (Betaseron)

2) Medications

a) Immunosuppressants: azathioprine (Imuran) or beta-interferon (Betaseron)

b) Muscle spasticity and tremors: baclofen (Lioresal), gabapentin (Neurontin), clonazepam (Klonopin)

c) Urinary problems and constipation: oxybutynin (Ditropan), tolterodine (Detrol), propantheline (Pro-Banthine), psyllium (Metamucil)

d) Depression: amitriptyline (Elavil), imipramine (Tofranil), sertraline (Zoloft), fluoxetine (Prozac)

e) Sexual difficulties: sildenafil (Viagra)

f) Fatigue: amantadine (Symmetrel), modafinil (Provigil)

10. Parkinson's disease: Chronic, progressive neurological disorder affecting the brain centers that are responsible for control and regulation of movement; extrapyramidal tract; loss of pigmented cells of substantia nigra and depletion of dopamine

a. Manifestations

1) Bradykinesia with rigidity

2) Resting tremor

3) Expressionless, fixed gaze; mask-like and depression

4) Drooling and slurred speech

5) Constipation

6) Retropulsion, propulsion

b. Stages

1) Unilateral flexion of upper extremity

2) Shuffling gait with progressive weakness and difficulty ambulating

3) Progressive, permanent disability

c. Collaborative Care

 1) **NURSING INTERVENTIONS**

a) Teach the client fall precautions.

b) Encourage the client to wear clothing that fosters independence (no snaps, buttons, or zippers).

c) Encourage a high-fiber diet.

2) Medications

a) Antiparkinsonian agent: levodopa (Dopar); levodopa (Sinemet); side effects include hypotension and gastrointestinal upset; administer on an empty stomach ½ to 1 hr before meals

b) Antiparkinsonian agent: carbidopa (Lodosyn); side effects include hypokinesia, hyperkinesia, and psychiatric manifestations

c) Dopamine agonist: bromocriptine mesylate (Parlodel)

d) Anticholinergic: benztropine (Cogentin); trihexyphenidyl (Artane); side effects include dry mouth, mydriasis, constipation, and confusion

e) Antiviral, antiparkinsonian: amantadine HCl (Symmetrel); side effects include tremor, rigidity, and bradykinesia

11. Amyotrophic lateral sclerosis (ALS): Rapidly progressive, invariably fatal neurological disease that attacks nerve cells (neurons) that control voluntary muscles; also known as Lou Gehrig's disease

    a. Progression

        1) Most commonly affects men 40 to 60 years of age.

        2) Presents with muscle weakness in extremities and slurred speech, and progresses to inability to swallow, chew, communicate, breathe, and perceive sensory or tactile stimulation.

        3) Greatest risk of respiratory failure or pneumonia is within 3 to 5 years of onset.

        4) Eventually the client loses the ability to breathe without ventilator support and dies from respiratory failure or pneumonia.

        5) ALS does not affect the client's sensory or cognitive abilities; all senses remain intact.

    b. Manifestations

        1) Twitching, cramping, and stiffness of muscles

        2) Muscle weakness affecting an arm or leg

        3) Slurred or nasal speech with difficulty forming words (dysarthria)

        4) Difficulty chewing and swallowing (dysphagia)

        5) Overactive gag reflex

        6) Fatigue

        7) Difficulty with manual dexterity

    c. Etiology unknown; no known cure; treatment is symptomatic

    d. **NURSING INTERVENTIONS**

        1) Speech therapy assists with communication and swallowing needs.

        2) Occupational therapy assists with adaptive devices to foster independence

        3) Physical therapy helps maintain muscle strength and tone.

        4) Support respiratory needs with mechanical respirator devices.

        5) Medication provides relief from excessive salivation, pain, muscle cramps, constipation, and depression.

        6) Provide supportive services to the client and family with anticipatory grieving.

12. Myasthenia gravis: Disorder of unknown origin affecting the neuromuscular transmission of the voluntary muscle of the body; loss of acetylcholine receptors on the postsynaptic membrane of the neuromuscular junction (probable autoimmune basis)

    a. Manifestations

        1) Extreme muscular weakness: increased with fatigue and relieved by rest

        2) Progressive deterioration, particularly the respiratory system, and muscle wasting

        3) Early manifestations: diplopia, ptosis, dysphagia

    b. Types of Crisis

        1) Cholinergic: usually from overmedication; causes severe tremors

        2) Myasthenic: spontaneous or from infection; drooling and severe ptosis; can actually cause respiratory arrest

        3) Differentiate between the two with the Tensilon test: edrophonium (Tensilon) injected; response expected in 30 seconds; if no response, it becomes a cholinergic crisis

    c. Collaborative Care

        1) **NURSING INTERVENTIONS**

           a) Maintain patent airway.

           b) Plan activities for the client early in the day to avoid fatigue.

           c) Teach the client manifestations of crisis.

           d) Give the client medications on time.

        2) Medications

           a) Anticholinesterase medications that increase the amount of acetylcholine in the neuromuscular function

           b) Pyridostigmine (Mestinon); neostigmine (Prostigmin)

           c) Atropine is antidote for medications.

           d) Steroids: prednisone (Deltasone)

        3) Therapeutic Measures

           a) Thymectomy (excision of the thymus)

13. Guillain-Barré syndrome: An acquired acute inflammatory disease of peripheral nerves resulting in demyelination characterized by ascending, reversible paralysis; severity determines verbal or motor manifestations

    a. Manifestations

        1) Disease is usually preceded by an infection (respiratory or gastrointestinal).

        2) Initial manifestations: tingling of the legs that may progress to upper extremities, trunk, and facial muscles; ascending paralysis is a classic disease presentation.

        3) Progresses to paralysis and possible respiratory failure.

        4) Recovery takes anywhere from several months to 1 year in descending form (the last lost is the first recovered).

        5) Immunotherapy prescribed; plasmapheresis; IV immune globulin

    b. **NURSING INTERVENTIONS**

        1) Maintain the client's airway; monitor respiratory status, oximetry.

        2) Monitor the client's blood pressure and heart rate.

        3) Provide nutrition, especially if the client has difficulty chewing and swallowing; may need parenteral feedings.

        4) Manage bowel and bladder problems.

5) Collaborate with physical therapy to maintain the client's muscle strength, flexibility, and contractures.

6) Prevent complications of immobility: pneumonia, deep vein thrombosis, urinary tract infection atelectasis, and skin breakdown.

D. Common Surgical Procedures

1. **Laminectomy**: A surgical procedure to remove a portion of vertebrae for the treatment of severe pain and disability resulting from compression of spinal nerves by a ruptured disk or bony compression; also an option to relieve persistent pain or to treat progressive neurological problems due to nerve compression

2. **Diskectomy**: A surgical procedure to remove a herniated disk

3. **Spinal Fusion**: A surgical procedure to stabilize spine after multiple laminectomies

   a. Collaborative Care (interventions for all procedures)
   1) Monitor the client for circulatory impairment.
   2) Assess the client for loss of sensation in lower extremities.
   3) Monitor the dressing for spinal fluid leakage, bleeding, or signs of infection.
   4) Log roll the client.
   5) Address the client's sexual concerns.

E. Sensory Assessment

1. Evaluation of visual acuity

   a. Assessment of the client's ability to see objects at specified distances
   1) Manifestation
      a) Myopia (nearsightedness): Distant objects appear blurred.
      b) Hyperopia (farsightedness): Close objects appear blurred.
      c) Presbyopia (farsightedness associated with aging): A progressive condition in which the lens of the eye loses its ability to focus.
      d) Macular degeneration (loss of visual acuity associated with aging): A progressive disorder of the retina causing decreased vision and potentially the loss of central vision.

2. Treatment of visual acuity problems

   a. Abnormal refractory findings are typically treated with corrective lens.

   b. Lasik surgery: This surgical procedure permanently changes the shape of the cornea and (in most cases) restores 20/20 vision.

3. Common optical problems

   a. Detached retina: Occurs when the sensory retina separates from the pigment epithelium of the retina; vitreous humor fluid flows between the layers when a tear occurs in the retina; can be related to age and trauma
   1) Manifestations
      a) Sudden visual disturbances
      b) Flashes of light
      c) Blurred vision with floaters
      d) Curtain or shadow over visual field

    2) **NURSING INTERVENTIONS** (preoperative)
      a) Ensure immediate bed rest with head of the bed elevated.
      b) Instruct the client to avoid coughing, sneezing, and straining.
      c) Surgical intervention includes scleral buckling, photocoagulation, cryosurgery.

    3) **NURSING INTERVENTIONS** (postoperative)
      a) Maintain bed rest with both of the client's eyes bandaged for 24 hr.
      b) Avoid jarring or bumping head.
      c) Teach regular self-administration of eye drops on schedule.

   b. Cataract: Slow, progressive clouding of the lens by development of thickening material
   1) Manifestations
      a) Diplopia, blurred vision, and photophobia
      b) Frequent change in eyeglasses prescription
      c) Halos around lights and colors appear pale

    2) **NURSING INTERVENTIONS** (preoperative—dilate the eye)
      a) Mydriatics
      b) Cycloplegics

    3) **NURSING INTERVENTIONS** (postoperative)
      a) Keep the client's operative eye covered.
      b) Elevate head of bed 30° to 45° and do not turn the client onto operative side.
      c) Instruct the client to avoid bending at the waist, lifting, sneezing, and coughing, and to not touch the eye area.
      d) Prevent vomiting or straining.
      e) Report severe pain immediately, as it may indicate the development of glaucoma.
   4) Therapeutic Measures
      a) Surgical treatment: removal of the lens under local anesthesia, with intraocular lens implant

c. Glaucoma: Increased intraocular pressure due to the inability of aqueous humor to drain; if uncorrected, glaucoma may lead to atrophy of the optic nerve and blindness.

   1) Manifestations

     a) Acute (closed angle)

      (1) Results from an obstruction to the outflow of aqueous humor

      (2) Severe pain in and around the client's eye

      (3) Lights appear to have a rainbow of colors around them

      (4) Cloudy and blurred vision with dilated pupils

      (5) Nausea and vomiting

      (6) Within hours, the client may develop gastrointestinal, sinus, neuro, and dental manifestations

     b) Chronic (open angle)

      (1) Insidious onset with slowly decreasing peripheral vision

      (2) Tired feeling in the client's eye

      (3) Halos around lights

      (4) Progressive loss of visual field

   2) Collaborative Care

      a) **NURSING INTERVENTIONS**

      (1) Administer medications consistently on time.

      (2) Avoid anticholinergic medications.

     b) Medications

      (1) Medication causes pupils to contract and the iris to pull away from the corneas.

      (2) Aqueous humor may drain through lymph spaces (meshwork) into Schlemm's canal.

       (a) Pilocarpine hydrochloride (Pilocar) lasts 6 to 8 hr; medication of choice for glaucoma.

       (b) Acetazolamide (Diamox) decreases production of aqueous humor; a side effect includes gastric distress.

       (c) Mannitol (Osmitrol), IV; reduces intraocular pressure by increasing blood osmolality; indications—treatment of acute attacks and preoperatively.

       (d) Isosorbide (Isordil), oral; cautions—safer than IV medication for cardiac clients; may cause diuresis, which is troublesome in men with prostatitis.

     c) Therapeutic Measures

      (1) Iridencleisis

      (2) Thermosclerectomy

     d) Client Education

      (1) Teach the client that glaucoma is controllable, but not curable.

      (2) Avoid emotional upsets, extreme exertion, lifting, and colds.

      (3) Encourage moderate exercise, regular bowel habits, daily use of medicines, medical checkups, and the importance of wearing a Medic-Alert bracelet; monitor fluid intake.

F. Auditory Assessment

1. Audiology exam (audiogram) tests the client's ability to hear sounds at varying intensity and decibels.

2. Presbycusis (hearing deficit associated with aging) is a progressive disorder characterized by a loss of the ability to hear sounds at high frequencies; may lead to deafness.

3. Client may need hearing aids to amplify desirable environmental sounds.

4. **Ménière's disease**: Disorder of the inner ear in which an increase in fluid causes change in sensory perception

   a. Manifestations

     1) Vertigo

     2) Tinnitus—hearing loss

     3) Pressure in the ear

   b. Collaborative Care

    1) **NURSING INTERVENTIONS**

     a) Encourage the client to implement a low-sodium diet.

     b) Instruct the client to eat six small meals per day.

     c) Initiate and teach the client fall precautions.

     d) Maintain a quiet environment for the client.

   2) Medications

     a) Meclizine (Antivert) to manage vertigo

     b) Hydrochlorothiazide (HCTZ) to reduce inner ear fluid volume and pressure

     c) Dexamethasone (Prednisone) to reduce inflammation

   3) Client Education

     a) Assist the client with identifying triggers such as bright lights, loud music, caffeine, stress, and nicotine.

     b) Encourage the client to avoid caffeine.

     c) Manage the client's anxiety and stress.

Oncology Nursing

> **!** **POINT TO REMEMBER:** Providing care to clients and families experiencing cancer can be complex and challenging. Treatment regimens (protocols) have been established for most types of cancer.

A. Overview of Cancer

1. Healthy cells transform into malignant cells upon exposure to certain etiological agents—viruses, chemicals, and physical agents.

2. Malignant cells metastasize and extend directly into adjacent tissue, moving through the lymph system, entering the blood circulation, and diffusing into body cavities.

B. General Disease-Related Consequences of Cancer

1. Decreased immunity and blood-producing function

   a. Occurs most often with leukemia and lymphoma or any cancer that invades the bone marrow and reduces the production of WBCs, RBCs, and platelets, causing thrombocytopenia.

   b. Clients are at increased risk for infection.

   c. Changes are caused by either the cancer or chemotherapy.

   d. Clients may experience weakness, fatigue, and bleeding.

2. Altered GI structure and function

   a. Impaired absorption and elimination related to tumor obstruction or compression.

   b. Tumors increase the metabolic rate, increasing the need for proteins, fats, and carbohydrates.

   c. Liver tumors reduce function and lead to malnutrition.

3. Motor and sensory deficits

   a. Occur when cancers invade the bone or brain or compress nerves.

   b. Bone metastases cause pain, fractures, spinal cord obstruction, and hypercalcemia, which decreases mobility.

   c. Sensory changes occur if the spinal cord is damaged by tumor pressure or compression.

   d. Sensory, motor, and cognitive functions are impaired when cancer is in the brain.

   e. Pain is often significant, especially in the terminal stages of the disease process.

4. Decreased respiratory function

   a. Disrupts respiratory function and gas exchange (i.e., tumors in an airway cause an obstruction).

   b. Lung capacity is decreased; gas exchange is impaired.

   c. Tumors can compress blood and lymph vessels in the chest, blocking blood flow through the chest and lungs, causing pulmonary edema and dyspnea.

C. Tumors

1. Classified according to type of tissue from which they evolve.

2. Carcinomas begin in epithelial tissue (skin, gastrointestinal tract lining, lung, breast, uterus).

3. Sarcomas begin in nonepithelial tissue (bone, muscle, fat, lymph system).

4. Cell type affects appearance, rate of growth, and degree of malignancy (epithelial basal cells are basal cell carcinoma; bone cells are osteogenic carcinoma; gland epithelium are adenocarcinoma).

D. Manifestations Suggesting Malignant Disease (American Cancer Society 7 Warning Signs)

C – Change in bowel or bladder habits

A – A sore that does not heal

U – Unusual bleeding or discharge

T – Thickening or lumps in breast or elsewhere

I – Indigestion or difficulty swallowing

O – Obvious change in wart or mole

N – Nagging cough or hoarseness

E. Cancer Management: Purpose is to prolong survival time or improve the quality of life. Therapies include chemotherapy, radiation, surgery, hormonal manipulation, photodynamic therapy, immunotherapy, gene therapy, and a variety of alternative therapies.

1. Chemotherapy

   a. Medications interfere with cell division; combination of medications usually given

   b. Classification (all cause bone marrow depression)
      1) Alkylating agents: uracil mustard (nitrogen mustard), cyclophosphamide (Cytoxan)
      2) Antimetabolite: fluorouracil (5-FU), methotrexate (MTX) (Folex)
      3) Antibiotics: doxorubicin hydrochloride (Adriamycin), bleomycin (Blenoxane), dactinomycin (actinomycin D)
      4) Plant alkaloids: vincristine (Oncovin), vinblastine (Velban)
      5) Hormones: estrogen, progesterone, tamoxifen citrate (Tamofen)
      6) Biological modifiers (Procrit, Neupogen)

   c. Common side effects and interventions to counteract
      1) Leukopenia (WBC less than 1,000 mm³):
         a) Interventions to enhance the immune system include a balanced diet, rest, and handwashing.
         b) Administer filgrastim (Neupogen) to increase WBC production.
         c) Implement protective isolation during hospitalization.
         d) Monitor lab and diagnostic results.

2) Anemia (Hgb less than 10)
   a) Administer oxygen therapy; provide iron-rich foods.
   b) Monitor CBCs and administer blood transfusions as needed.
   c) Administer erythropoietin (Epogen) and epoetin alfa (Procrit) to increase RBCs.
3) Thrombocytopenia (platelets less than 50,000)
   a) Administer prescribed platelet transfusions; oprelvekin (Neumega) to increase platelets.
   b) Implement bleeding precautions; avoid use of aspirin.
4) Alopecia (hair loss 2 weeks after start of treatment)
   a) Apply ice to the client's scalp during chemotherapy to slow hair loss. Use gentle shampoo, hats, scarves, and sunscreen.
   b) Refer client to the American Cancer Society, which provides wigs and supportive services.
5) Anorexia, nausea, and vomiting
   a) Administer antiemetic prior to therapy; ondansetron (Zofran).
   b) Administer loperamide (Imodium A-D) to manage diarrhea.
   c) The client should drink cool beverages and eat small, favorite meals high in potassium with high-calorie supplements. Avoid unpleasant odors.
   d) Provide soft, bland, high-protein foods at room temperature for stomatitis, and use a straw for fluids. Rinse mouth with a topical anesthetic, may need topical steroids and zinc supplements.
6) Elevated uric acid, crystal, and urate stone formation
   a) Administer allopurinol (Zyloprim) therapy; increase fluid intake.
7) Mucositis: Often develops in the GI tract especially in the mouth (stomatitis). Mucous membranes, because they undergo rapid cell division, are killed more rapidly than the cells are replaced.
   a) Provide frequent mouth assessment and oral hygiene including teeth cleaning and mouth rinsing.
   b) Avoid traumatizing oral mucosa due to risk of bleeding; use soft-bristled toothbrush or swabs.
   c) Use plain water or saline for oral rinses
8) Specific medications have specific toxic effects.
   a) Doxorubicin hydrochloride (Adriamycin): irreversible cardiomyopathy
   b) Cisplatinum (Platinol): renal toxicity
   c) Vincristine sulfate (Oncovin): peripheral neuropathy

2. Radiation: Therapy destroys cancer cells with minimal exposure of normal cells to the damaging actions of radiation. Cells damaged by radiation either die or become unable to divide. Gamma rays are used most commonly because of their ability to penetrate tissues and damage cells.
   a. Radiation Delivery
      1) Teletherapy: distance treatment; the radiation source is external to the client.
      2) Brachtherapy: short or close therapy; radiation comes into direct, continuous contact with the tumor tissues. Provides a high dose of radiation with a limited amount to surrounding tissues.

 b. **NURSING INTERVENTIONS**
      1) Client must always be in the same position for all radiation treatments; ensure that the client can get into and maintain the same position during treatment; fixing devices and markings must be in the correct position for each treatment.
      2) Assess condition of skin and cleanse the area gently each day with water or mild soap.
      3) Wet reaction: skin's response to radiation; skin becomes dry or develops blisters that may break, causing pain and the potential for infection. If dry reaction, keep clean and lubricated. If wet reaction, clean and cover to prevent infection.
      4) Instruct client to not remove skin markings; avoid powders, lotions, and creams.
      5) Instruct client to wear soft loose clothing and avoid exposure to the sun.
      6) For clients with sealed implants of radioactive sources:
         a) Assign clients to a private room.
         b) Place "Caution Radioactive Material" sign on the client's door in hospital setting.
         c) Wear a lead apron while providing care; pregnant nurses should not care for these clients.
         d) Limit visitors to ½ hour each day, and instruct to remain at least 6 feet from the source.
         e) Do not touch the radioactive source with bare hands.
         f) Save all radioactive dressings and linens until the radioactive source is removed.
         g) Follow institution guidelines for radiation containment.

3. Managing Cancer Pain: Adequate pain control can make a significant difference in improving the client's quality of life. Oncology clients are often under-treated for pain. As a client advocate, it is the nurse's responsibility to ensure that the client is receiving adequate pain control (see Opioid Analgesics in the Pharmacology section)

SECTION 12

Review of Immunologic Disorders

! Point to Remember: Immunity is composed of many cell functions that protect individuals against the effects of injury or microscopic invasion. Immune function can be reduced by disease, injury, or medical therapies. When the functions of the immune system are working well, an individual is considered immunocompetent.

A. Acquired Immune Deficiency Syndrome (AIDS)

1. A chronic, potentially life-threatening condition caused by the human immunodeficiency virus (HIV); infectious disease characterized by severe deficits and destruction of cellular immune function; manifested clinically by opportunistic infection and/or unusual neoplasms. HIV destroys CD4 cells.

2. Contributing Factors: exposure to individual infected with HIV; infected blood, semen, or vaginal secretions during unprotected intercourse; and needle sharing or blood transfusions. Infected mothers can infect their babies during pregnancy or delivery, or through breast-feeding.

3. Manifestations
   a. Flu-like symptoms
   b. Swollen lymph glands
   c. Weight loss with wasting syndrome
   d. Chronic diarrhea and fever
   e. Night sweats
   f. CD4 lymphocyte count less than 200 (800–1,200 is normal)
   g. Dementia complex
   h. Opportunistic infection
      1) Pneumocystic pneumonia, cytomegalovirus, tuberculosis, toxoplasmosis, cryptosporidiosis, *Candida albicans*
   i. Kaposi's sarcoma is a cancer in the advanced stage of infection (purplish or brown skin lesions)

4. Diagnostic Procedures
   a. ELISA (antibody assay): Positive within 3 weeks to 3 months following infection. Most common and least expensive.
   b. Plasma HIV-1 RNA viral load is > 1500 copies.
   c. CD4+ cell count: Decreased < 750 cells/mm³. Clients with values < 200 cells/mm³ have an 85% likelihood of progressing to AIDS within 3 years.
   d. CBC and platelets are decreased.
   e. Brain, lung, or CT scans may be abnormal.

5. Collaborative Care

 a. **NURSING INTERVENTIONS**
   1) Assess for risk factors; Monitor I&O, vital signs, electrolytes, respiratory status, skin, weight, nutritional intake, and pain.
   2) Depending on stage of the disease, administer oxygen as needed and provide analgesia.
   3) Prevent the spread of infection by using standard precautions and blood and body fluid precautions.

b. Medications
   1) Medication therapy: World Health Organization; highly active antiretroviral therapy guidelines (HAART) (research findings are constantly being updated)
   2) Efavirenz (Sustiva), azidothymidine (AZT), and lamivudine (Epivir)
      a) Common adverse effects: neutropenia, gastrointestinal distress, anemia, insomnia
   3) Zidovudine (AZT) recommended for protecting the unborn fetus of women who are HIV positive
   4) Interferon (Roferon)
   5) Pneumocystis pneumonia prophylaxis : pentamidine (Pentam 300)
   6) Antifungals: metronidazole (Flagyl) and amphotericin B (Fungizone)
   7) Antituberculosis medications as needed
   8) Acyclovir (Zovirax) herpes treatment
   9) Protease inhibitors: saquinavir (Fortovase), ritonavir (Norvir)
   10) Antivirals: zalcitabine, dideoxycytidine (Hivid)

c. Client Education
   1) Transmission, control measures, and safe sex practices
   2) Nutritional needs, self-medication of prescribed medications, and potential side effects
   3) Symptoms that need to be reported immediately (infection, bleeding)
   4) Need for follow-up monitoring CD4+ and viral load counts

B. Lupus Erythematosus (SLE)

1. Definition: a chronic inflammatory disease that occurs when the body's immune system attacks the tissues and organs. Inflammation caused by lupus can affect multiple organ systems such as the joints, skin, kidneys, blood cells, heart, and lungs.

2. Contributing Factors:
   a. Lupus is more common in women.
   b. Age: most often diagnosed between the ages of 15 and 40
   c. Race: more common in blacks, Hispanics, and Asians
   d. Sunlight: exposure to the sun may bring on lupus skin lesions or trigger an internal response in susceptible people

e. Certain prescription medications: drug-induced lupus results from the long-term use of certain prescription drugs, which include the antipsychotic chlorpromazine; high blood pressure medications, such as hydralazine (Apresoline); the tuberculosis drug isoniazid; and the heart medication procainamide (Pronestyl, Procanbid)

f. Exposure to chemicals: some studies have shown that people who work in jobs that involve exposure to mercury and silica may have an increased risk of lupus

3. Manifestations:

a. Insidious onset characterized by remissions and exacerbations

b. Erythematosus "butterfly rash" on both cheeks and across the bridge of the nose; rash deepens on exposure to sunlight

c. Polyarthralgia; also Raynaud's phenomena (arterial vasospasm in response to cold and stress)

d. Fever, malaise, and weight loss; alopecia

e. Anemia, lymphadenopathy; joint pain, swelling, and tenderness

f. Positive for antinuclear antibodies

g. Depression

4. Collaborative Care

 a. **NURSING INTERVENTIONS**

1) Assess for pain, mobility, and fatigue and manifestations associated with alterations in organ functions.

2) Assess vital signs, especially blood pressure (elevated due to edema from renal compromise).

3) Supportive care depends on organs involved.

4) Encourage uninterrupted sleep and daytime naps.

b. Medications

1) NSAIDs to reduce inflammation: contraindicated for clients with renal compromise

2) Corticosteroids for immunosuppression and to reduce inflammation

3) Immunosuppressant agents: methotrexate, azathioprine (Imuran)

4) Antimalarial (hydroxychloroquine) for suppression of synovitis, fever, and fatigue

c. Client Education and Referral

1) Instruct the client to use sunscreen and wear protective clothing.

2) Encourage small, frequent meals if anorexia is present.

3) Limit salt intake for fluid retention secondary to steroid therapy and renal involvement.

4) Refer to support groups as appropriate.

SECTION 13
Burns

A. Overview

1. Thermal, chemical, electrical, and radioactive agents can cause burns, resulting in cellular destruction of the skin layers and underlying tissue. The type and severity of the burn impact the treatment plan.

2. Burn injuries can result in the loss of temperature regulation, sweat and sebaceous gland function, and sensory and organ function.

3. Assessment and severity of the burn is based upon the following:

a. Percentage of total body surface area (TBSA)

b. Depth of the burn

c. Body location

d. Client's age

e. Causative agent

f. Presence of other injuries

g. Respiratory involvement and overall health of the client

B. Burn Assessment

1. Extent of body surface

! **Point to Remember:** The rule of nines assesses the percentage of burn and is used to help guide treatment decisions including fluid resuscitation; it is part of the guidelines to determine burn management.

Rule of Nines for Establishing Extent of Body Surface Burned in Adults

Anatomic Surface	Percentage of Total Body Surface
Head and neck	9%
Anterior trunk	18%
Posterior trunk	18%
Arms, including hands	9% each
Legs, including feet	18% each
Genitalia	1%

Rule of Nines for Establishing Extent of Body Surface Burned in Infants and Young Children

Anatomic Surface	Percentage of Total Body Surface
Anterior head	9%
Posterior head	9%
Anterior torso	18%
Posterior torso	18%
Anterior leg	6.5%
Posterior leg	6.5%
Anterior arm	4.5%
Posterior arm	4.5%
Genitilia/perineum	1%

2. Depth of burn and manifestations

Burn Descriptions

Classifica-tion	Superficial	Superficial Partial Thickness	Deep Partial Thickness	Full-Thickness	Deep Full-Thickness
Degree (old term)	First degree	Second degree	Third degree	Same as deep partial	
Layer Involved	Epidermis	Epidermis and parts of dermis	Epider-mis and deep into dermis	Same as partial—may extend into sub-cutaneous tissue; nerve damage	All layers plus muscles, tendons, bones
Appear-ance	Pink to red, tender, no blis-ters, mild edema, no eschar	Red to white with blisters, mild to moderate edema, no eschar	Red to white with moderate edema, no blisters, soft/dry eschar	Red to tan, black, brown, white. No blisters; severe edema, hard inelastic eschar	Black with no edema

3. Diagnostic testing

   a. CBC, serum electrolytes, BUN, creatinine and myoglobin for deep burns, ABGs, fasting blood glucose, liver studies, urinalysis, clotting studies, and chest x-ray

      1) Initial fluid shift (first 24 hours after injury)

         a) Hct/Hgb elevated due to fluid shifts into interstitial spacing and fluid loss

         b) Sodium < secondary to third spacing

         c) Potassium > due to cell destruction

      2) Fluid mobilization

         a) Hct/Hgb < due to fluid shift from intersti-tial back into vascular fluid

         b) Sodium remains decreased; potassium < due to renal loss and movement back into the cells

   b. WBC count: initial increase then decrease with a shift to the left (an increase in the percentage of neutrophils having only one or a few lobes)

      a) Blood glucose: elevated due to stress response

      b) ABGs: slight hypoxemia and metabolic acidosis

      c) Total protein and albumin: low due to fluid loss

C. Collaborative Care

 1. **NURSING INTERVENTIONS** for moderate and major burns

   a. Maintain airway and ventilation.

   b. Provide humidified oxygen as prescribed.

   c. Monitor vital signs.

   d. Maintain cardiac output and provide IV fluid replacement using Parkland formula:

      1) Give 4 mL/kg/% burn.

      2) Give half of total fluids in first 8 hr.

      3) Give second half over remaining 16 hr.

      4) Deduct any fluid given prehospital from the amount to be infused in the first 8 hr.

   e. Maintain urine output of 30–50 mL/hour for a burn client.

   f. Monitor for manifestations of shock.

   g. Provide pain management.

   h. Assess for and prevent infection.

   i. Provide nutritional support.

      1) Client with a large burn injury will be in a hypermetabolic state and may need up to 5,000 calories per day.

      2) Increase protein intake to prevent tissue breakdown and promote healing.

      3) Enteral or total parenteral therapy is often necessary.

   j. Promote restoration of mobility.

   k. Provide psychological support to both client and family members.

2. Medications: Antimicrobial creams and pain manage-ment (PCA infusion pump preferred to deliver con-tinuous dosing.)

   a. Silver nitrate 0.5%

   b. Silver sulfadiazine 1% (Silvadene): broad-spectrum coverage; water soluble

   c. Mafenide acetate (Sulfamylon): broad-spectrum coverage; penetrates tissue wall; never use a dress-ing; breakdown of medication causes a heavy acid load, which may cause acidosis; painful

   d. Bacitracin

3. Treatments

   a. Wound care

   b. Biologic skin coverings

   c. Permanent skin coverings

4. Methods of Treating Burns

   a. Open-exposure method

      1) Allows for drainage of burn exudate

      2) Eschar forms hardened crust (may constrict circulation, requiring escharotomy)

      3) Use of topical therapy; asepsis crucial

      4) Skin easily visualized and assessed

      5) Range of motion easier

      6) Disadvantages

         a) Increases pain and heat loss

         b) Difficult to manage burns of hands and feet

b. Closed method
   1) Gauze dressing wrapped distal to proximal
   2) Decreased fluid and heat loss
   3) Limited mobility may result in contractures
   4) Wound assessment only during dressing changes

c. Topical antimicrobials (see Medications above)

d. Biologic dressings and tissue grafts
   1) Homograft or allograft (human tissue donors)
   2) Xenograft or heterograft (animal sources)
   3) Amniotic membrane
   4) Biosynthetic (Biobrane) or synthetic (transparent film)

5. Client Education

a. Skin care following discharge
   1) Wear pressure garment 23.5 hr/day to reduce scarring and controil swelling.
   2) Engage in regular exercise per physical therapy.
   3) Elevate affected areas as much as possible.
   4) Keep skin moisturized.
   5) Control itching with cool baths and loose, cotton fabric.
   6) Avoid sun exposure.
   7) Change in appearance of skin as scars fade from red to near natural coloration.
   8) Encourage the client to take in extra calories and protein.

SECTION 14

End-of-Life Care

Definition: Care and management of the client and caregivers facing end-of-life care issues with the outcome of providing "good death"

A. Contributing Factors

1. Chronic terminal illness
2. Hospice care
3. Palliative care

B. Manifestations

1. Anorexia
2. Decreased peripheral circulation (mottled skin)
3. Disorientation and somnolence
4. Cheyne-Stokes respirations
5. Increased respiratory secretions
6. Decreased metabolic function
7. Incontinence
8. Restlessness
9. Weakness and fatigue

C. Collaborative Care

 1. **NURSING INTERVENTIONS**

a. Assess for an end-of-life care plan, advanced directives, and caregiver support.
b. Do not force client to eat or drink.
c. Talk to the client even if the client does not respond.
d. Keep perineal area clean and dry.
e. Position for comfort.
f. Elevate head of bed.
g. Administer medications to manage symptoms of pain, restlessness, excess secretions.
h. Avoid noxious stimuli.

2. Symptom Management

a. **NOTE:** Pain is the symptom dying clients "fear the most."
   1) Long-acting opioid narcotics
   2) Massage
   3) Music therapy
   4) Aromatherapy

b. **NOTE:** Dyspnea and gurgling are the "most distressing" symptoms noted by caregivers.
   1) Morphine elixir
   2) Scopolamine (transdermal or parenteral)
   3) Oxygen via nasal cannula
   4) Avoid deep suctioning

c. Restlessness and agitation
   1) Lorazepam (Ativan)
   2) Haloperidol (Haldol)

d. Nausea and vomiting
   1) Prochlorperazine (Compazine)

e. Psychosocial management
   1) Offer physical and emotional support by "being with" client and caregivers.
   2) Assess cultural and/or religious preferences.
   3) Encourage reminiscence.
   4) Communicate with the client.
   5) Provide palliative care needs.

D. Referral and Follow-up

1. Hospice care
2. Chaplain
3. Social services

E. Postmortem Care

1. Notify provider, chaplain, and mortuary as defined by end-of-life care plan.
2. If no autopsy is planned, remove any tubes or lines.
3. Clean and prepare client for immediate viewing as desired by family or significant other.
4. Provide family or significant other the opportunity to participate in care as desired.

5. Verify the completion of death certificate and required facility documents.

6. Prepare client for transport to morgue, funeral home, or mortuary per facility protocol (ensure client identification tags are present).

SECTION 15

Nutrition: Therapeutic Diets

A. Overview

1. Nutrients absorbed and utilized by the body determine, to a large degree, the health of the body.

2. The process of ingestion, digestion, absorption, and metabolism of food and fluids is essential for life. Disease processes and altered clinical conditions involving the GI tract can prevent either all or some of these processes from taking place.

3. The nurse reviews the medical history and conducts a nutritional assessment to determine the possibility of increased metabolic needs, sources of potential problems with ingestion, digestion, or absorption.

4. Contributing factors may include chronic disease, trauma, recent surgery of the GI tract, drug and alcohol abuse, significant weight loss or gain, and altered cognitive and functional processes that may affect nutritional status.

5. The nurse assesses for:

   a. Decreased appetite; weight loss

   b. History of recent illness

   c. Poor-fitting or no dentures, or poor dental health; poor eyesight; dry mouth or mucous membranes; in infants, shrunken fontanels or absence of tears

   d. Cognitive or functional decline; chronic physical illness

   e. Acute or chronic pain; history of substance abuse

   f. Altered mental health conditions, economic, and/or environmental factors that may impact nutritional requirements

   g. Weight gain or subjective complaints of lack of satiety

6. Older adults in any health care or community setting are at increased risk for altered nutrition due to the physiologic changes of aging, cognitive and functional decline, environmental factors, and social isolation.

B. Guidelines for Healthy Eating (The U.S. Department of Agriculture [USDA] and the U.S. Department of Health)

1. Protein: 0.8–1 g/kg daily

2. Fat: < 30% of total kcal

3. Carbohydrates: 40–55% of daily caloric intake

4. Calcium: 1,000 mg/daily

   a. Postmenopausal women: 1,500 mg/day

5. Potassium: 2,300 mg/day

6. Iron:

   a. Men (19 years and older) 8 mg/day

   b. Women (19 to 50 years old) 18 mg/day

   c. Women (> 51 years old) 8 mg/day

7. Daily fluid requirement in mL = body weight in lb × 15

8. Fiber: 30–38 g/day

9. Sodium: ~2 mg/day (~1 teaspoon)

10. Recommendations differ for pregnant/lactating women, children, and teens.

Foods with Increased Levels of Fat and Water-Soluble Vitamins

Foods Rich in Fat-Soluble Vitamins	
Vitamin A	Liver, egg yolk, whole milk, butter, green and yellow vegetables
Vitamin D	Fish oils, fortified milk and margarine
Vitamin K	Egg yolks, liver, cheese, green leafy vegetables
Foods Rich in Water-Soluble Vitamins	
Vitamin C	Citrus fruits, tomatoes, broccoli, cabbage
Thiamine (B_1)	Lean meats (beef, pork, liver), whole grain cereals, legumes
Riboflavin (B_2)	Milk, organ meats, enriched grains
Niacin	Meat, beans, peas, peanuts, enriched grains
Pyridoxine (B_6)	Products containing yeast, wheat, corn, organ meats
Cobalamin (B_{12})	Lean meats, liver, kidneys
Folic acid	Leafy green vegetables, eggs, liver

C. Therapeutic and Modified Diets

1. Overview

   a. Therapeutic nutrition is often an essential component in the treatment of disease and clinical disorders.

   b. The diet becomes therapeutic when modifications are made to meet client needs. Modifications may include increasing or decreasing caloric intake, fiber, or other specific nutrients; omitting specific foods; and often modifying the consistency of foods.

   c. Nurses often collaborate with or refer clients to the dietician for nutritional or dietary concerns.

2. Clear-Liquid Diet

   a. Indicated for resting the gastrointestinal tract, maintaining fluid balance; immediately postoperative; for diarrhea, nausea, and vomiting; acute illness and reduction of colon fecal material before and after a diagnostic test.

   b. Consists of foods that are clear and liquid at room temperature; water, tea, coffee, fat-free broth, carbonated beverages, clear juices, and gelatin. Limit caffeine consumption, as it can lead to dehydration and increased hydrochloric acid and nausea.

   c. Consists primarily of water and carbohydrates; requires minimal digestion, leaves minimal residue, and is non-gas forming. The diet is nutritionally inadequate and is used on a short-term basis.

3. Full-Liquid Diet

   a. Typically, after surgery, when clear liquids are tolerated well, clients may progress to full liquids; prescribed for febrile illness, acute gastritis, and intolerance of solid foods.

   b. Diet offers more variety and nutritional support than the clear liquid diet and can provide adequate amounts of energy and nutrients. If used for more than 3 days, high protein, high calorie may be indicated.

   c. Consists of foods that are liquid at room temperature: clear liquids; milk and milk products, such as custard, pudding, creamed soups, ice cream, and sherbet; strained fruits and vegetables; vegetable and fruit juices; and refined or strained cereals.

   d. Diet contraindicated for clients who have lactose intolerance or hypercholesterolemia.

4. Pureed Diet

   a. Indicated for clients with chewing or swallowing difficulties, oral or facial surgeries, and wired jaws.

   b. The composition and consistency of the diet varies according to the client's dietary needs.

   c. Can be modified to increase or decrease calories, nutrients such as vitamins and minerals, carbohydrates, fat, and protein.

   d. Consists of food and fluids that have been pureed to a liquid or thick liquid form.

5. Soft Diet (Bland or Low-Fiber)

   a. Indicated for clients transitioning between full liquid and regular diets, acute infections, chewing difficulties, or gastrointestinal disorders such as gastric or duodenal ulcers. Promotes healing of gastric mucosa by eliminating chemically and mechanically irritating food sources.

   b. Contains foods that are low in fiber, lightly seasoned, and easily digested. Foods may be smooth, creamy, or crisp. Fruits, vegetables, coarse breads, cereals, beans, and other gas-forming foods are excluded.

   c. Foods are often introduced in stages with gradual addition of foods; provided in small, frequent feedings to assist in diluting or neutralizing stomach acid; protein foods are effective at neutralizing; fat has some ability to inhibit the secretion of acid and delays stomach emptying.

6. Mechanical Soft Diet

   a. Indicated for clients with limited chewing or swallowing difficulty, dysphagia, poor-fitting dentures, or no teeth; surgery to the head, neck, or mouth; or strictures of the intestinal tract. May also be used during initiation of feeding post CVA and after swallow studies are performed.

   b. Consists of a regular diet that has been modified in texture; altered to meet specific nutritional needs.

   c. Foods require minimal chewing such as ground meats, canned fruits, and softly cooked vegetables.

   d. Dried fruits, most raw fruits and vegetables, and foods containing seeds and nuts are excluded.

7. Low-Protein Diet

   a. Indicated for renal impairment, hepatic coma, and advanced cirrhosis. Protein intake is modified according to disease severity and progression of illness.

   b. Modifies end products of protein metabolism by limiting protein intake.

   c. Limit foods high in protein such as eggs, meat, milk, and milk products.

   d. Additional high-carbohydrate foods to meet energy requirements.

8. High-Protein Diet

   a. Indicated for nutritional and protein deficiencies, tissue building, burns, correction of malabsorption syndromes, and pregnancy.

   b. Encourage high biological value (HBV) protein foods such as fish, fowl, organ and meat sources, soy, and dairy products. Egg whites are considered the gold standard in HBV protein sources.

   c. May include protein supplements.

   d. Ensure clients consume adequate fluid when protein consumption increases. Increased protein can strain renal capillaries, and additional fluid aids in elimination of by-products.

9. Diet for Alteration in Amino-Acid Metabolism

   a. Use for phenylketonuria (PKU), galactosemia, and lactose intolerance.

   b. Diet components reduce or eliminate the offending enzyme.

   c. Avoid milk and milk products for all three diets; include soy-based supplements.

   d. For PKU, milk, eggs, and aspartame (Nutrasweet®) should be avoided.

e. For galactosemia, the simple sugar in lactose must be avoided. Educate families to read labels carefully, as galactosemia can be life threatening.

f. Supplement calcium and vitamin D in those with lactose-restricted or -eliminated diets.

10. Low-Cholesterol Diet

a. Indicated for cardiovascular diseases, diabetes mellitus, and high-serum cholesterol levels.

b. Attempts to modify and decrease cholesterol levels by limiting cholesterol intake.

c. Limit foods high in low-density lipoproteins, saturated fats, and trans-fatty acids such as animal products (egg yolks, organ meats, bacon, fatty meats, and butter).

d. Consists of low-cholesterol foods containing high-density lipoproteins, omega-3 fatty acids, and unsaturated fats. Includes fatty fish such as sardines and salmon; olive and flaxseed oils, shellfish, walnuts, raw or cooked vegetables, fruits, lean meats, and skinless fowl.

11. Modified-Fat Diet

a. Indicated for malabsorption syndromes, malabsorption of fats, cystic fibrosis, gallbladder disease, obstructive jaundice and liver disease, and obesity.

b. Fat content in the diet is decreased.

c. Avoids gravies, fatty meat and fish, cream, fried foods, rich pastries, whole milk products, cream, soups, polyunsaturated salad and cooking oils, nuts, and chocolate.

d. Consists of two to three eggs per week, lean meat, vegetables, fruits, lean meats, fowl, fish, bread, cereal, and limited amounts of butter and margarine.

e. A fat-free diet attempts to dramatically decrease intake of fats by restricting all fatty meats and fat, while consisting of vegetables, fruits, lean meats, fowl, fish, bread, and cereal.

f. Reduce saturated fats and trans-fatty acids by avoiding foods from animal sources, whole milk products, egg yolks, organ meats, bacon, fatty meats, tropical oils, and partially hydrogenated vegetable oils.

12. Potassium-Modified Diets

a. Increase potassium intake for diabetic acidosis.

b. Reduce potassium intake for kidney disease and failure.

c. Foods high in potassium include fruits (and their juices) such as oranges, grapefruits, bananas, apples, and dried apricots and prunes; avocados, dried beans, soy beans, lima beans, kidney beans, squash, baked potatoes, milk, and broiled meats.

d. Foods low in potassium include breads, cereals, sugar, fats; vegetables such as alfalfa, asparagus, cabbage; fruits such as apples, apricots, blackberries, blueberries, cherries, and cranberries.

13. Sodium-Restricted Diets

a. Sodium is restricted in hypertension, heart failure, MI, hepatitis, adrenal cortical diseases, kidney disease, lithium carbonate therapy, cystic fibrosis, and conditions such as cirrhosis of the liver and pre-eclampsia, which cause persistent edema. Sodium restrictions are generally classified according to the amount of sodium allowed per day:

   1) Moderate restriction includes 1 g of sodium daily.
   2) Strict restriction includes 500 mg of sodium daily.
   3) Severe restriction includes 250 mg of sodium daily.
   4) No added salt is a term used for a mild sodium restriction.

b. Limit foods high in sodium, such as potato chips and other salted snack foods; canned soups and vegetables; baked goods that contain baking powder or soda; cereals; seafood; beef; processed meats such as bologna, ham, and bacon; dairy products, especially cheese; pickles; olives; and condiments such as soy sauce, steak sauce, Worcestershire sauce, and salad dressings.

c. Encourage clients to become "label savvy" for sodium.

14. Iron Alterations

a. Increased iron intake is indicated for correction or prevention of iron deficiency anemia, which is most likely to occur in infants, toddlers, adolescents, and pregnant women.

b. Food sources high in iron include fish, meats (particularly organ meats), green leafy vegetables, enriched breads, cereals and macaroni products, whole grain products, dried fruits such as raisins and apricots, and egg yolks.

c. Vitamin C enhances absorption of iron from the gastrointestinal tract.

d. Oral iron supplementation can cause constipation and GI distress, so adequate iron intake through foods is ideal.

15. Calcium Alterations

a. Increased calcium intake is indicated for growing children and adolescents, pregnant and lactating women, and postmenopausal women (to help prevent osteoporosis and osteopenia).

b. Food sources high in calcium include milk and milk products such as yogurt and cheese; dark green vegetables such as collard greens, kale, and broccoli; dried beans and peas; shellfish and canned salmon; and antacids such as Tums, Rolaids, and Titralac.

c. No more than 500–600 mg of calcium can be absorbed at one time, so supplements should be taken 3 times daily; no more than 2,500 mg should be taken per day.

d. Vitamin D is required for absorption of calcium from the gastrointestinal tract.

SECTION 16

"Need to Know" Laboratory Values*

A. Serum Electrolytes

1. Sodium (Na^+): 135–145 mEq/L
2. Potassium (K^+): 3.5–5 mEq/L
3. Calcium (Ca^{++}): 8.5–10 mg/dL 4
4. Magnesium (Mg^{++}): 1.8–3 mg/dL
5. Phosphorus (PO_4): 2.5–4.5 mg/dL
6. Glucose (fasting): 70–110 mg/dL

B. Arterial Blood Gases (ABGs)

1. pH: 7.35–7.45; over 90 years: 7.25–7.45
2. $PaCO_2$: 35–45 mm Hg (arterial)
3. PaO_2: > 80–100 mm Hg (arterial)
4. HCO_3 (bicarbonate): 22–26 mEq/L
5. Cl^- (chloride): 85–115 mEq/L

C. CBC

1. RBCs males: 4.7–6.1 mm³
2. RBCs females: 4.2–5.4 mm³
3. Hgb males: 14–18 g/dL; females: 12–16 g/dL
4. Hct males: 42–52%; females 37–47%
5. WBCs: 4,800–10,800 mm³
6. Erythrocyte sedimentation rate: < 20 mm/hr

D. Blood Lipid Levels

1. Total serum cholesterol: desirable less than 200 mg/dL; risk for cardiac or stroke event with levels greater than 150 mg/dL is the target range for therapy and has been shown to be the cut point to decrease CV or arterial incidences.
2. LDL (low-density lipids): desirable less than 100 mg/dL
3. HDL (high-density lipids): desirable greater than 40 mg/dL for men, 50 mg/dL for women
4. Triglycerides: desirable less than 150 mg/dL (< 100 mg/dL if on medication)

E. Anticoagulant Therapy Coagulation Times

1. Therapeutic INR: 2.0–3.0
2. PT: 11–14 seconds. Therapeutic range for anticoagulant therapy is 1.5–2 × the normal or control value.
3. Partial thromboplastin time: 16–40 range; remain < 40 seconds. Therapeutic range for anticoagulant therapy is 1.5–2.5 × the normal or control value.

4. INR
   a. Normal INR is 0.9–1.2.
   b. The INR is a corrected ratio of a client's protime to normal.
   c. Universal test is not affected by variations in laboratory norms.
   d. If the client requires anticoagulation, the desired value is increased to approximately 2 to 3.
5. Platelets: 150,000–450,000 cu/mm

F. Liver Function Tests

1. Albumin: 3.8–5 g/dL
2. Ammonia: 35–65 mcg/dL
3. Total bilirubin: 0.0–1.5 mg/dL
4. Total protein = 6–8 gm/dL

G. Urinalysis

1. Specific gravity = 1.010–1.030
2. pH = average 6.0; range 4.6–8.0
3. Glucose = negative
4. RBCs = negative
5. WBCs = negative
6. Albumin = negative
7. Bacteria: < 1000 colonies/mL

H. Renal Function

1. Serum creatinine: males 0.6–1.2 mg/dL; women 0.5–1.1 mg/dL
2. BUN: 10–20 mg/dL
3. Glomerular filtration rate (GFR): 90–120 mL/min

I. Therapeutic Medication Monitoring

1. Digoxin level: 0.8–2 ng/mL
2. Lithium level: 0.4–1.0 mEq/L
3. Magnesium sulfate: Levels are obtained 1 hour after the loading dose and then every 6 hours, and the maintenance dosage should be titrated to maintain a serum level of 4–8 mg/dL.
4. Phenobarbital: 10–30 mcg/mL
5. Theophylline: 10–20 mcg/mL

J. Blood Glucose Levels

1. Glucose (fasting) = 70 – 110 mg/dL
2. Glycosylated hemoglobin: (HbA1c) 5% (up to 7% in clients who have diabetes mellitus)

---

* *Note:* "Need to know" values are those listed in the 2010 Detailed Test Plan for the NCLEX-RN® examination under the heading of "Physiological Adaptation: Reduction of Risk Potential, Laboratory Values."

UNIT THREE ❖ ADULT MEDICAL-SURGICAL NURSING

UNIT FOUR

Mental Health Nursing

Mental Health: A personal state of being in which an individual has a positive self-perception, is able to cope adaptively with stressors, and is able to consistently develop toward autonomy and self-actualization. Mental health nurses use a holistic approach when applying the nursing process to clients in mental health settings.

A. Mental Health Nursing

1. Interpersonal process
   a. Communication
   b. Caring
2. Expected Client outcomes
   a. Coping with emotional responses to stress and crisis
   b. Satisfying basic needs
   c. Learning more effective ways of behaving
   d. Developing a healthy lifestyle
   e. Achieving a realistic and positive self-concept
3. Responsibilities of the nurse
   a. Developing a therapeutic relationship
   b. Creating and maintaining a therapeutic environment
4. Nursing process
   a. Assessment
   b. Diagnosis
   c. Planning
   d. Implementation
   e. Evaluation
5. Roles of the nurse
   a. Counselor
   b. Teacher
   c. Advocate
   d. Leader, coordinator, manager

B. Assessment

1. Psychosocial history
   a. Perception of own health needs
   b. Stress level and perceived coping abilities
   c. Cultural beliefs and practices
   d. Spiritual beliefs
   e. Use/history of substance abuse
   f. Activity/leisure time
   g. Mental Status Examination (MSE)
2. Physical
   a. Level of consciousness/Glasgow Coma Scale
   b. Physical appearance and general health status

3. Behavior
   a. Voluntary/involuntary body movements
   b. Eye contact, mood, and affect
4. Cognitive ability
   a. Orientation × 4
   b. Short- and long-term memory
   c. Level of knowledge/perception of illness

C. Theoretical Models of Treatment

1. Medical-biologic model
   a. Oriented to diagnosing mental disturbances as medical diseases with specific classifiable manifestations
      1) Contributing Factors
         a) Biochemical
         b) Psychological conditions
         c) Psychophysiological conditions
         d) Structural problems
      2) Diagnosis
         a) History
         b) Physical
         c) *Diagnostic and Statistical Manual of Mental Disorders* (*DSM-IV*)
      3) Focus
         a) Accurate diagnosis
         b) Selection of treatment modalities
         c) Nurse's role is supportive
   b. Treatment
      1) Physical or somatic
      2) Interpersonal
   c. Psychoanalytical model (Sigmund Freud)
   d. Oriented to uncovering childhood trauma and repressed feelings that cause conflicts in later life
      1) Psychopathology
         a) Alterations in psychosocial behavior
         b) Stress-related behaviors
      2) Structure of the mind
         a) Id: contains instinctual primitive drives
         b) Ego: mediates demands of primitive id and self-critical superego
         c) Superego: values and mores that guide behavior
         d) Conscious: ability to recall or remember events without difficulty
         e) Unconscious: memories and thoughts that do not enter awareness
      3) Freud's psychosexual stages
         a) Oral: 0–1 year
         b) Anal: 1–3 years
         c) Phallic (oedipal): 3–6 years
         d) Latency: 6–12 years
         e) Genital: 12 years to young adult

e. Treatment modalities: oriented to clarifying the meaning of unconscious and conscious events, feelings, and behavior to gain insight
  1) Transference (unconscious projection of feelings onto others)
  2) Countertransference
  3) Free association
  4) Dream analysis
  5) Catharsis (talking it out)

 f. **NURSING INTERVENTIONS**
  1) Establish guidelines for understanding human behavior.
  2) Determine adaptive/maladaptive personality traits.
  3) Individualize teaching based on psychosexual development.

2. Psychosocial developmental model (Erik Erikson): oriented to psychosocial tasks that are accomplished throughout the life cycle; an individual who experiences failure in any stage is likely to have greater difficulty achieving success in future stages of development.

  a. Uses an interdisciplinary approach to treatment; wellness is on a continuum

  b. Developmental stages (see following table)

 c. **NURSING INTERVENTIONS**
  1) Identify client's present stage of psychosocial development.
  2) Assist client to complete that stage.
  3) Set goals toward advancing through next stage(s).

3. Basic human needs model (Maslow): a hierarchy of needs; a belief that needs are fulfilled in a progressive order

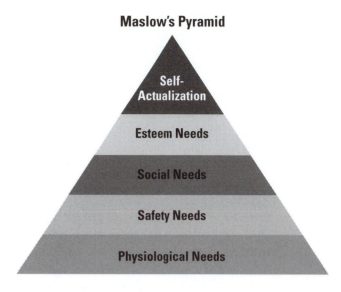

Maslow's Pyramid

a. Levels
  1) Physiological
    a) Oxygen
    b) Food
    c) Sleep
    d) Sexual expression
  2) Safety
    a) Avoiding harm
    b) Feeling secure

Erikson's Stages of Development

Stage	Task	Behavior	Definition
Newborn/infant (birth to 1 year)	Trust vs. mistrust	Hopefulness, trusting vs. withdrawn, alienated	Newborns/infants learn to trust one consistent parent (not necessarily the mother).
Toddler (1 to 3 years)	Autonomy vs. shame, doubt	Self-control vs. compliance and compulsiveness, uncertainty	Toddlers learn independence and self-control; learn how to affect the environment with direct manipulation.
Preschooler (3 to 6 years)	Initiative vs. guilt	Realistic goals—explores, tests reality vs. strict limits on self-worry	Preschoolers engage in personal exploration and set goals that influence the environment. Begins to initiate, not imitate, activities; develops conscience and sexual identity.
School-age child (6 to 12 years)	Industry vs. inferiority	Explores, persistent, competes vs. incompetent, low self-esteem	School-age children develop a sense of self and competency; they learn to create and interact.
Adolescent (12 to 20 years)	Identity vs. role confusion	Sense of self vs. confusion, indecision	Adolescents integrate life experiences that allow them to seek a sense of self (try new roles to see what fits); peer pressure creates tumultuous rebellions. Adolescents also examine their own sexual identity.
Young adult (20 to 35 years)	Intimacy vs. isolation	Commitment in love/work/play vs. superficial, impersonal	Young adults develop intimate or committed relationships, between work and family life; seek balance in life.
Middle adult (35 to 65 years)	Generativity vs. stagnation	Productivity, caring about others vs. self-centered and indulgent	Middle adults establish and guide the next generation by giving back to society in terms of volunteering and being productive through reminiscing.
Older adult (over 65 years)	Integrity vs. despair	Sense of accomplishment vs. hopelessness, depression	Older adults undergo a review of life (necessary); they learn to accept one's life as purposeful, worthwhile, and/or successful; want to provide a legacy.

3) Love and belonging
   a) Group identity
   b) Being cared about
   c) Caring for others
   d) Play
4) Self-esteem
   a) Self-confidence
   b) Self-acceptance
5) Self-actualization
   a) Self-knowledge
   b) Satisfying, interpersonal relationships
   c) Environmental mastery
   d) Stress management

b. Treatment
1) Interdisciplinary: shared roles
2) Developmental: interpersonal view of the self
3) Goal: needs fulfilled in progressive manner

c. **NURSING INTERVENTIONS**
1) Utilize Maslow stages as assessment guidelines.
2) Identify the client's current stage of psychosocial development.
3) Prioritize client care based on Maslow's hierarchy of needs.
4) Assist the client to successfully progress through the current stage.
5) Set goals to advance to the next stage.

4. Behaviorist model (behavior modification): "Maladaptive behavior is learned."

a. Changes behavior by using learning theory: replaces nonadaptive behavior with more adaptive behavior

b. Treatment
1) Reconditioning: unlearning learned or maladaptive behavior
2) Reinforcement: increases the probability of positive behavior recurring
   a) Positive reinforcement: per contract, use rewards to increase or reinforce desired behavior (e.g., adding something such as food, attention, phone privileges)
   b) Negative reinforcement: per contract, extinguish undesirable behavior by removing aversive consequences (e.g., removal of imposed restrictions)
3) Positive punishment: decrease behavior by adding aversive consequences (e.g., quiet time)
4) Negative punishment: decrease behavior by withdrawing a reward (e.g., privilege, such as an outing or calls)

c. Main uses
1) Children
2) Clients who are severely regressed
3) Personality disorders
4) Anxiety disorders such as phobias
5) Eating disorders
6) Clients who are mentally disabled

d. **NURSING INTERVENTIONS**
1) Assess behavior.
2) Implement specific behavioral interventions, either negative or positive reinforcement (contracts, role-play, progressive relaxation).
3) Place emphasis on positive reinforcement as a primary nursing intervention.
4) Evaluate progress and change behavioral interventions according to client's needs.

5. Community mental health model (psychosocial rehabilitation): individual interacting with environment

a. Uses interdisciplinary team approach; nurse works as case manager and supervises the team

b. Emphasis on providing treatment services in the least restrictive setting

c. Treatment modalities
1) Primary prevention: maintenance and promotion of health by teaching (e.g., risk factors, medication management, health promotion and wellness)
2) Secondary prevention: early diagnosis and treatment (e.g., crisis intervention, partial hospitalization, acute care hospitalization)
3) Tertiary prevention: rehabilitation, follow-up to avoid permanent disability (e.g., psychiatric day care)

d. **NURSING INTERVENTIONS**
1) Provide holistic care.
2) Practice therapeutic use of self in the nurse/client relationship.
3) Use primary, secondary, and tertiary prevention.
4) Identify client needs, strengths, and community resources.

D. Treatment Modes

1. Group therapy

a. Definition: group of individuals interacting together with a shared purpose

b. Dynamics and concepts
1) Content: work done to problem solve and fulfill the group functions and goals
2) Process: what is happening in the group; interactions, seating, participation
3) Cohesiveness: feeling of belonging, helpfulness, problem solving, sharing
4) Norms: standards of behavior adhered to by group

c. **NURSING INTERVENTIONS**
1) Assume leadership role.
2) Promote problem solving.
3) Direct group toward common goals and tasks.
4) Set limits and prevent scapegoating within group.
5) Clarify issues and promote consistency.
6) Support group members.

d. Types of groups
  1) Supportive, therapeutic
  2) Task groups
  3) Teaching groups
  4) Psychotherapy
  5) Peer support
  6) Self-help groups
    a) 12-step (Alcoholics Anonymous [AA], Al-anon, Alateen, Overeaters Anonymous, Gamblers Anonymous)
    b) Recovery, Inc.
    c) Ostomy Clubs

2. Family therapy

  a. Definition: psychotherapy in which the focus is on the family as the unit of treatment, not just one individual

  b. Concepts
    1) Systems approach: member with the manifestations, illness
    2) Scapegoating: the object of blame or displaced aggression, usually one member of the family
    3) Family involvement necessary for treatment

   c. **NURSING INTERVENTIONS**
    1) Help family reestablish communication between members.
    2) Help family redefine roles and rules.
    3) Clarify ambiguous communication patterns between family members.
    4) Support individual family members.
    5) Teach family problem-solving techniques.
    6) Help the family accept differences among the members.

3. Milieu therapy

  a. Definition: management of the client's environment to promote a positive living experience and facilitate recovery (holistic approach)

  b. Concepts
    1) Client government: groups and meetings between client and staff to promote shared responsibility and cooperation
    2) Environment in the facility as close to the "real world" as possible and has potential for therapeutic value

  c. **NURSING INTERVENTIONS**
    1) Provide for client safety and protection.
    2) Provide guidance in developing new ways of helping the client relate and learn to cope more effectively.
    3) Help client maintain strengths.
    4) Manage the client's day-to-day activities.
    5) Provide a positive, therapeutic environment through environmental manipulation.
    6) Assist in developing effective relationship and coping skills.

4. Adjunctive therapies

  a. Definition: therapies used to aid assessment, increase social skills, encourage expression of feelings, and provide opportunities to raise self-esteem, relieve tension, and be creative

  b. Types
    1) Dance: movement
    2) Recreational: picnic, volleyball
    3) Occupational: painting, hand work
    4) Art: clay, painting, drawing
    5) Alternative therapies: pet therapy, reminiscence therapy, music therapy

5. Interdisciplinary team approach

  a. Definition: a team with members of different disciplines involved in a formal arrangement to provide client services while maximizing educational interchange

  b. Members of the team
    1) Nurse
    2) Primary care provider
    3) Social worker
    4) Psychologist
    5) Case manager
    6) Occupational therapist
    7) Recreational therapist
    8) Job coaches
    9) Mental health technicians.

E. **Nurse/Client Relationship:** An interpersonal and collaborative process characterized by a sequence of events leading to a mutually identified goal

  1. Phases

    a. Pre-interaction phase
      1) Review available data including medical and nursing history.
      2) Anticipate health concerns or issues.
      3) Identify location to promote privacy and comfort; plan adequate time for initial interaction.

    b. Orientation phase
      1) Establish confidentiality, trust, honesty, and empathy with the client.
      2) Clarify client's and nurse's roles.
      3) Assess the client's physical and emotional status.
      4) Prioritize client problems and client goals.
      5) Formulate contracts when appropriate.
      6) Begin discussions related to termination of the relationship.

    c. Working phase
      1) Explore thoughts and feelings related to client's health status.
      2) Take action to meet goals set with the client.
      3) Use therapeutic communication to facilitate interactions.

d. Termination phase
      1) This phase is initially addressed on admission or first contact with the client.
      2) Evaluate goal achievement with the client.
      3) Transfer care to other support systems.
      4) Separate from the client by relinquishing responsibility.
      5) Facilitate a smooth transition for the client to other caregivers as needed.

F. **Therapeutic Nurse–Client Communication:** Therapeutic communication between the nurse and client promotes the attainment of health-related goals. The nurse establishes and directs therapeutic interactions knowing that the client's needs take priority over the nurse's needs.

   1. Communication tools: Method of using conversation to enhance a client's verbalization of thoughts and feelings in a nonjudgmental environment.
      a. Listening: Use nonverbal cues and eye contact, and face the client with proactive body language.
      b. Offering self: "I will stay with you."
      c. Broad openings: "Tell me what you would like to talk about."
      d. Clarifying: "What does that mean to you?"
      e. Reflecting: Verbalize ideas back to the client, or feelings conveyed such as, "You say you feel tense when you fight?"
      f. Showing empathy: State a feeling implied by the client.
      g. Summarizing: "Today we have discussed..."
      h. Silence: Convey interest through the use of body language.
      i. Making observations: "You seem angry."
      j. Restating main idea: "You are sad?"
      k. Validating: "I hear you saying that..."

   2. Communication blocks: Statements or questions that can be answered with "yes" or "no," or verbal interactions that prevent the client from freely verbalizing his own feelings or thoughts
      a. False reassurance: "Don't worry."
      b. Agreeing and disagreeing: "I think you did the right thing."
      c. Advising: "You should..."
      d. Judging: "That was good."
      e. Belittling: "Everyone feels like that."
      f. Defending: "All of our doctors are great."
      g. Approving: Classify an action as good or bad.
      h. Focusing on the nurse: "I feel that way, too."
      i. Changing the subject or ignoring the client.

    3. **NURSING INTERVENTIONS**
      a. Avoid communication blocks and negative nonverbal communication.
      b. Use open-ended statements or questions.

   c. Avoid asking "why" questions.
   d. Limit client questions to one idea at a time.
   e. Mention nonverbal cues observed: "I notice your hands are shaking."
   f. Do not invade the client's space (3 to 6 ft).
   g. Use touch cautiously because it can often be misinterpreted as a threat.

SECTION 2
Anxiety and Defense Mechanisms

A. **Defense Mechanisms**
   1. Overview
      a. Individuals normally use different defense mechanisms throughout life. An ego defense mechanism becomes pathological only when its persistent use leads to maladaptive behavior and the physical and/or mental health of the individual is adversely affected.
      b. Adaptive use of defense mechanisms can protect the mind/self/ego from anxiety or provide a refuge from a situation with which one cannot currently cope.
      c. Maladaptive dysfunctional behavior may occur when defense mechanisms are used as a response to anxiety, which interferes with functioning, relationships, and orientation to reality
   2. Unconscious mechanisms
      a. Denial: The avoidance of an unpleasant reality by ignoring or refusing recognition ("I can quit drinking any time I want.").
      b. Rationalization: Offering a socially acceptable explanation for unacceptable impulses ("I failed the exam because it was a bad test.").
      c. Displacement: Transferring feelings to a neutral object (had a bad day at work, so go home and yell at family).
      d. Projection: Blaming one's own thoughts or actions on another person ("You made me angry; you made me hit you.").
      e. Compensation: Putting more effort toward achievements in areas of real or imagined deficiency (a student who fails a class later becomes the valedictorian).
      f. Reaction formation: Displaying behaviors or attitudes directly opposite of unacceptable conscious or unconscious thoughts (being friendly with an individual you dislike).
      g. Identification: Subconsciously adopting the characteristics of an individual who is admired (Elvis impersonator).
      h. Sublimation: Directing unacceptable behaviors into a socially acceptable area (individual with violent thoughts writes a murder mystery novel).

i. Regression: Going back to an earlier developmental level (becoming dependent on another for all decisions).

j. Undoing: Compulsive, unconscious act meant to reverse previous unacceptable impulses (mother spanks child, then begins to bake cookies).

k. Introjection: Incorporating the emotions of another (a nurse becomes depressed while caring for a client who is depressed).

l. Isolation: A splitting-off response in which the psyche blocks unpleasant feelings (an individual is inappropriately calm when told of the death of a loved one).

m. Repression: Involuntary forgetting of painful memories, feelings, or actions (denying occurrence of child abuse).

n. Splitting: A viewpoint of absolutes in which individuals are all bad or all good.

3. Conscious defense mechanism

a. Suppression: Deliberately forgetting or delaying painful acts or thoughts (an individual repeatedly cancels dentist appointments).

B. Anxiety

1. Definition: a stress-based sense of apprehension in response to a perceived physiological or psychological threat, resulting in feelings of fear and helplessness

2. Levels of anxiety

3. Manifestations

a. Psychological
   1) Sense of fear and helplessness
   2) Poor self-confidence and insecurity
   3) Anger or guilt

b. Physiological
   1) Elevated blood pressure, heart and respiratory rates
   2) Palpitations, diaphoresis
   3) Dry mouth, sweaty palms
   4) Hyperventilation, diarrhea
   5) Fidgeting, giggling, talkative
   6) Maladaptive physiological manifestations

c. Panic attacks: sudden onset of intense apprehension, fear, or terror that is out of proportion to occurring external events (may last from minutes to hours)

d. Dyspnea and faintness

e. Chest pain with palpitations

f. Hyperventilation and choking.

g. Fear of dying or going crazy

! **POINT TO REMEMBER:** The initial nursing priority is to reduce the client's anxiety to levels that are tolerable. Progress cannot be made until the anxiety is manageable.

Levels of Anxiety

Level	Physiological Responses	Cognitive State and Behavioral Changes	Nursing Interventions
Mild	Slight discomfort, GI "butterflies," restlessness, tension relief, fidgeting, tapping	Perceptual field can be heightened; learning can occur	• Listen to the client. • Promote insight and problem solving. • Discuss alternatives with the client.
Moderate	Increased pulse, respirations, shakiness, voice tremors, difficulty concentrating, pacing	Perceptual field narrows; client is selective in attention, focusing on immediate events; benefits from the guidance of others	• Remain calm and rational in discussion. • Encourage the client to engage in relaxation exercises.
Severe	Elevated blood pressure, tachycardia, reports somatic symptoms, hyperventilation, confusion	Perceptual field greatly reduced; attention scattered and unable to focus; feelings of increasing threat; purposeless activity; feelings of impending doom	• Listen to the client. • Encourage the client to express his feelings. • Establish concrete activity with the client. • Reduce the client's stimuli with simple tasks.
Panic Level	Immobility or severe hyperactivity, cool, clammy skin, pallor, dilated pupils, chest pain and palpitations	Prolonged anxiety can lead to exhaustion; perceptual field diminished; hallucinations or delusions may occur; effective decision making is impossible; mute or psychomotor agitation; may strike out physically or withdraw; loss of control	• Isolate the client from stimuli. • Stay with the client. • Remain very calm. • Protect the client's safety. • Do not touch the client.

C. Crisis Intervention

1. Definitions

   a. Crisis: overwhelming feelings of helplessness when coping mechanisms are inadequate in response to an event

   b. Crisis intervention: response to a crisis in which the nurse focuses on safety, support, and the strengths of the client (crises are self-limiting—4 to 8 weeks)

2. Types of crisis

   a. Situational: unanticipated (e.g., death, divorce, termination from job)

   b. Transitional: maturational, anticipated (e.g., birth, marriage)

   c. Cultural/social (e.g., disaster, war)

3. Responses to crisis

   a. Physiological (nervous system)

   b. Psychological (panic, fear, helplessness)

   c. Behavioral (extremes, talkative to withdrawn)

4. Principles of crisis management

   a. Requires prompt intervention in calm, controlled atmosphere

   b. Focus on client strengthens positive coping skills

   c. Time limited (4 to 8 weeks)

5. **NURSING INTERVENTIONS**

   a. Provide therapeutic interventions to keep client focused on immediate problem.

   b. Set specific goals for resolution.

   c. Help client develop more adaptive coping behaviors, sense of mastery.

   d. Use simple, concrete sentences with step-by-step direction to promote effective communication.

D. Anxiety Disorders

1. Generalized anxiety disorder (GAD): A pattern of frequent, constant worry and tension over many different activities and events; occurs for more than 6 months

   a. Contributing Factors

      1) Often begins at an early age; chronic; symptoms may develop more slowly than other anxiety disorders, substance abuse, and mood disorders; commonly occurs with major depression

   b. Manifestations

      1) Constant worrying or obsession about small or large concerns

      2) Restlessness and feeling keyed up or on edge

      3) Fatigue

      4) Difficulty concentrating or your mind "going blank"

      5) Irritability

      6) Muscle tension or muscle aches

      7) Trembling, feeling twitchy, or being easily startled

      8) Trouble sleeping

      9) Sweating, nausea, or diarrhea

      10) Shortness of breath or rapid heartbeat

   c. Diagnostic Testing

      1) Hamilton Rating Scale for Anxiety

      2) Modified Spielberger State Anxiety Scale

   d. Collaborative Care

      1) **NURSING INTERVENTIONS**

         a) Assess for safety concerns and promote client safety.

         b) Encourage the client to discuss concerns.

         c) Assist the client to identify the source of the anxiety.

         d) Help the client to identify personal strengths.

         e) Teach the client how to develop positive coping skills.

      2) Medications

         a) Antidepressants: sertraline (Zoloft), fluoxetine (Prozac), paroxetine (Paxil), escitalopram (Lexapro), sertaline (Zoloft), venlafaxine (Effexor), and imipramine (Tofranil)

         b) Anti-anxiety medication: buspiron (BuSpar); may be used on an ongoing basis

         c) Benzodiazepines; clonazepam (Klonopin), lorazepam (Ativan), diazepam (Valium), chlordiazepoxide (Librium), and alprazolam (Xanax); generally used for managing acute anxiety on a short-term basis

      3) Therapeutic Measures

         a) Cognitive behavioral therapy: Type of psychotherapy for generalized anxiety disorder. Generally a short-term treatment that focuses on teaching the client specific skills to identify negative thoughts and behaviors and replace them with positive ones.

      4) Client Education

         a) Teach signs and symptoms of anxiety.

         b) Notify provider of worsening symptoms; do not stop or change medications.

         c) Methods of alternative stress relief and effective coping mechanisms.

2. Phobic disorders: Irrational fear of a specific object, activity, or situation that leads to avoidance (e.g., fear of flying).

   a. Contributing Factors

      1) There is no one specific known cause for phobias, and it is thought that phobias run in families, are influenced by culture and how one is parented, and can be triggered by life events and conditioning.

   b. Types (manifestations depend on the type of phobia)

      1) Agoraphobia: fear of being places outside of the home

      2) Arachnophobia: fear of spiders

3) Social phobia (most common): also referred to as social anxiety disorder, which is an irrational fear of embarrassment or ridicule in any social setting or event

c. Manifestations (common with all types)
1) Feeling of uncontrollable anxiety when exposed to the source or fear
2) Attempts made to avoid source and, when exposed, an inability to function normally
3) Awareness that fear is unreasonable or exaggerated but client is powerless to control it
4) Physical symptoms such as diaphoresis, rapid heart rate, difficulty breathing, and feeling of intense panic and anxiety

d. Collaborative Care
1) **NURSING INTERVENTIONS**
   a) Use gradual desensitization experiences.
   b) Employ behavior modification techniques.
   c) Teach relaxation techniques and biofeedback.
   d) Avoid decision making or competitions.
   e) Discuss use of positive coping strategies.
2) Medications
   a) Antidepressants (SSRIs)
   b) Beta blockers: propranolol (Inderal); decreases the physical symptoms associated with panic by blocking the effects that adrenaline has on the body
   c) Benzodiazepines
3) Therapeutic Measures
   a) Cognitive therapy
   b) Behavior modification

3. Obsessive-compulsive disorder: Obsession is a persistent recurring fixed idea or thought that cannot be voluntarily removed from consciousness, and compulsion is an irresistible impulse to perform an action, regardless of its logic (may occur together or separately).

a. Contributing Factors
1) Psychological and biological factors play a role in causing the disorder.

b. Manifestations
1) Repeated, persistent, and unwanted ideas, thoughts, images, or impulses.
2) Impulses are involuntarily and seem to make no sense.
3) Obsessions typically intrude when client is attempting to think of or do other things.
4) Feelings of inferiority, low self-esteem.
5) Irrational coping to handle guilt.

c. Collaborative Care
1) **NURSING INTERVENTIONS**
   a) Do not interrupt the client's compulsive act.
   b) Schedule time for the client to complete his ritual (client may perform ritual slowly).
   c) Decrease the time and frequency of the client's rituals.

d) Distract and substitute self-esteem–building activities.
e) Provide safety, structure, and activities.
f) Demonstrate acceptance of the client's feelings.
2) Medications
   a) Antidepressants including clomipramine (Anafranil), fluvoxamine (Luvox), fluoxetine (Prozac), paroxetine (Paxil, Pexeva), sertraline (Zoloft)
3) Therapeutic Measures
   a) Cognitive behavioral therapy
   b) Psychotherapy
4) Client Education
   a) Teach relaxation techniques.
   b) Teach importance of maintaining medication regimen at home.
   c) Identify triggers that enhance symptoms and develop a plan when symptoms return.
   d) Avoid drug and alcohol use.

4. Posttraumatic stress disorder (PTSD): A severe anxiety disorder that occurs following exposure to a major traumatic event, which results in repeated flashbacks, nightmares, or emotionally crippling fear responses. PTSD changes the body's response to stress. It affects the stress hormones and chemicals that carry neurotransmitters.

a. Contributing Factors
1) Cause of PTSD is unknown.
2) Psychological, genetic, physical, and social factors are involved.
3) History or recent trauma may increase risk: assault, domestic abuse, prison stay, rape, terrorism, and war.

b. Manifestations
1) Flashback episodes, where the event seems to be happening again and again
2) Repeated upsetting memories of the event; repeated nightmares of the event
3) Emotional "numbing"; feeling detached; inability to remember important aspects of the trauma
4) Having a lack of interest in normal activities
5) Avoiding places, people, or thoughts that remind you of the event
6) Difficulty concentrating
7) Agitation or excitability; insomnia

c. Collaborative Care
1) **NURSING INTERVENTIONS**
   a) Teach stress reduction techniques to the client.
   b) Identify community support systems for the client.
   c) Encourage the client to attend a support group.

2) Medications
   a) Antidepressants such as sertraline (Zoloft) and paroxetine (Paxil)
   b) Anti-anxiety medications
   c) If manifestations include nightmares or insomnia, prazosin (Minipress) has been prescribed. Normally used to treat hypertension, prazosin blocks the brain's response to norepinephrine and has been effective in suppressing nightmares.
3) Therapeutic Measures
   a) Cognitive therapy
   b) Exposure therapy.

5. Somatoform disorders: A group of disorders characterized by reports of physical symptoms, with no organic pathology (e.g., a soldier paralyzed during a war, but who has no physical injury) (See Conversion disorders below.)

6. Conversion disorders (hysteria): Alteration in physical function that is an expression of an unconscious psychological need

   a. Contributing Factors
      1) Freud suggested that the emotional charge of painful experiences are consciously repressed as a way of managing the pain; the emotional charge is then "converted" into the neurological symptoms. Both somatoform and conversion disorders are used to suppress emotional pain and anxiety.

   b. Manifestations
      1) Sensory: blindness, deafness, and/or loss of sensation in extremities
      2) Motor: mutism, ataxia, paralysis
      3) Visceral: migraines, dyspnea
      4) "La belle indifférence": a condition in which the person is unconcerned with symptoms caused by a conversion disorder. A naive, inappropriate lack of emotion or concern for the perceptions by others of one's disability, usually seen in persons with conversion disorder

   c. Collaborative Care
      1) **NURSING INTERVENTIONS**
         a) Redirect the client away from manifestations.
         b) Encourage the client to express his feelings.
         c) Teach the client relaxation and stress-reduction techniques.
         d) Schedule daily activities for the client to decrease the time focused on symptoms.
      2) Medications (no FDA-approved medications at this time to treat this disorder)
         a) Antidepressant medications: can be effective with depression, anger, impulsivity, irritability, or hopelessness, which may be associated with personality disorders

      b) Mood-stabilizing medications: can be effective to even out mood swings or reduce irritability, impulsivity, and aggression
      c) Anti-anxiety medications: may be effective to control anxiety, agitation, or insomnia. Can, in some cases, increase impulsive behavior
      d) Antipsychotic medications: may be effective if symptoms include losing touch with reality (psychosis), anxiety, or anger problems
   3) Therapeutic Measures
      a) Psychotherapy
      b) Physical therapy
      c) Hypnosis
   4) Client Education
      a) Instruct client that stress-relieving activities such as meditation and yoga may help reduce reactions to the events that prompt symptoms of conversion disorder.

7. Hypochondriasis: Exaggerated preoccupation with physical health; no organic pathology

   a. Contributing Factors
      1) Suggested that personality, life experiences, upbringing, and inherited traits may all play a role.
      2) Similarities exist between hypochondria and anxiety disorders such as panic disorder and obsessive-compulsive disorder.

   b. Manifestations
      1) Varies with the individual and changes frequently
      2) Client ponders manifestations
      3) Constantly seeks medical care from multiple health care providers

   c. Collaborative Care
      1) **NURSING INTERVENTIONS**
         a) Set limits on pondering.
         b) Do not support the client's manifestations.
         c) Help the client express his feelings.
      2) Medications
         a) SSRIs including fluoxetine (Prozac), fluvoxamine (Luvox), and paroxetine (Paxil)
         b) Tricyclic antidepressants such as clomipramine (Anafranil) and imipramine (Tofranil)
      3) Therapeutic Measures
         a) Cognitive behavioral therapy

SECTION 3
Schizophrenia

A. Definition: A chronic mental disorder characterized by regression, thought disturbances, and bizarre dress that may be accompanied by delusions, hallucinations, and/or abnormal motor behaviors; requires lifelong treatment

B. Contributing Factors
1. Cause is unknown, but researchers believe that a combination of genetics and environment contributes to development of the disease.
2. Having a family history of schizophrenia, fetal exposure to viruses, toxins or malnutrition, stressful life circumstances, older paternal age, and taking psychoactive drugs during adolescence and young adulthood are thought to be risk factors.

C. Types
1. Disorganized: incoherent, severe thought disturbance with inappropriate behaviors
2. Catatonic (psychomotor): stupor, excitement, waxy flexibility or bizarre posturing, negativism, and mutism
3. Paranoid: hallucinations, delusions, anger, suspiciousness, mistrust
4. Undifferentiated: mixed characteristics; meets criteria of more than one type

D. Manifestations
1. Delusions: fixed false beliefs of grandeur
2. Hallucinations: visual or auditory
3. Perceptions without environmental stimuli
4. Illusions: misinterpretation of actual stimuli, such as believing an extension cord is a snake
5. Ideas of reference: only personalizing environmental stimuli to self
6. Neologisms: self-coined words
7. Circumstantiality: cannot come to a point
8. Blocking: sudden interruption of speech due to distraction of thoughts
9. Echolalia: the repetition of words or phrases heard from another individual
10. Echopraxia: imitation of movement or gestures of another individual
11. Pressured speech: speaking rapidly

E. Collaborative Care
1. **NURSING INTERVENTIONS**
   a. Provide physical care and promote safety.
   b. Increase client trust while developing a one-on-one nurse/client relationship.
   c. Orient client to reality.
   d. Provide structure; keep interactions simple and concrete; often nonverbal and short.
   e. Help client cope with regressive or bizarre behavior, anxiety, and irritation.
   f. Intervene with hallucinations:
      1) Promote therapeutic communication and establish a trusting relationship with the client.
      2) Provide for client safety.
      3) Do not confront; do not deny.
      4) Point out that others do not share the same perception, but acknowledge that the hallucination is real to the client.
      5) Encourage to verbalize auditory hallucinations.
      6) Engage client in activities and encourage participation in group work (e.g., current events discussion groups).
      7) Provide least restrictive environment and avoid restraining.
      8) Provide consistency, positive reinforcement, and acceptance.
2. Medications
   a. Atypical antipsychotics: aripiprazole (Abilify), clozapine (Clozaril), olanzapine (Zyprexa), paliperidone (Invega), quetiapine (Seroquel), risperidone (Risperdal), ziprasidone (Geodon)
   b. Typical antipsychotics include chlorpromazine (Thorazine), haloperidol (Haldol)
3. Therapeutic Measures
   a. Psychosocial therapy
4. Client Education and Referral
   a. Importance of group work and psychotherapy
   b. Importance of self-care activities
   c. Compliance with medication regimen
   d. Avoidance of alcohol and drugs
   e. Case management to provide follow-up for the client and family.

SECTION 4
Pervasive Developmental Disorders

A. Autism: A severe developmental disorder of varying degrees. Children with autism generally have problems in three crucial areas of development—social interaction, language, and behavior.
1. Contributing Factors
   a. Has no single cause; thought to be caused from both genetic and environmental factors

2. Manifestations (social, behavioral, and language skills are affected)

 a. Lack of interest in human contact

 b. Lack of effective daily living skills

 c. No social play or interaction

 d. Performs repetitive movements, such as rocking, spinning, or hand-flapping

 e. Develops specific routines or rituals

 f. Becomes disturbed at the slightest change in routines or rituals

 g. Autoerotic behaviors (rocking)

 h. Self-mutilation (head-banging)

 i. Moves constantly

 j. May be fascinated by parts of an object, such as the spinning wheels of a toy car

 k. May be unusually sensitive to light, sound, and touch and yet oblivious to pain

 l. Starts talking later than age 2 and has other developmental delays by 30 months

 m. Loses previously acquired ability to say words or sentences

 n. Doesn't make eye contact when making requests

 o. Speaks with an abnormal tone or rhythm—may use a singsong voice or robot-like speech

3. Collaborative Care

 a. **NURSING INTERVENTIONS**

 1) Assess the client's physical and psychological status.

 2) Determine the ability of the client's family to understand and cope.

 3) Facilitate communication between the client and family.

 4) Assist the client and family to reach optimal level of function.

 b. Medications

 1) There are no specific medications identified to treat autism.

 c. Therapeutic Measures

 1) Creative therapies; dietary modifications

 2) Special education classes and language/communication therapies

 d. Client Education and Referral

 1) Encourage parents and family members to collaborate with trusted professionals, seek out support groups, and learn about the disorder.

B. Asperger's Syndrome: A developmental disorder that displays mild cognitive and/or language delay, and is generally identified late in childhood. Affects an individual's ability to socialize and communicate effectively with others. Children with Asperger's syndrome typically exhibit social awkwardness and an all-absorbing interest in specific topics.

1. Contributing Factors

 a. The disorder seems to be linked to changes in the structure of the brain.

 b. Boys are far more likely to develop Asperger's syndrome than are girls.

2. Manifestations

 a. Engaging in one-sided, long-winded conversations, without noticing if the listener is listening or trying to change the subject

 b. Unusual nonverbal communication, such as lack of eye contact, few facial expressions, or awkward body postures and gestures

 c. Showing an intense obsession with one or two specific, narrow subjects, such as baseball statistics, train schedules, weather, or snakes

 d. Appearing not to understand, empathize with, or be sensitive to others' feelings

 e. Having a hard time "reading" other people or understanding humor

 f. Speaking in a voice that is monotonous, rigid, or unusually fast

 g. Moving clumsily, with poor coordination

3. Collaborative Care

 a. **NURSING INTERVENTIONS**

 1) Encourage one-on-one interactions with the client.

 2) Use positive reinforcement to encourage desired behaviors.

 3) Encourage the client to communicate with family/significant others.

 b. Administer Medications

 1) Aripiprazole (Abilify): may be effective for treating irritability

 2) Guanfacine (Intuniv): may be helpful for the problems of hyperactivity and inattention

 3) Selective serotonin reuptake inhibitors (SSRIs): fluvoxamine (Luvox) may be used to treat depression or to help control repetitive behaviors

 4) Risperidone (Risperdal): may be helpful for agitation and irritability

 c. Therapeutic Measures

 1) Cognitive behavioral therapy and social skills training

 d. Client Education and Referral

 1) Refer to a team of trusted professionals

 2) Community support groups

C. Attention Deficit Hyperactivity Disorder: A chronic conduct disorder that is usually diagnosed in children and characterized by a lack of attention, impulsiveness, and excessive hyperactivity

1. Contributing Factors

   a. Maternal exposure to toxins

   b. Smoking, drinking alcohol, or using drugs during pregnancy

   c. A family history of ADHD or certain other behavioral and mood disorders

   d. Low birth weight

2. Manifestations

   a. Difficulty concentrating and easily distracted

   b. Poor attention span, failure to complete a task

   c. Often has problems organizing tasks or activities

   d. Avoids or dislikes tasks that require sustained mental effort, such as schoolwork or homework

   e. Impulsive actions without thought of possible consequences

3. Collaborative Care

    a. **NURSING INTERVENTIONS**

      1) Encourage effective communication in the client.

      2) Assist the client to learn adaptive coping behaviors.

      3) Assess the client's safety and intervene as needed.

      4) Provide positive feedback when appropriate

      5) Initiate educative techniques between the parent(s) and child by using play therapy, family therapy, and/or cognitive behavioral therapy.

   b. Medications

      1) Stimulant medications for ADHD include methylphenidate (Ritalin, Concerta, Daytrana), dextroamphetamine (Dexedrine, Dextrostat), amphetamine (Adderall)

      2) Stimulants are considered the preferred option; if not effective or if intolerable side effects are experienced, antidepressants are the second option.

   c. Therapeutic Measures

      1) Behavior therapy; psychotherapy

      2) Parenting skills training; family therapy, social skills training, and support groups

   d. Client Education and Referral

      1) Teach importance of medication compliance and side effects of stimulant medications.

      2) Initiate educative techniques between the parent(s) and child by using play therapy, family therapy, and/or cognitive behavioral therapy.

      3) Teach behavior-changing strategies to cope with difficult situations and behaviors.

      4) Refer to community and school support groups.

Mood Disorders

A. Major Depressive Disorder: A single or recurrent episode of unipolar depression lasting 2 or more weeks (not associated with mood swings from depression to mania). Depression is a mood state of gloom, despondency, and dejection, accompanying physical, cognitive, and behavioral responses.

1. Contributing Factors

   a. Biological relatives with depression

   b. Females are more likely to experience

   c. Traumatic experiences as a child

   d. Biological relatives with a history of alcoholism

   e. Family members who have committed suicide

   f. Experiencing stressful life events, such as the death of a loved one

   g. Having few friends or other personal relationships

   h. Recently given birth (postpartum depression)

   i. Presence of serious illness, such as cancer, heart disease, Alzheimer's, or HIV/AIDS

   j. Personality traits, such as having low self-esteem and being overly dependent, self-critical, or pessimistic

   k. Abusing alcohol, nicotine, or illicit drugs

2. Manifestations

   a. Feelings of sadness or unhappiness

   b. Irritability or frustration, even over small matters

   c. Loss of interest or pleasure in normal activities

   d. Reduced sex drive

   e. Insomnia or excessive sleeping

   f. Changes in appetite—depression often causes decreased appetite and weight loss

   g. Indecisiveness, distractibility, and decreased concentration

   h. Fatigue, tiredness, and loss of energy—even small tasks may seem to require a lot of effort

   i. Feelings of worthlessness or guilt, fixating on past failures, or blaming self when things aren't going right

   j. Frequent thoughts of death, dying, or suicide

   k. Unexplained physical problems, such as back pain or headaches

3. Diagnostic Testing

   a. Physical exam: height and weight; vital signs

   b. Laboratory tests: complete blood count (CBC); TSH (can identify underlying disorders)

   c. Psychological evaluation: Hamilton Depression Scale, Beck Depression Inventory

4. Collaborative Care

 a. **NURSING INTERVENTIONS**

  1) Maintain a safe environment and assess for suicidal tendencies.

  2) Monitor client's ability to perform ADLs; encourage independence.

  3) Relate therapeutically to the client to identify thoughts and feelings; make observations and use open-ended statements and questions.

b. Medications

  1) SSRIs

  2) Tricyclic antidepressants

  3) Monoamine oxidase inhibitors

  4) SNRIs

c. Therapeutic Measures

  1) Counseling to enhance problem solving, coping abilities, and self-esteem; assertiveness training

  2) Alternative and complimentary therapies

    a) St. John's wort

    b) Light therapy

    c) Electroconvulsive therapy: a medical procedure in which a small amount of electricity is quickly passed through the brain, inducing a grand mal seizure; used for clients who are severely depressed or have not responded to other therapeutic modalities; used after other methods have failed

      (1) Overview

        (a) Electric current is passed through the client's temporal lobe and hypothalamus for 0.1 seconds.

        (b) The nurse may observe a slight grimace or plantar flexion in the client.

        (c) The client may undergo 6 to 10 treatments; three per week.

        (d) Requires consent of the client.

       (2) **NURSING INTERVENTIONS**

        (a) The day prior to the procedure, instruct the client to remain NPO after midnight.

        (b) Assess and document pre-procedural vital signs.

        (c) Verify that the client has signed the informed consent.

        (d) Remove the client's jewelry/prosthetics.

        (e) Have the client empty bladder.

        (f) Instruct the client and family that short-term memory loss is temporary for up to 2 months.

        (g) Administer preoperative medications as prescribed.

        (h) Understand that general anesthesia will be used.

d. Client Education and Referral

  1) Offer follow-up case management to client and/or family as needed

  2) Chronicity of the disorder and need for long-term medication management and psychological support

  3) Precipitating factors, indications of relapse, and ways to manage crisis

  4) Importance of maintaining regular sleep, eating, and activity patterns

B. Grief: Strong, occasional overwhelming emotion in response to loss. Duration can be up to 24 months; known as dysfunctional grief when the client is unable to accept loss after a 24-month period.

  1. Contributing Factors

    a. Death in family

    b. Separation

    c. Divorce

    d. Physical illness; loss of limb

    e. Work failure

    f. Disappointment

  2. Stages (Kübler-Ross)

    a. Denial: "I feel fine."

    b. Anger: "Why is this happening to me?"

    c. Bargaining: "I'll do anything to make this go away."

    d. Depression: "I am so sad. Why bother with anything?"

    e. Acceptance: "I will be okay. This is happening for a reason."

  3. **NURSING INTERVENTIONS**

    a. Provide for client's safety needs.

    b. Accept client's stage of grief and offer empathy.

    c. Encourage expression of feelings.

    d. Assist through stages by providing anticipatory guidance.

C. Bipolar Disorder: Sometimes called manic-depressive disorder; causes mood swings that range from the lows of depression to the highs of mania. Mood shifts may only occur a few times a year, or as often as several times a day. In some cases, bipolar disorder causes symptoms of depression and mania at the same time.

  1. Contributing Factors

    a. Thought to be a combination of physical, neurological, genetic, and environmental factors.

    b. Having blood relatives such as a parent or sibling with bipolar disorder.

    c. Risk factors may include periods of high stress, drug or alcohol abuse, major life changes, such as the death of a loved one, and being between the ages of 15 and 30.

2. Manifestations: Divided into several subtypes. Each has a different pattern of symptoms. Types include:

a. Bipolar I disorder: The client has at least one episode of mania alternating with major depression.

b. Bipolar II disorder: The client has one or more hypomanic episodes (must last all day for a period of 4 days) alternating with major depressive episodes.

c. Cyclothymia: The client has at least 2 years of repeated hypomanic episodes alternating with minor depressive episodes.

   1) Depression

      a) Feelings of sadness or unhappiness

      b) Irritability or frustration, even over small matters

      c) Loss of interest or pleasure in normal activities

      d) Reduced sex drive

      e) Insomnia or excessive sleeping

      f) Changes in appetite—depression often causes decreased appetite and weight loss

      g) Indecisiveness, distractibility, and decreased concentration

      h) Fatigue, tiredness, and loss of energy—even small tasks may seem to require a lot of effort

      i) Feelings of worthlessness or guilt, fixating on past failures, or blaming self when things aren't going right

      j) Frequent thoughts of death, dying, or suicide

      k) Unexplained physical problems, such as back pain or headaches

   2) Mania or elation

      a) Extroversion

      b) Flight of ideas

      c) Accelerated speech

      d) Accelerated motor activity

      e) Anger turned outward

      f) Impulsivity

      g) Arrogant, demanding, controlling behavior with underlying feelings of vulnerability and inadequacy

      h) Delusions of grandeur

3. Collaborative Care

 a. **NURSING INTERVENTIONS** for depression

   1) Initiate suicide precautions.

   2) Promote client's physical well-being.

   3) Structure environment and time.

   4) Build trust, and arrange for short, frequent nurse-client communications.

   5) Encourage client to focus on strengths and promote ADLs.

   6) Schedule leisurely or recreational activities.

   7) Encourage goal setting to provide success.

 b. **NURSING INTERVENTIONS** for mania

   1) Protect client from impulsive activity to promote safety.

   2) Provide for physical welfare.

   3) Provide frequent, small feedings.

   4) Reduce external stimuli (client responds to environment).

   5) Communicate calmly to client.

   6) Initiate milieu activities such as walks, ball tossing, creative writing, and drawing; avoid competitive games.

c. Medications

   1) Mood stabilizers: lithium carbonate (Eskalith)

   2) Antiepileptic agents that act as mood stabilizers: valproic acid (Depakote), clonazepam (Klonipin), lamotrigine (Lamictal), gabapentin (Neurontin), and topiramate (Topax)

   3) Benzodiazepines used on a short-term basis for insomnia related to mania: lorazepam (Ativan)

   4) Antidepressants used to manage a major depressive disorder: SSRI fluoxetine (Prozac)

d. Therapeutic Procedures

   1) Electroconvulsive therapy (ECT)

   2) Cognitive behavioral therapy

   3) Family therapy

e. Client Education and Referral

   1) Offer follow-up case management to client and/or family as needed

   2) Chronicity of the disorder and need for long-term medication management and psychological support

   3) Precipitating factors and indications of relapse and ways to manage crisis

   4) Importance of maintaining regular sleep, eating, and activity patterns

   5) Medication administration

D. Suicide: Self-imposed death stemming from depression, especially hopelessness and negative feelings about the future

1. Contributing Factors

a. History of depression, hallucinating, or delusional patterns of behavior

b. Organic mental disorders, substance abuse

c. Adolescence or elderly adulthood

d. Chronic or painful illness; sexual identity conflicts

2. Warning Signs

a. Client has a specific plan

b. Giving away personal items, completing wills, finalizing personal or business matters

c. Making amends

d. Sudden changes in behavior

e. Gesture or history of attempt

f. States, "Everything is figured out."

3. Collaborative Care

 a. **NURSING INTERVENTIONS**

 1) Initiate suicide precautions.

 2) Establish a no-suicide contract with the client.

 3) Initiate one-on-one constant supervision.

 4) Take all of the client's gestures seriously.

 5) Remove potentially harmful objects.

 6) Understand that it is impossible to "sterilize" the client's environment.

 7) Encourage the client to verbalize feelings.

 8) Nurture and maintain positive goals with the client.

b. Administer Medications

 1) Antidepressants (SSRIs): citalopram (Celexa), fluoxetine (Prozac), sertraline (Zoloft)

 2) Benzodiazepines: diazepam (Valium), lorazepam (Ativan)

 3) Mood stabilizers: lithium carbonate (Eskalith)

 4) Atypical antipsychotics: risperidone (Risperdal), olanzapine (Zyprexa)

c. Therapeutic Measures

 1) Cognitive behavioral therapy

 2) Group therapy

 3) Family therapy

 4) ECT

d. Client Education

 1) Assist client to develop a support system list with specific names, agencies, and emergency phone numbers.

 2) Ask the client to agree to a no-suicide contract emphasizing the need to not harm self and to seek help in crisis.

SECTION 6

Personality Disorders

A. Overview

1. A client with a personality disorder demonstrates long-term maladaptive behavior that prevents accomplishment of desired goals in relationships and other efforts.

2. Maladaptive behaviors are not experienced as uncomfortable by the individual, and some areas of functioning may be very adequate.

3. Disorders are predisposing factors for many other mental health disorders.

B. Antisocial/sociopath: Unstable personality traits reflecting maladaptive chronic inflexibility with impaired social and emotional functioning

1. Contributing Factors

 a. Biologic and genetic abnormalities

 b. Environmental influences such as past physical or emotional abuse

 c. Often comorbid substance use disorders

 d. Deficient ego/superego development

 e. Inappropriate or nonexistent parent and child relationship

2. Manifestations

 a. Lack of remorse or guilt

 b. Disregard for other with exploitation

 c. Inability or refusal to accept responsibility

 d. Failure at school/work/relationships

 e. Superficial, but manipulative charm/wit

 f. Reckless disregard for rights of others

 g. Delinquency and violation of rules

 h. Does not seek treatment and behavior does not change with punishment

C. Borderline Personality: A behavioral disorder characterized by instability of moods and an altered sense of self

1. Contributing Factors

 a. Mostly seen in women

 b. Can be learned responses

 c. Poor parental relationships

 d. History of emotional or sexual abuse

2. Manifestations

 a. Impulsive, unpredictable, and self-destructive behaviors (sex/gambling)

 b. Intense, unstable relationships

 c. Manipulative, splitting behaviors

 d. Intolerance of being alone, easily bored

 e. Identity disturbance, poor self-image

 f. Self-mutilation, suicidal gestures

3. Collaborative Care

 a. **NURSING INTERVENTIONS**

 1) The nurse should be aware of own feelings.

 2) Confront the client regarding behaviors.

 3) Set clear rules and boundaries with the client.

 4) Reinforce consequences with the client for rule violations.

 5) Protect other clients from the client's physical and verbal abuse.

 6) Establish a contract for behavioral changes.

b. Therapeutic Measures

 1) Dialectical behavior therapy (DBT): designed specifically to treat borderline personality disorder through individual, group, and phone counseling. Uses a skills-based approach to teach clients to regulate emotions, tolerate distress, and improve relationships.

 2) Group therapy to identify the client's manipulative behaviors and encourage accountability.

c. Client Education

    1) Education about the disorder and compliance treatment plan

    2) Reinforce importance to attend therapy sessions

    3) Practicing healthy ways to ease painful emotions, rather than inflicting self-injury

    4) Identifying factors that may trigger angry outbursts or impulsive behavior

SECTION 7

Substance Abuse

A. Substance-Related Disorders: A client's use of psychotropic drugs, including alcohol, to the extent of significant interference where his physical, social, and/or emotional well-being is characterized by a preoccupation with obtaining and/or using a particular substance(s)

1. Terms

    a. Substance abuse: repeated use of chemical substances, leading to clinically significant impairment over a 12-month period

    b. Substance dependence: presence of tolerance, phenomenon of withdrawal, substance taken in larger amounts, persistent desire to control use of a substance, and continued use of a substance despite the problems it has caused

    c. Non-substance-related dependency (process addictions): dependence on a behavior such as gambling, sex, shopping, or Internet usage, including pornography

    d. Addiction: characterized by loss of control, whether on a substance or a process (e.g., sex), participation in the dependency despite continuing associated problems, and a tendency to relapse back into the dependency

2. Contributing Factors

    a. Genetic predisposition

    b. Peer pressure and availability; risk-taking tendencies

    c. Low self-esteem or socioeconomic status

    d. Inappropriate coping skills; history of life stressors, loss, or social isolation

    e. Family, work, and/or relationship problems

3. Manifestations

    a. Life events perceived as stressful

    b. Sleep problems and chronic pain

    c. Concern over abuse and attempts to decrease consumption of the substance

    d. CNS: progresses from mild dysphoria to impaired motor activities, psychosis, stupor, seizures, and Wernicke-Korsakoff syndrome (also called wet brain or alcoholic encephalopathy), which is a manifestation of thiamine (vitamin B_1) deficiency. This is usually secondary to alcohol abuse. It mainly causes vision changes, ataxia, and impaired memory.

    e. Neurological system: memory loss, ataxia, and confusion secondary to thiamine and niacin deficiencies

    f. Cardiac system: arrhythmias, myopathy, and hypertension

    g. Gastrointestinal system: gastritis, cirrhosis, pancreatitis, ulcers, and esophageal varices

    h. Respiratory system: COPD (secondary to the use of cigarettes while drinking), pneumonia, and cancer

    i. Genitourinary system: fetal alcohol syndrome (in pregnant women) and decreased libido

    j. Skin: spider angiomas and fractures

4. Collaborative Care (based on type of substance, length of addiction, and presence of multiple drugs or comorbidities)

    a. **NURSING INTERVENTIONS**

        1) Nurse must assess own feelings concerning abuse; an objective, nonjudgmental approach by the nurse is imperative.

        2) Maintain a safe environment.

        3) Observe closely for withdrawal symptoms and need for one-on-one supervision.

        4) Orient client to time, person, and place.

        5) Maintain adequate nutrition.

        6) Monitor for covert substance abuse.

        7) Educate the client and family about addiction.

        8) Encourage self-responsibility and provide referral to 12-step recovery groups.

    b. Medications

        1) Alcohol withdrawal: diazepam (Valium), lorazapam (Ativan), carbamazepine (Tegretol), clonidine (Catapres)

        2) Alcohol abstinence: disulfram (Antabuse), naltrexone (Revia), acamprosate (Campral)

        3) Opoid withdrawal: methadone (Dolphine), clonidine (Catapres), buprenorphine (Sobutrex), buprenorphine combined with naloxone (Suboxone)

        4) Nicotine withdrawal: bupropion (Zyban), nicotine replacement therapy (nicotine gum and nicotine patch)

    c. Therapeutic Measures

        1) Individual psychotherapy including relaxation techniques and cognitive reframing

        2) Group therapy; participation in 12-step recovery support groups

d. Client Education

    1) Encourage the client to adhere to treatment plan.

    2) Educate about addiction and need for abstinence.

    3) Educate client and family about codependent behaviors.

    4) Instruct to remove alcohol and prescription medications from the home.

    5) Encourage self-responsibility.

    6) Assist client to develop an emergency plan when tempted to use drug of choice.

    7) Support attendance and participation in 12-step groups.

B. Alcohol Withdrawal Syndrome: Physical manifestations that develop within 6–8 hours after abstinence from alcohol. Intensify and diminish over 24–48 hours.

1. Manifestations

    a. Confusion and elevated vital signs

    b. Nausea, vomiting, heightened sensitivity to light and sound

    c. Shakiness and tremors; headache

    d. Anxiety and mood swings/insomnia

2. Collaborative Care (based on the degree of intoxication and addiction)

    a. **NURSING INTERVENTIONS**

        1) Provide for client safety.

        2) Monitor viral signs.

        3) Initiate fluid replacement (generally IV).

        4) Replace depleted vitamins (thiamine/niacin).

        5) Decrease stimuli and reorient the client frequently.

        6) Avoid restraining the client.

        7) Implement a high-protein, low-fat, low-salt, high-carbohydrate diet.

    b. Medications

        1) Antianxiety medications: benzodiazepines, such as chlordiazepoxide (Librium), diazepam (Valium), or oxazepam (Serax)

        2) Administer antidiarrheal medication as needed

    c. Therapeutic Measures and Client Education (see Nursing Interventions for Substance-Related Disorders above)

C. Delirium Tremens: Acute state of advanced withdrawal that occurs within 72 hours after a client's last drink of alcohol but can occur up to 7–10 days after the last drink. Occurs in approximately 5% of individuals experiencing withdrawal.

1. Manifestations

    a. Elevated B/P, heart and respiratory rates; sweating, nausea and vomiting, diarrhea; may experience chest pain, fever, and stomach pain

    b. Severe agitation, disorientation, and confusion

    c. Persistent visual and auditory hallucinations

    d. Seizures are most common in the first 24–48 hours after the last drink and are most common in clients with past complications from alcohol withdrawal; usually generalized tonic-clonic seizures

2. Lab and Diagnostic Testing

    a. Electrolytes, BUN, creatinine, blood glucose, CBC, and drug screens

3. Collaborative Care

    a. **NURSING INTERVENTIONS**

        1) Provide for client safety.

        2) Monitor the client for depression and suicide.

        3) Monitor vital signs frequently.

        4) Provide for physical and nutritional needs.

        5) Administer IV fluids with 5% glucose for rehydration.

        6) Observe the client for physical complications.

        7) Provide an environment conducive to rest.

        8) Provide a quiet, dimly lit room.

        9) Provide firm limits and monitor the client's visitors.

    b. Medications:

        1) Antianxiety: diazepam (Valium), lorazapam (Ativan), carbamazepine (Tegretol), clonidine (Catapres). Seizures are prevented and treated with benzodiazepines.

        2) Antipsychotic agent: haloperidol (Haldol) is sometimes used in addition to first-line measures such as benzodiazepines to control agitation or psychosis.

        3) Vitamins: prophylactic administration of thiamine IV (high-risk clients should receive parenteral thiamine at 100–250 mg once daily for several days). Alcoholics are often vitamin and nutrient deficient, which can cause the development of Wernicke-Korsakoff syndrome. Thiamine and folic acid should always be administered before any glucose is administered, otherwise Wernicke-Korsakoff syndrome can be precipitated.

        4) Disulfiram (Antabuse) is given to deter the use of alcohol, which is a type of aversion therapy to sensitize the client to alcohol. If the client ingests alcohol while taking disulfiram, nausea and vomiting occurs; shock, chest pain, dyspnea, confusion with circulatory collapse can cause death. Antabuse cannot be initiated until 2 weeks after the client's last drink. If the client stops medication, no alcohol can be consumed for at least 2 weeks.

    c. Therapeutic Measures

        1) Cognitive behavioral therapy and motivational enhancement therapy are used successfully to prevent relapse.

        2) Refer to group therapy and 12-step support groups.

d. Client Education

    1) Encourage the client to adhere to treatment plan.

    2) Educate about addiction and need for abstinence.

    3) Educate client and family about codependent behaviors.

    4) Instruct to remove alcohol and prescription medications from the home.

    5) Encourage self-responsibility.

    6) Assist client to develop an emergency plan when tempted to use drug of choice.

    7) Support attendance and participation in 12-step groups.

SECTION 8

Cognitive Disorders

A group of conditions characterized by the disruption of thinking, memory, processing, and problem solving

A. Delirium: A serious disturbance in a person's mental abilities that results in a decreased awareness of one's environment and confused thinking. The onset of delirium is usually sudden, often within hours or a few days, and frequently has an identifiable cause.

1. Contributing Factors

  a. Dementia

  b. Older age

  c. Limited ability to perform everyday activities

  d. Visual or hearing impairment

  e. Poor nutrition or dehydration

  f. Severe, chronic, or terminal illness

  g. Multiple medical problems

  h. HIV/AIDS

  i. Alcohol or drug abuse

  j. Medication interactions

  k. Fever/infection

  l. Acid/base or electrolyte imbalances

  m. Anesthesia/blood loss

B. Dementia: A chronic, progressive deterioration of the cognitive processes, personality, and motor skills, as well as a loss of behavioral control. Indicates problems with at least two brain functions, such as memory loss and impaired judgment or language. There are three stages: mild, moderate, and severe.

1. Contributing Factors

  a. Age, family history

  b. History or current use of alcohol and drugs

  c. Atherosclerosis, hypertension, elevated cholesterol levels

  d. Depression, diabetes, smoking

  e. Chronic disease such as Alzheimer's disease

2. Manifestations

  a. Memory loss

  b. Aphasia and difficulty communicating

  c. Apraxia: difficulty with coordination and motor functions

  d. Agnosia: inability to recognize or name objects despite intact sensory abilities

  e. Inability to learn or remember new information

  f. Difficulty with planning and organizing

  g. Personality changes

  h. Inability to reason

  i. Inappropriate behavior

  j. Paranoia

  k. Agitation

  l. Hallucinations

C. Alzheimer's Disease: A disease process characterized by brain changes that gradually get worse. It is the most common cause of dementia—a group of brain disorders that cause progressive loss of intellectual and social skills, severe enough to interfere with day-to-day life.

1. Contributing Factors

  a. Age; family history or genetics.

  b. Females have a higher incidence.

  c. No lifestyle factor has been conclusively shown to reduce the risk of Alzheimer's disease.

2. Manifestations and Stages

  a. Stage 1: No impairment; normal function

  b. Stage 2: Very mild cognitive decline, which may appear to be normal age-related changes

  c. Stage 3: Mild cognitive decline—losing or misplacing objects; short-term memory loss; difficulty remembering words or names; difficulty in work or social situations

  d. Stage 4: Moderate cognitive decline—personality changes; withdrawal; obvious memory loss; difficulty performing tasks requiring planning or organizing; difficulty with complex cognition such as math

  e. Stage 5: Moderately severe cognitive decline—inability to remember important details; disorientation to time and place

  f. Stage 6: Severe cognitive decline—loss of awareness of events or surroundings; significant personality changes such as hallucinations, delusions, compulsive behaviors; assistance required with ADLs; incontinence

  g. Stage 7: Very severe cognitive decline—loss of ability to respond to environment; unrecognizable speech; incontinence; decreased mobility; death frequently related to infection or choking

D. Lab and Diagnostic Studies for Cognitive Disorders

1. Chest and skull x-rays, EEG, ECG

2. Standardized screening tools

   a. Functional Dementia Scale: provides information regarding the client's ability to perform self-care, the extent of memory loss, mood changes, and degree of danger to self or others

   b. MSE—Mental Status Examination

E. Collaborative Care

 1. **NURSING INTERVENTIONS**

   a. Provide for a safe and therapeutic environment.

   b. Monitor ongoing health status, assessing for signs of infection such as respiratory, urinary, or skin.

   c. Assess food and fluid intake, monitoring for weight loss.

   d. Ensure adequate food and fluid intake.

   e. Communicate in calm, reassuring tone; avoid arguing or questioning delusions or hallucinations; reinforce reality and orientation to time, place, and person.

   f. Encourage reminiscence about happy times; talk about familiar things.

   g. Establish eye contact and use short, simple sentences.

   h. Maintain consistent caregivers if possible.

2. Medications

   a. Alzheimer's: donepezil (Aricept), rivastigmine (Exelon), and galantamine (Razadyne); memantine (Namenda) blocks the entry of calcium into nerve cells, thus slowing down brain cell death.

   b. Estrogen for females may help to prevent development of Alzheimer's disease.

   c. Gingko biloba may be used to enhance memory.

3. Therapeutic Measures

   a. Provide support for caregivers and referral to community resources for long-term care.

4. Client Education

   a. Determine teaching needs for family and caregivers and refer to support groups for caregivers.

   b. Educate family and caregivers about disease processes, methods of care, and home adaptation for safety.

   c. Establish a care routine and need for caregivers to apply the routine.

   d. Attempt to provide consistency of caregivers.

A. Anorexia Nervosa: An eating disorder characterized by an extreme fear of obesity and altered perception of one's own body weight

1. Two types

   a. Restricting: Client drastically restricts food intake and does not binge or purge.

   b. Binge eating–purging: Client engages in binge eating or purging behaviors.

2. Contributing Factors

   a. Adolescent struggles with independence

   b. Poor self-image, loss of control/introvert

   c. Family issues (conflict, chaos, denial)

   d. Type-A personality/manipulative

3. Manifestations

   a. Usually manifests between ages 13 and 22

   b. Preoccupied with food/weight

   c. More than 20% under normal body weight

   d. Electrolyte imbalances (hypokalemia), anemia, osteoporosis, hypoglycemia

   e. Muscle atrophy, emaciated, no fatty tissue

   f. Dryness of hair/presence of lanugo

   g. Hypotension/amenorrhea

4. Lab and Diagnostic Testing

   a. Electrolytes, CBC, glucose, ECG, bone density

   b. Eating Disorders Inventory, Body Attitude Test, Diagnostic Survey for Eating Disorders (Diagnostic tools are designed for use in a clinical setting to assess the presence of an eating disorder.)

5. Collaborative Care

 a. **NURSING INTERVENTIONS**

   1) Monitor the client for the need to be hospitalized.

   2) Monitor food and fluid intake, electrolytes, and vital signs.

   3) Monitor the client for 30–60 min after meals.

   4) Do not allow the client to exercise after meals.

   5) Initiate a behavior modification plan.

   6) Provide positive reinforcement for weight gain.

   b. Medications

   1) SSRIs: fluoxetine (Prozac)

   c. Therapeutic Measures

   1) Individual cognitive behavioral therapy

   2) Family and group therapy

d. Client Education and Referral

    1) Encourage client to maintain treatment regimen.

    2) Inform provider about intake of vitamin and mineral supplements.

    3) Encourage client to resist urge to weigh self.

    4) Refer to a registered dietician to provide nutritional and dietary guidance.

    5) Encourage follow-up treatment in an outpatient setting.

    6) Encourage participation in a support group.

    7) Continue individual and family therapy as indicated.

B. Bulimia: An uncontrollable compulsion to consume large amounts of food in a short period of time (binging), followed by a compensatory need to rid the body of the calories consumed, usually accomplished by inducing vomiting (purging).

1. Two Types

  a. Purging: Client uses self-induced vomiting, laxatives, diuretics, and enemas to lose or maintain weight.

  b. Nonpurging: Client may also compensate for binging through other means such as excessive exercise and the misuse of laxatives, diuretics, and/or enemas.

2. Contributing Factors

  a. Family genetics/family problems

  b. Excessive parental and peer pressure

  c. Distorted body image/feelings of ineffectiveness/extrovert

3. Manifestations

  a. Onset between ages 15 and 26

  b. Admits eating behavior is abnormal

  c. Dental caries/gingival infections

  d. Hides/hoards high-calorie foods

  e. Binges, then purges—induces vomiting

  f. Uses laxatives, diuretics, drugs

  g. May have calluses on back of hands

4. Lab and Diagnostic Testing

  a. Similar to anorexia with an emphasis on identifying hypokalemia, hyponatremia, and hypochloremia

  b. Eating Disorders Inventory, Body Attitude Test and Diagnostic Survey for Eating Disorders (Diagnostic tools are designed for use in a clinical setting to assess the presence of an eating disorder.)

5. Collaborative Care

 a. **NURSING INTERVENTIONS**

    1) Monitor the client for the need to be hospitalized.

    2) Monitor food and fluid intake, electrolytes, vital signs.

    3) Monitor the client for 30–60 min after meals.

    4) Do not allow the client to exercise after meals.

    5) Initiate a behavior modification plan.

    6) Provide positive reinforcement for weight gain.

b. Therapeutic Measures

    1) Individual cognitive behavioral therapy

    2) Family and group therapy

c. Client Education

    1) Encourage client to maintain treatment regimen.

    2) Inform provider about intake of vitamin and mineral supplements.

    3) Encourage client to resist urge to weigh self.

! POINT TO REMEMBER: Clients who have eating disorders are extremely resistant to change, and progress may be slow. However, eating disorders are life-threatening and may place clients at risk for suicide. The nurse must focus on reinforcing the seriousness of the disorder to both the client and family.

SECTION 10
Family Violence

Purposeful infliction of physical, verbal, or emotional harm occurring within families of all socioeconomic levels, across all races, and cultural lines.

A. Contributing Factors

1. History of previous family violence.

2. Caregiver is experiencing family stress.

3. Victim is physically or cognitively impaired.

4. Victim is isolated.

B. Types of Abuse

1. Physical: unsolicited use of force that results in injury, pain, or impairment

2. Emotional: inflicting mental anguish through threats, humiliation, or intimidation

3. Sexual: nonconsensual or illegal sexual contact

4. Neglect: failure to provide essential food, clothing, shelter, or medical care, including abandonment

5. Social isolation: from other family members or outside support systems

6. Economic: (particularly among older adults) includes theft, embezzlement, or misuse of life savings

C. Characteristics of Perpetrator

1. Possible use of threats and intimidation to control the victim
2. Usually an extreme disciplinarian who believes in physical punishment
3. Frequent history of drug or alcohol abuse
4. Poor coping skills/low self-esteem
5. Victim of previous childhood abuse
6. Impulsive/immature/poor anger management

D. Characteristics of Victim

1. Feelings of helplessness/hopelessness/suicide
2. Submissive/fearful of being harmed
3. Emotionally dependent on abuser; demonstration of low self-esteem
4. Codependency issues; attempts to protect the abuser and accept responsibility for the abuse.
5. Possible denial of the severity of the situation.

E. Manifestations

1. Frequent emergency room visits in which explanation of injuries does not fit the pathology of the injury
2. Unexplained symptoms such as fractures (especially spiral), burns, bite marks, bruises, or difficulty walking in which the physical appearance does not match the history or mechanism of injury
3. Poor hygiene/hunger/dehydration
4. Venereal disease or STDs, especially in children
5. Anxiety/fear/hesitant to speak openly
6. Depression/runaway behaviors/anger
7. Suicidal ideation or attempts

F. Collaborative Care

 1. NURSING INTERVENTIONS

   a. Identify signs of abuse in all clients, particularly those who are younger than 18 or older than 65.
   b. Be aware that most adult victims will deny being abused due to the fear of reprisal or shame.
   c. Build trust; be nonjudgmental toward the client.
   d. Provide privacy when conducting interviews with the client; use open-ended statements to elicit descriptive responses.
   e. Ask client for specific details and look for inconsistencies.
   f. Offer assistance in seeking a safe shelter.
   g. Report all suspected cases of child and/or older adult abuse to the appropriate group (the nurse does not have to prove that abuse occurred). The burden of proof belongs to the legal system.
   h. Attempt to ensure that clients are physically and psychologically safe from harm.
   i. Assist the client to identify support systems and crisis intervention resources.
   j. Encourage the client to keep clothes, money, and important papers in a safe location.

2. Therapeutic Measures

   a. Encourage participation in support groups.
   b. Use crisis intervention techniques to help resolve family or community situations where abuse or violence has been psychologically devastating.

3. Client Education and Referral

   a. Help client develop a safety plan.
   b. Instruct client regarding normal growth and development.
   c. Teach self-care and empowerment skills.
   d. Teach methods to manage stress.
   e. Initiate case management to coordinate community, medical, criminal justice, and social services.

SECTION 11

Sexual Assault (Rape)

A pressured or forced sexual contact, including sexually inappropriate talk or actions, inappropriate touching, or intercourse, incest, or rape (forced, nonconsensual sexual intercourse).

A. False Concepts Regarding Rape

1. The victim is promiscuous.
2. The victim provoked the event through a mode of dress or actions.
3. Only women are raped.
4. Victims cannot be raped against their will.
5. Only young adults are raped.

B. Manifestations

1. Experiences rape trauma syndrome.
2. Fear and disorganized thinking.
3. Physical and emotional stress.
4. May have nightmares and flashbacks.

C. Collaborative Care

a. **NURSING INTERVENTIONS**

   b. Nurse must initially perform a self-assessment in order to approach the client with an empathetic, objective, and nonjudgmental attitude.
   c. The client will initially need a safe, secure, and private environment for assessment and rape exam by a sexual assault nurse examiner (SANE).
   d. Collect evidence in the presence of law enforcement and according to the facility policy to preserve the chain of evidence.
   e. Arrange for a follow-up to check for STDs/AIDS.
   f. Stay with the client to offer emotional support/empathy.

g. Encourage the client to verbalize feelings.

h. Allow for choices to help the client regain her sense of control.

1. Therapeutic Measures

   a. Initiate appropriate referrals for counseling and short-/long-term support

SECTION 12

Legal Aspects of Mental Health Nursing

A nurse who works in a mental health setting is responsible for providing ethical, competent, and safe care consistent with local, state, and federal laws.

A. Types of Admissions

1. Voluntary

   a. Admits self

   b. Consents to all treatment

   c. Can refuse treatment, including medications, unless a danger to self or others

   d. Can demand and receive discharge

2. Involuntary

   a. Client deemed by lawful authority to be a danger to self or others

   b. At the end of a specified time, the client must have a hearing or be released

B. Informed Consent Required for:

1. Electroconvulsive therapy

2. Medications

3. Seclusion

4. Restraints

C. Client Rights

1. Clients diagnosed and/or hospitalized with a mental health disorder are guaranteed the same civil rights as any other citizen. These include:

   a. Right to receive or refuse treatment

   b. Access to stationery and postage

   c. Receipt of unopened mail

   d. Visits by health care provider, attorney, or clergy

   e. Daily interaction with visitors or phone access

   f. Right to have and/or spend money

   g. Storage space for personal items

   h. Right to own property, vote, and marry

   i. Right to make wills and contracts

   j. Access to educational resources

   k. Right to sue, or be sued, including challenging one's hospitalization

! **POINT TO REMEMBER:** A nurse's priority is to promote and provide care to a client in the least restrictive environment possible.

D. Mental Health Terms

Mental Health Terms

Terms	Definitions
Affect	Mood or feeling tone
Akathisia	Regular restless movements or pacing
Anhedonia	Inability to experience pleasure
Apraxia	Loss of purposeful motor movements
Associative Looseness	Disturbance of thinking in which ideas shift from one subject to another in unrelated themes
Binge	Ingestion of large quantities of food in a short period of time
Blackout	Experience in which a person drinks heavily and appears to function normally, but later is unable to recall prior events
Catatonia	State of psychological immobilization that can revert to episodes of extreme agitation
Clanging	Meaningless rhyming of words
Comorbidity	The presence of one or more disorders (or diseases) in addition to a primary disease or disorder; often used to identify when a client has manifestations of both physical illness and a psychiatric illness
Compulsion	Repetitive purposeless ritualistic behavior performed in accordance with specific rules or in a routine manner in an attempt to reduce anxiety
Concrete Thinking	Thinking characterized by immediate experiences rather than abstract thought
Confabulation	A compensatory mechanism for memory loss; filling in the memory gaps with imaginary stories the teller believes to be true
Countertransference	Experience where the therapist transfers his or her feelings for significant others onto the client
Crisis	A conflict that cannot readily be resolved by using usual coping mechanisms
Defense Mechanisms	Mental strategies used to help cope with areas of conflict
Delusion	A fixed false belief held to be true even with evidence to the contrary
Denial	Unconscious attempt to escape unpleasant realities by denying their existence
Desensitization	Gradual systematic exposure of the client to feared situations under controlled conditions

(continues)

Mental Health Terms (continued)

Terms	Definitions
Dissociation	Disturbance in the integrated organization of memory, identity, perception, or consciousness
Echolalia	Repetition by one person of what is said by another
Echopraxia	A meaningless imitation of movement
Enabling	Helping a chemically dependent person avoid experiencing the consequence of his or her drinking or drug use
Extrapyramidal Reaction	A reversible side effect of some psychotropic drugs characterized by muscle rigidity, drooling, restlessness, shuffling gait, and blurred vision
Flight of Ideas	Rapid flow of speech in which the person jumps from one idea to another before the first idea has been concluded
Grandiosity	Exaggerated belief or claim about one's importance or identity
Grief	An emotional response to a recognized loss
Hallucination	False sensory perception without external stimuli that can involve any of the senses
Hypomania	An elevated mood with symptoms less severe than those of mania
Ideas of Reference	False impressions that outside events have special meaning for oneself
Illusions	Misinterpretation of a real, external sensory experience
Insight	Understanding and awareness of the reasons and meanings behind one's motives and behaviors
Judgment	The ability to make logical or rational decisions
Labile	Having rapidly shifting emotions
Limit Setting	Clear statement of rules with consistent reinforcement
Mania	Unstable elevated mood
Manipulation	Behavior that is self-directed to get needs met at the expense of others
Milieu Therapy	Management of the client's environment to promote a positive living experience and facilitate recovery
Narcissism	Self-involvement with lack of empathy for others

Terms	Definitions
Neologism	Coined word with special meaning to the user
Neuroleptic Malignant Syndrome	A rare and sometimes fatal reaction to high-potency antipsychotic medications. Symptoms include muscle rigidity, fever, and elevated WBC
Obsession	Repetitive, uncontrollable thought
Paranoia	Irritable suspicions or distrust that is defended without basis in reality
Phobia	A persistent, irrational fear of a specific object, activity, or situation as the result of severe unrelieved anxiety
Premorbid	Occurring before development of a disease
Psychosis	State in which there is impairment in a person's ability to recognize reality, communicate, and relate to others appropriately
Purging	Purposeful vomiting or elimination of a substance that has been ingested
Reframing	A technique that involves changing one's viewpoint of a situation and replacing it with another viewpoint that alters the entire meaning
Secondary Gains	Benefits from being ill, such as attention
Self-esteem	The degrees of feeling worthwhile or valued
Self-image	One's thoughts about oneself
Somatization	The expression of a psychological stress through physical symptoms
Splitting	The tendency to label individuals into "all good" or "all bad" categories
Tardive Dyskinesia	Irreversible, involuntary tonic muscular spasms of the tongue, fingers, toes, neck, and pelvis that result from long-term use of antipsychotic medications
Transference	Unconscious phenomenon in which feelings, attitudes, and wishes toward significant others in one's early life are linking to and projected onto others, usually a therapist in one's current life
Waxy Flexibility	Condition in which the extremities remain in a fixed position for a long period of time
Word Salad	Spoken words and phrases having no apparent meaning or logic

UNIT 5

Maternal and Newborn Nursing

Female Reproductive Organs

A. Contributing Factors

1. Ovaries
2. Fallopian tubes
3. Uterus
4. Cervix
5. Vagina

B. Fertilization and Fetal Development

1. Conception (fertilization): union of sperm and ovum
2. Conditions necessary for fertilization

   a. Mature egg and sperm

   b. Timing of deposit of sperm
      1) Lifetime of ovum is 24 hr.
      2) Lifetime of sperm in female genital tract is 72 hr.
      3) Menstruation begins approximately 14 days after ovulation if conception has not occurred.

   c. Climate of the female genital tract

   d. Vaginal and cervical secretions—less acidic during ovulation (sperm cannot survive in a highly acidic environment)

   e. Cervical secretions—thinner during ovulation (sperm can penetrate more easily)

   f. Process of fertilization (7–10 days)
      1) Ovulation occurs.
      2) Ovum travels to fallopian tube.
      3) Sperm travels to fallopian tube.
      4) One sperm penetrates the ovum.
      5) Zygote forms (fertilized egg).
      6) Zygote migrates to uterus.
      7) Zygote implants in uterine wall.
      8) Progesterone and estrogen are secreted by the corpus luteum to maintain the lining of the uterus and prevent menstruation until the placenta starts producing these hormones (note: progesterone is a thermogenic hormone that raises body temperature, an objective sign that ovulation has occurred).

   g. Placental development
      1) Chorionic villi develop that secrete human chorionic gonadotropin (HCG), which stimulates production of estrogen and progesterone from the corpus luteum (production of HCG begins on the day of implantation and can be detected by day 6).
      2) Chorionic villi burrow into the endometrium, forming the placenta.
      3) The placenta secretes HCG, human placental lactogen (HPL), and (by week 3) estrogen and progesterone.

   h. Fetal membranes develop and surround the embryo and fetus.
      1) Amnion: inner membrane
      2) Chorion: outer membrane

   i. Umbilical cord
      1) Two arteries carrying deoxygenated blood to the placenta
      2) One vein carrying oxygenated blood to the fetus
      3) No pain receptors
      4) Encased in Wharton's jelly (thick substance that surrounds the umbilical cord that acts as a buffer, preventing pressure on the vein and arteries in the umbilical cord)
      5) Covered by chorionic membrane

   j. Amniotic fluid
      1) Production origins
      2) Maternal serum during early pregnancy
      3) Replaced every 3 hr
      4) 800–1,200 mL at end of pregnancy

Prenatal Nursing

Prenatal period: Pregnancy, antepartum. Begins with conception and ends before birth.

A. Contributing Factors

1. **Female Anatomy**: Hormones, ovulation, organs
2. **Male Anatomy**: Sperm, vas deferens, seminal fluid
3. **Products of Conception**: Placenta, umbilical cord, amniotic fluid and membranes
4. **Fetal/Maternal Circulation**
5. **Assisted Fertilization**: Various methods and fertility can affect the number of fetuses.
6. **Physiological Changes During Pregnancy**: Recognizing changes during pregnancy is helpful for both a client and a nurse. The nurse and health care provider will assess these findings during the client's initial prenatal visit.

B. Manifestations (see table below)

Adaptations in Pregnancy

Adaptation	Trimester			NURSING INTERVENTIONS
	1	2	3	
Ambivalence	X			Assess meaning of pregnancy to the client/partner and socioeconomic supports; refer if needed.
Accepting		X		Assess if ambivalence is increased and how the client views the fetus.
Preparing for birth			X	Review/teach birthing plan. A infant feeding methods , birth control. and home preparations for baby.

Adaptation	Trimester 1	Trimester 2	Trimester 3	🩺 NURSING INTERVENTIONS
Skin: striae, linea nigra, chloasma		X	X	Discuss that commercial treatments are not useful; pigmentation usually disappears after pregnancy; striae may fade.
Breasts: size, striae, tenderness	X			Assess for injury and infection. Discuss supportive bra. OTC products do not reduce stretch marks.
Breasts: colostrum, pigment changes		X	X	Teach regarding colostrum; pads; nipple care; keep dry. Pigment may fade after delivery.
Respiratory: dyspnea		X	X	Sleep propped or sitting up. Teach about lightening.
Cardiovascular: varicose veins		X	X	Assess activity: sitting/standing; constrictive clothing; crossing legs. Teach leg elevation, position changes, support hose, exercise.
GI: nausea/ vomiting	X			Teach diet: dry crackers, 5–6 small meals, ginger, raspberry, check any OTC/herbs, avoid spice, smells. Assess weight, UO, and signs of hyperemesis. Teach to call if cannot eat/drink for > 24 hr, urine becomes scant and dark, heart pounds, or becomes dizzy.
GI: constipation		X	X	Teach about activity, fluids, fiber; check OTC/herbs.
GI: heartburn		X	X	Encourage small meals; sit upright for ≥ 30 min after eating; avoid spicy, fatty foods; check OTC/herbs.
GU: frequency	X		X	Assess for UTI. Teach frequent voiding; do not decrease fluids; Kegels; urinate after intercourse. Call provider if dysuria, cloudy or foul-smelling urine, flank pain.
GU: leukorrhea		X	X	Assess for infection. Teach not to douche. Review hygiene. Call if itching and curdled discharge.
GU: Braxton Hicks		X	X	Teach possible benefit of Braxton Hicks; teach difference between Braxton Hicks and true labor. See Table: False vs. True Labor, page 128.
Nutrition	X	X	X	Assess/teach weight gain patterns; caloric increase 300–400 kcal/d; protein increase by 25 g/d; iron intake 30 mg/d; folate intake 600 mg/d; prenatal vitamins.

Diagnostic Procedures

A. Signs of pregnancy are classified into three groups.

1. Signs of Pregnancy

Presumptive— changes felt by the client	Probable— changes observed by an examiner	Positive— attributable only to the presence of a fetus
• Amenorrhea • Fatigue • Nausea and vomiting • Urinary frequency • Breast changes: Darkened areola, enlarged Montgomery's tubules • Quickening: slight fluttering movements of the fetus felt by a woman, usually between 16 to 20 weeks of gestation. • Uterine enlargement • Linea nigra • Chloasma (mask of pregnancy) • Striae gravidarum	• Abdominal enlargement related to changes in uterine size, shape, and position • Cervical changes • Hegar's sign: softening and compressibility of lower uterus • Chadwick's sign: deepened violet-bluish color of vaginal mucosa secondary to increased vascularity of the area. • Goodell's sign: softening of cervical tip • Ballottement: rebound of unengaged fetus • Braxton Hicks contractions – false contractions, painless, irregular, and usually relieved by walking • Positive pregnancy test • Fetal outline felt by examiner	• Fetal heart sounds • Visualization of fetus by ultrasound • Fetal movement palpated by an experienced examiner

B. Verifying Possible Pregnancy: Serum and urine tests provide an accurate assessment for the presence of human chorionic gonadotropin (hCG).

1. hCG can be detected 6–11 days in serum and 26 days in urine after conception following implantation.

   a. Production of hCG begins with implantation, peaks at about 60–70 days of gestation, and then declines until around 80 days of pregnancy, when it begins to gradually increase until term.

   b. Higher levels of hCG can indicate multifetal pregnancy, ectopic pregnancy, hydatidiform mole (gestational trophoblastic disease), or a genetic abnormality such as Down syndrome.

c. Lower blood levels of hCG may suggest a miscarriage or ectopic pregnancy. Some medications (anticonvulsants, diuretics, tranquilizers) can cause false-positive or false-negative pregnancy results.

d. Urine samples should be first-voided morning specimens.

C. Calculating Delivery Date and Determining Number of Pregnancies for Pregnant Client

1. Nagele's rule: Take the first day of the woman's last menstrual cycle, subtract 3 months, and then add 7 days and 1 year.

2. McDonald's method: Measure uterine fundal height in centimeters from the symphysis pubis to the top of the uterine fundus (between 18 and 30 weeks of gestation). Estimate gestational age to be equal to that of the fundal height.

D. Diagnostic Tests

1. Ultrasound: Doppler ultrasound blood flow analysis

   a. Indications for the use of an ultrasound during pregnancy
      1) Confirm pregnancy and possible multiple gestation
      2) Confirm gestational age by biparietal diameter (side-to-side) measurement
      3) Site of fetal implantation (uterine or ectopic)
      4) Assess fetal growth and development
      5) Assess fetal well-being in normal and high risk pregnancies
      6) Assess maternal structure
      7) Rule out or verifying fetal abnormalities
      8) Locate the site of placental attachment
      9) Evaluate amniotic fluid volume
      10) Fetal movement observation (fetal heartbeat, breathing, and activity)
      11) Placental grading (evaluating placental maturation)
      12) Adjunct for other procedures (e.g., amniocentesis, biophysical profile)

    b. **NURSING INTERVENTIONS** for an ultrasound
      1) Preparation of a client
         a) Explain the procedure and any potential risks to the client.
         b) Ensure that the client has a full bladder.

2. Non-stress test (NST): most widely used technique for antepartum evaluation of fetal well-being performed during the third trimester. It is a noninvasive procedure that monitors response of the fetal heart rate (FHR) to fetal movement.

   a. Indications for the use of a NST during pregnancy
      1) Assess for fetal well being and an intact CNS during the third trimester.
      2) Ruling out the risk for fetal death in clients who have high risk pregnancies such as Diabetes Mellitus.
      3) Hypertension related disorders

b. Interpretation of findings
   1) Reactive NST: An NST is interpreted as reactive if the FHR is a normal baseline rate with moderate variability, *accelerates to 15 beats/min for at least 15 sec, and occurs two or more times during a 20-min period.*
   2) Non-reactive NST indicates that the FHR does not accelerate adequately with fetal movement. *It does not meet the above criteria after 40 min.* If this is so, a further assessment such as a *contraction stress test (CST) or biophysical profile (BPP)* is indicated.

 c. **NURSING INTERVENTIONS**
   1) Prepare the client.
   2) Seat the client in a reclining chair or place in a semi-Fowler's or left-lateral position.
   3) Apply conduction gel, two belts and transducers, to the client's abdomen.

3. Contraction stress test (CST)

   a. Nipple-stimulated CST consists of a woman lightly brushing her palm across her nipple for 2 or 3 minutes. The same process is repeated after a 5-min rest period.
      1) Stimulates contractions and analyzes the FHR in conjunction with the contractions to determine how the fetus will tolerate the stress of labor.
      2) A pattern of at least three contractions within a 10-min period with duration of 40–60 sec each must be obtained to use for assessment data.
      3) Hyperstimulation of the uterus should be avoided.

   b. Oxytocin (Pitocin) administration CST is used if nipple stimulation fails and consists of the IV administration of oxytocin to induce uterine contractions. Contractions started with oxytocin may be difficult to stop and can lead to preterm labor.

   c. Indications for the use of a CST during pregnancy:
      1) Non-reactive stress test
      2) Decreased fetal movement
      3) Intrauterine growth restriction
      4) Postmaturity
      5) Gestational diabetes mellitus
      6) Gestational Hypertension
      7) Maternal chronic hypertension
      8) History of previous fetal demise
      9) Advanced maternal age
      10) Sickle-cell disease

   d. Interpretation of findings
      1) A negative CST (normal finding) is indicated if within a 10-min period, with three uterine contractions, there are no late decelerations of the FHR.

2) A positive CST (abnormal finding) is indicated with persistent and consistent late decelerations on more than half of the contractions. This is suggestive of uteroplacental insufficiency. Variable decelerations may indicate cord compression, and early decelerations may indicate fetal head compression. Based on these findings, the primary care provider may determine to induce labor or perform a cesarean birth.

e. **NURSING INTERVENTIONS**

1) Prepare the client.
2) Obtain a baseline of the FHR, fetal movement, and contractions for 10–20 min and document.
3) Explain the procedure to the client and obtain an informed consent form from her.
4) Complete an assessment without artificial stimulation if contractions are occurring spontaneously.
5) Initiate nipple stimulation if there are no contractions. Instruct the client to roll a nipple between her thumb and fingers or brush her palm across her nipple.
6) The client should stop when a uterine contraction begins.
7) Monitor and provide adequate rest periods for the client to avoid hyperstimulation of the uterus.
8) Initiate IV oxytocin administration if nipple stimulation fails to elicit a sufficient uterine contraction pattern. If hyperstimulation of the uterus and/or preterm labor occurs:
    a) Monitor for contractions lasting longer than 90 sec and/or occurring more frequently than every 2 min.
    b) Administer tocolytics as prescribed.
    c) Maintain bed rest during the procedure.
    d) Observe the client for 30 min afterward to see that contractions have ceased and preterm labor does not begin.

4. Biophysical profile (BPP) uses a real-time ultrasound to visualize physical and physiological characteristics of the fetus and observes for fetal biophysical responses to stimuli.

   a. BPP assesses the fetal well-being by measuring the following five variables with a score of 2 for each normal finding and 0 for each abnormal finding for each variable.

Biophysical Profile

Variables	Normal Score = 2	Abnormal score = 0
Fetal breathing movements	At least 1 episode of 30 sec in 30 min) = 2	Absent or less than 30 sec duration = 0.
Gross body movements	At least 3 body or limb extensions with return to flexion in 30 min = 2	Less than 3 episodes = 0.
Fetal tone	At least 1 episode of extension with return to flexion) = 2	Slow extension and flexion, lack of flexion, or absent of movement = 0
Reactive FHR	(reactive NST) = 2	nonreactive = 0
Amniotic fluid volume	At least 1 pocket of fluid that measures at least 1 cm in 2 perpendicular planes = 2	Pockets absent or less than 1 cm = 0
Total Score Each variable is assigned a score of 0 or 2. The score will be even numbers only ranging from 0–10	Total score of 8–10 is normal. 6 is equivocal/ borderline	Total score of < 4 is abnormal

5. Amniocentesis
   a. Fetal anomalies
      1) Genetic anomalies (e.g., Down syndrome, trisomy 18, and trisomy 13)
      2) Assess amniotic alfa-fetoprotein for detection of neural tube defects.
   b. Fetal maturity
   c. LS ratio to assess fetal lung maturity.

d. **NURSING INTERVENTIONS** for amniocentesis
   1) Preprocedure: Explain procedure and risks to patient and obtain informed consent.
   2) Ensure client has a patent IV and has a full bladder
   3) Postprocedure:
      a) Monitor FHR, fetal activity
      b) Assess for signs of labor.
      c) Assess for vaginal bleeding or hemorrhage.
      d) Administer Rho(D) immune globulin (RhoGAM) if client is Rh-negative.
   4) Educate patient on what to notify physican immediately of any:
      a) Bleeding
      b) Contractions
      c) Signs and symptoms of infection

Note: According to the NCLEX® scope of practice only RNs may administer Rhogam IM. It is a blood product!

6. Percutaneous Umbilical Blood Sampling (PUBS): The most common way to obtain a fetal blood sample or administer an intrauterine blood transfusion. A needle is placed into the amniotic sac and into the umbilical vein for blood sampling ubder ultrasound guidance

   a. Indications

      1) Kleihauer-Betke-ensures blood was obtained from fetus

      2) CBC

      3) Indirect coombs to test for Rh antibodies

      4) Karyotyping of chromosomes

   b. Nursing Interventions

      1) Pre-procedure

         a) Provide client education and ensure a consent form is signed

         b) Administer any medications ordered

      2) Post-procedure

         a) Monitor for bleeding, preterm labor, fetal distress and amnionitis

         b) Inform client to notify health care provider of any bleeding, contractions, lack of fetal movement, elevated temperature, or abdominal pain or tenderness.

7. Chorionic villi sampling: Assess fetal anomalies and genetic defects. Can be done as early as 8–10 weeks.

    a. **NURSING INTERVENTIONS**

      1) Same as with amniocentesis for pre and post procedure

8. Maternal Alphafetoprotein screening (MSAFP) is recomenned for women between 16 & 28 weeks gestation.

   • Lower than normal levels—recommended follow-up to detect Down syndrome

   • Higher than normal levels—recommended follow-up to detect neural tube defects

E. Fetal Assessment

1. FHR

2. Fundal height

3. Fetal activity: kick counts or daily fetal movement counts

   a. Contact if fetal movement decreases.

   b. Contact if less than 10 kicks/2 hr.

   c. Try to do at the same time each day.

   d. Most active after meals and in the evening.

   e. Fetal movement may be decreased by drugs including alcohol and cigarette smoke.

   f. Obesity may hinder the sensation of fetal activity

Terms

A. Number of Pregnancies, Terms, and Guidelines

1. Gravidity: number of pregnancies

   a. Nulligravida: a woman who has never been pregnant

   b. Primigravida: a woman in her first pregnancy

   c. Multigravida: a woman who has had two or more pregnancies

2. Parity: number of pregnancies in which the fetus or fetuses reach viability. Any fetus delivered after 20 weeks or fetal weight of more than 500 g [2 lb], regardless of whether the fetus is born alive or not, is counted as a para.

   a. Nullipara: no pregnancy beyond the stage of viability

   b. Primipara: has completed one pregnancy to stage of viability

   c. Multipara: has completed two or more pregnancies to stage of viability

3. GTPAL

   a. **G**ravidity

   b. **T**erm births (38 weeks or more)

   c. **P**reterm births (from viability up to 37 weeks)

   d. **A**bortions/miscarriages (prior to viability)

   e. **L**iving children

4. Fetal age

   a. Preterm

   b. Term

   c. Posterm

Collaborative Care

A. Prenatal Care

1. Initial exam

   a. Psychosocial assessment

   b. Complete history including medications; pertinent history from partner; family history of genetic concerns

   c. Complete physical

   d. Baseline laboratory values:

      1) CBC

      2) Blood type and Rh

      3) Urinalysis

      4) STI screen, including:

         a) HIV

         b) Rubella titer

         c) Streptococcus B hemolytic

   e. Nutritional counseling (see Adaptations in Pregnancy table on pages 116–117)

f. Teratogens
   1) Medications
      a) Category A: Have not shown a negative side effect on fetus.
      b) Category B: Considered safe, but there have not been controlled studies in women. There may be animal studies that did not show any problem to the animals.
      c) Categories C and D: Studies show risks, but may be used if the benefits outweigh the risks.
      d) Category X: No benefit outweighs the risks.
   2) Cigarette smoke
      a) Maternal active smoking or secondhand smoke
      b) Spontaneous abortion; prematurity; SGA; SIDS
   3) Thermal risks
      a) Avoid hot tubs, long baths, or hot showers
   4) Infections
      a) Group B strep
      b) Herpes
      c) See the Sexually Transmitted Diseases table in the Reproductive Health Nursing section, pages 152–153.

2. Initial and subsequent exams
   a. Weight
   b. Fundal height
   c. FHR
   d. Fetal activity (include date of quickening)
   e. Urine check for glucose and protein
   f. Anticipatory guidance. See Adaptations in Pregnancy table, pages 116–117. Review when to contact provider:
      1) Rupture of membranes prior to 37 weeks
      2) Abdominal pain
      3) Vaginal bleeding
      4) Elevated temperature
      5) Dysuria, oliguria
   g. Provide education for signs of preeclampsia:
      1) Edema on face or hands
      2) Upper right quadrant pain
      3) Decreased urinary output
      4) Severe headache
      5) Blurred vision
      6) Seizures

3. 16 weeks
   a. Screen for NTDs with maternal serum alpha fetoprotein.
   b. Offer genetic testing:
      1) For mother with advanced maternal age (> 35 years)
      2) For clients with a history of genetic or chromosomal anomalies
      3) For clients with an elevated or low MSAFP

4. 28 weeks
   a. Screen for diabetes.
   b. Administer Rho(D) immune globulin (RhoGAM) if Rh-negative.
   c. Begin NST testing twice a week for any pregnancy at risk for intrauterine fetal death
5. 35 weeks
   a. Test for group B strep.

B. Anticipatory Care: Do not assume symptoms are normal adaptations of pregnancy—assess. See Adaptations in Pregnancy table, pages 116–117.

1. Physiological changes
   a. Physiologic Changes in Pregnancy are the result of hormone production and from the enlarging uterus.

Physiologic Changes

System	Changes
Reproductive	Uterus increases in size, shape, position Ovulation and menses cease
Cardiovascular	Increased cardiac output and blood volume (45-50% at term) Increased heart rate Increased coagulation
Respiratory	Increased maternal oxygen needs Uterine enlargement displaces diaphragm causing increased respiratory rate and decreased total lung capacity
Musculoskeletal	Pelvic joint relaxation Body alterations require adjustment in posture Separation of rectus abdominis muscles
Gastrointestinal	N & V, slowed digestive processes, Constipation
Renal	Increased glomerular filtration, urinary frequency
Endocrine/Metabolic	Increased hormone production (hCG, progesterone, estrogen, hPL and prostaglandins; Increased thyroid and parathyroid activity; Insulin resistance
Integument	Hyperpigmentation causing chloasma, linea nigra, striae gravidarum and palmar erythema

Changes in physical appearance may lead to a negative body image. The client may make statements of resentment toward the pregnancy and express anxiousness for the pregnancy to be over soon.

2. Expected vital signs

  a. Blood pressure

    1) Measurements are within the prepregnancy range during the first trimester.

    2) Blood pressure decreases 5–10 mm Hg for both the diastolic and the systolic during the second trimester.

    3) Blood pressure should return to the pre-pregnancy baseline range after approximately 20 weeks of gestation.

    4) **Position of the pregnant woman** may also affect her blood pressure. In the supine position, blood pressure may appear to be lower due to the weight and pressure of the gravid uterus on the vena cava, which decreases venous blood flow to the heart.

    5) **Maternal hypotension and fetal hypoxia** may occur, which are referred to as supine hypotensive syndrome or supine vena cava syndrome. Signs and symptoms include dizziness, lightheadedness, and pale, clammy skin.

    6) **Encourage the client to engage in maternal positioning** on the left-lateral side, semi-Fowler's position, or, if supine, with a wedge placed under one hip to alleviate pressure to the vena cava.

  b. **Pulse** increases 10–15/min around 20 weeks of gestation and remains elevated throughout the remainder of the pregnancy.

  c. **Respirations** increase by 1 to 2/min. Respiratory changes in pregnancy are attributed to the elevation of the diaphragm by as much as 4 cm as well as changes to the chest wall to facilitate increased maternal oxygen demands. Some shortness of breath may be noted.

3. Fetal heart tones

  a. Fetal heart tones are heard at a normal baseline rate of 110–160/min with reassurance.

  b. FHR accelerations noted, which indicate an intact fetal CNS.

SECTION 3

Complications During the Prenatal Period

Medical Problems

Preexisting conditions may complicate pregnancy. Some medical conditions develop during pregnancy and cause complications.

Note: Remember that the RN only may care for or assess High Risk or unstable clients, according to the NCLEX® scope of practice.

A. Cardiac Disease: Cardiovascular disease in pregnancy warrants early identification and monitoring to decrease incidence of maternal or fetal complications. Congenital cardiac anomaly and valvular disorders are the most commonly seen cardiovascular diseases in a client who is pregnant.

1. Contributing Factors

  a. Pregnancy expands maternal plasma volume and increase cardiac output.

  b. Preexisting heart conditions can be exacerbated.

  c. Heart failure, death may occur.

  d. Greatest risks:

    1) End of 2nd trimester when blood volume peaks

    2) During labor when blood volume increases during uterine contractions (blood is squeezed out of myometrium during contractions)

    3) After delivery when volume is suddenly increased by complete uterine contraction

2. Manifestations

  a. Subjective data

    1) Dizziness

    2) Shortness of breath

    3) Weakness

    4) Fatigue

    5) Chest pain on exertion

    6) Anxiety

  b. Objective data: physical assessment findings

    1) Arrhythmias

    2) Irregular heart rate

    3) Tachycardia

    4) Heart murmur

    5) Distended jugular veins

    6) Cyanosis of nails or lips

    7) Pallor

    8) Generalized edema

    9) Diaphoresis

    10) Increased respirations

    11) Cough

    12) Hemoptysis

    13) Intrauterine growth restriction

    14) Decreased amniotic fluid

    15) FHR with decreased variability

3. Lab and Diagnostic Testing

  a. Laboratory tests

    1) Hgb

    2) Hct

    3) WBC

    4) Chemistry profile

    5) Sedimentation rate

    6) Maternal ABGs

    7) Clotting studies

b. Other diagnostic procedures
   1) Echocardiogram
   2) Holter monitoring
   3) Chest x-ray
   4) Ultrasound
   5) Pulse oximetry
   6) NST
   7) Biophysical profile

4. Collaborative Care

  a. **NURSING INTERVENTIONS**
   1) Assess for signs/symptoms of fatigue/anemia, weight gain more than 1–2 pounds/week, pulmonary edema, peripheral edema, palpitations, tachycardia, angina
   2) Prevent infection
   3) Provide nutritional counseling

  b. **Medications**: pharmacological management is determined by the client's cardiac diagnoses and clinical presentation.
   1) Propranolol (Inderal): beta blocker; used to treat tachyarrhythmia's and to lower maternal blood pressure
   2) Gentamicin (Garamycin): aminoglycoside antibiotic; prophylaxis that is given to prevent endocarditis
   3) Ampicillin (Polycillin): antibiotic; prophylaxis given to prevent endocarditis
   4) Heparin sodium: anticoagulant used in treating clients with pulmonary embolus, deep vein thrombosis, prosthetic valves, cyanotic heart defects, and rheumatic heart disease
   5) Digoxin (Lanoxin): cardiac glycoside; used to increase cardiac output during pregnancy, and may be prescribed if fetal tachycardia is present
   6) Anticoagulant therapy (Heparin)
    a) Teach bleeding precautions
    b) Report any bleeding

B. Preexisting, or Chronic, Hypertension: Hypertensive disease in pregnancy is divided into clinical subsets of the disease based on end-organ effects and progresses along a continuum from mild gestational hypertension; mild and severe preeclampsia; eclampsia; to hemolysis, elevated liver enzymes, and low platelets (HELLP) syndrome.

1. **Vasospasm** contributing to poor tissue perfusion is the underlying mechanism for the signs and symptoms of pregnancy hypertensive disorders.

2. **Gestational hypertension (GH)**, which **begins after the 20th week** of pregnancy, describes hypertensive disorders of pregnancy whereby the woman has an elevated blood pressure at 140/90 mm Hg or greater, or a systolic increase of 30 mm Hg or a diastolic increase of 15 mm Hg from the prepregnancy baseline. There is no proteinuria or edema. The client's blood pressure returns to baseline by 12 weeks postpartum.

3. **Mild preeclampsia is GH** with the addition of proteinuria of 1 to 2+ and a weight gain of more than 2 kg (4.4 lb) per week in the second and third trimesters. Mild edema will also begin to appear in the upper extremities or face.

4. **Severe preeclampsia** consists of blood pressure that is 160/100 mm Hg or greater, proteinuria 3 to 4+, oliguria, elevated serum creatinine greater than 1.2 mg/dL, cerebral or visual disturbances (headache and blurred vision), hyperreflexia with possible ankle clonus, pulmonary or cardiac involvement, extensive peripheral edema, hepatic dysfunction, epigastric and right upper-quadrant pain, and thrombocytopenia.

5. **Eclampsia** is severe preeclampsia symptoms along with the onset of seizure activity or coma. Eclampsia is usually preceded by headache, severe epigastric pain, hyperreflexia, and hemoconcentrations, which are warning signs of probable convulsions.

6. **HELLP** syndrome is a variant of GH in which hematologic conditions coexist with severe preeclampsia involving hepatic dysfunction. HELLP syndrome is diagnosed by laboratory tests, not clinically.

  a. **H: hemolysis** resulting in anemia and jaundice

  b. **EL: elevated liver enzymes** resulting in elevated (ALT) or (AST), epigastric pain, and nausea and vomiting

  c. **LP: low platelets (< 100,000/mm³)**, resulting in thrombocytopenia, abnormal bleeding and clotting time, bleeding gums, petechiae, and possibly DIC

Note: Gestational hypertensive disease and chronic hypertension may occur simultaneously. Gestational hypertensive diseases are associated with placental abruption, acute renal failure, hepatic rupture, preterm birth, and fetal and maternal death.

7. Contributing Factors
  a. No single profile identifies risks for gestational hypertensive disorders, but some high risks include:
   1) Maternal age younger than 20 or older than 40
   2) First pregnancy
   3) Morbid obesity
   4) Multifetal gestation
   5) Chronic renal disease
   6) Chronic hypertension
   7) Familiar history of preeclampsia
   8) Diabetes mellitus
   9) Rh incompatibility
   10) Molar pregnancy
   11) Previous history of GH.

8. Manifestations
   a. Severe continuous headache; nausea
   b. Blurring of vision; flashes of lights or dots before the eyes
   c. Hypertension; proteinuria
   d. Periorbital, facial, hand, and abdominal edema
   e. Pitting edema of lower extremities
   f. Vomiting; oliguria
   g. Hyperreflexia
   h. Scotoma (partial alteration in one's field of vision)
   i. Epigastric pain; right-upper quadrant pain
   j. Dyspnea; diminished breath sounds
   k. Seizures
   l. Jaundice
   m. Rapid weight gain (2 kg [4.4 lb]) per week in the second and third trimesters
   n. Elevated liver enzymes (LDH, AST); increased creatinine
   o. Increased plasma uric acid; thrombocytopenia; decreased Hgb
   p. Hyperbilirubinemia
      1) Signs of progression include worsening liver involvement, renal failure, worsening hypertension, cerebral involvement, and developing coagulopathies

9. Lab and Diagnostic Testing
   a. Urinalysis to detect proteinuria,
   b. 24-hr urine collection for protein and creatinine clearance
   c. NST, contraction stress test, biophysical profile, and serial ultrasounds to assess fetal status
   d. Doppler blood flow analysis to assess fetal well-being
   e. Liver enzymes, serum creatinine, BUN, uric acid, and magnesium increase as renal function decreases.
   f. CBC, clotting studies, chemistry profile

10. Collaborative Care
     a. **NURSING INTERVENTIONS**
       1) Chronic hypertension
          a) Monitor BP.
          b) Assess medications.
          c) Discuss nutrition, exercise.
          d) Monitor for signs of preeclampsia.
       2) Gestational hypertension
          a) Monitor BP.
          b) Assess medications.
          c) Discuss nutrition, exercise.
          d) Monitor for signs of preeclampsia.
       3) Preeclampsia
          a) Assess client's psyche.
          b) Assess routine maternal/fetal assessments.

   c) Assess symptoms:
      (1) Weight
      (2) I&O
      (3) Reflexes
      (4) Blood pressure
      (5) CNS
   d) Discuss diet: high protein; 48–64 ounces of fluid/day; fiber; limit salt to 6 g/day; no alcohol, cigarettes, or caffeine
   e) Bed rest on left side
   f) Seizure precautions
   g) Monitor for HELLP and DIC.
       (1) **NURSING INTERVENTIONS** for HELLP: Monitor:
         (a) Lab values
         (b) Symptoms of malaise, epigastric or RUQ pain, bleeding
       (2) **NURSING INTERVENTIONS** for DIC: Monitor:
         (a) Lab values
         (b) Bleeding
         (c) Tachycardia
       (3) **NURSING INTERVENTIONS** for HELLP and DIC:
         (a) Correct preeclampsia.
         (b) Replace blood component.
         (c) Administer vitamin K.
         (d) Monitor urinary output.

NOTE: Remember, only RNs may administer blood products!

   b. Medications
      1) Magnesium sulfate: anticonvulsant
         a) Administer IV magnesium sulfate, which is the medication of choice for prophylaxis or treatment. It will lower blood pressure and depress the CNS.
       b) **NURSING INTERVENTIONS**
         (1) Use an infusion control device to maintain a regular flow rate.
         (2) Inform the client that she may initially feel flushed, hot, and sedated with the magnesium sulfate bolus.
         (3) Monitor the client's blood pressure, pulse, respiratory rate, deep-tendon reflexes, level of consciousness, urinary output (indwelling urinary catheter for accuracy), presence of headache, visual disturbances, epigastric pain, uterine contractions, and FHR and activity.
         (4) Place the client on fluid restriction of 100–125 mL/hr, and maintain a urinary output of 30 mL/hr or greater.

(5) Monitor the client for signs of magnesium sulfate toxicity:
   (a) Absence of patellar deep tendon reflexes
   (b) Urine output less than 30 mL/hr
   (c) Respirations less than 12/min
   (d) Decreased level of consciousness
   (e) Cardiac dysrhythmias
(6) If magnesium toxicity is suspected:
   (a) Immediately discontinue infusion.
   (b) Administer antidote calcium gluconate.
   (c) Prepare for actions to prevent respiratory or cardiac arrest.

C. Diabetes Mellitus

1. Types
   a. Pregestational diabetes mellitus: Client had diabetes prior to pregnancy
   b. Gestational diabetes mellitus: An impaired tolerance to glucose with the first onset or recognition during pregnancy. The ideal blood glucose level during pregnancy should fall between 70 and 110 mg/dL. Client develops diabetes mellitus during pregnancy, usually in the 2nd or 3rd trimester.

2. Contributing Factors
   a. Obesity
   b. Maternal age older than 25 years
   c. Family history of diabetes mellitus
   d. Previous delivery of an infant that was large or stillborn

3. Manifestations
   a. Hypoglycemia (nervousness, headache, weakness, irritability, hunger, blurred vision, tingling of mouth or extremities)
   b. Hyperglycemia (thirst, nausea, abdominal pain, frequent urination, flushed dry skin, fruity breath)
   c. Hypoglycemia, shaking, clammy pale skin, shallow respirations, rapid pulse, hyperglycemia, vomiting, excess weight gain during pregnancy

4. Laboratory Testing and Diagnostic Procedures
   a. Routine urinalysis with glycosuria
   b. Glucose tolerance test (50 g oral glucose load, followed by plasma glucose analysis 1 hr later performed at 24–28 weeks of gestation—fasting not necessary; a positive blood glucose screening is 140 mg/dL or greater; additional testing with a 3-hr glucose tolerance test is indicated).
      1) A 3-hr glucose tolerance test (following overnight fasting, avoidance of caffeine, and abstinence from smoking for 12 hr prior to testing; a fasting glucose is obtained, a 100 g glucose load is given, and serum glucose levels are determined at 1, 2, and 3 hr following glucose ingestion).

c. Monitor HbA1c
d. Monitor for ketones
e. BPP to ascertain fetal well-being
f. Amniocentesis with alpha-fetoprotein
g. NST to assess fetal well-being

5. Collaborative Care
   a. Risks to newborn increase with poor glucose control:
      1) Congenital anomalies
      2) Spontaneous abortions
      3) Macrosomia: birth trauma and dystocia
      4) Death
      5) Hypoglycemia after birth
   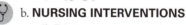 b. **NURSING INTERVENTIONS**
      1) Diet
      2) Exercise
      3) Blood glucose monitoring
      4) Insulin if medication required
   c. Medications
      1) Oral hypoglycemics are not used in pregnancy.
      2) Insulin
         a) a) May need insulin if not already using.
         b) Insulin needs may decrease during 1st trimester.
         c) Insulin needs may increase during the 2nd and 3rd trimester.

D. Hyperemesis Gravidarum: A severe form of morning sickness, with unrelenting, excessive pregnancy-related nausea and/or vomiting that prevents adequate intake of food and fluids. Women experiencing hyperemesis gravidarum often are dehydrated and lose weight despite efforts to eat. Nausea and vomiting begins in the first or second month of pregnancy. It is extreme and is not helped by normal measures.

1. Contributing Factors
   a. Believed to be caused by high levels of human chorionic gonadotropin (hCG)
   b. At times may have a psychological cause

2. Manifestations
   a. Loss of 5% or more of prepregnancy body weight
   b. Dehydration, causing ketosis and constipation
   c. Nutritional deficiencies
   d. Metabolic imbalances

3. Collaborative Care
    a. **NURSING INTERVENTIONS**
      1) Assess psyche; refer as needed.
      2) Assess weight.
      3) Assess for dehydration, electrolyte imbalance, and metabolic alkalosis.
      4) Monitor I&O.
      5) Administer IV fluids.
      6) Small meals per client preference.

    b. Medications
        1) Antiemetics such as ondansetron (Zofran) are considered safe and effective to treat nausea.
        2) Vitamin B_6 (no more than 100 mg daily) has been shown to decrease the nausea in early pregnancy.
    c. Therapeutic Measures
        1) Accupressure; relaxation techniques
    d. Client Education
        1) Nausea and vomiting usually peaks between 2 and 12 weeks of pregnancy and goes away by the second half of pregnancy.
        2) **Eat small, frequent meals**; eating dry foods such as crackers may help relieve uncomplicated nausea.
        3) Increase fluid intake to prevent dehydration; teach to increase fluids during the times of the day when the client feels the least nauseated; seltzer, ginger ale, or other sparkling waters may be helpful.

Placental Problems

A. Abruptio Placenta

1. Contributing Factors
    a. Trauma
    b. Preeclampsia
    c. Multiparity
    d. Cocaine use

B. Placenta Previa

1. Contributing Factors
    a. Placenta implants completely or partially over cervical os

Placenta Previa and Abruptio Placenta

	Placenta Previa	Abruptio Placenta
Vaginal Bleeding	Usually bright red. Can range from minimal to severe and life threatening. Color of beeding bright red.	Can range from absent to moderate dependant on the grade of abruption. Blood usually dark red in color.
Pain	Often none	Abdomen "boardlike" and very tender
Maternal Effect	Hemorrhage, shock, death	
Fetal Effect	Anoxia, CNS trauma, death	
Treatment	Partial previa might be treated with bed rest. Complete previa will be treated as with abruptio placenta.	Emotional support; immediate C-section; blood transfusions, monitoring for DIC

C. Hydatidiform Mole/Molar Pregnancy: Benign abnormal growth of chorionic villi. Appears as avascular transparent grapelike clusters. Complete molar pregnancy: Egg is fertilized but there is no fetus. Partial molar pregnancy: Egg fertilizes and some fetal parts may be present, but there is no complete fetus. Occurs in about 1/1200 fertilizations. About 1/5 clients will develop choriocarcinoma.

1. Contributing Factors
    a. Previous use of ovulation-stimulating drugs
    b. Age extremes: very young or over 40
    c. History of spontaneous abortion
    d. Poor nutrition
    e. Often unknown
2. Manifestations
    a. Early
        1) As with pregnancy
    b. Later
        1) Vaginal bleeding
            a) Brown
            b) Grape-like clusters
            c) Anemia
        2) Rapid uterine growth (increase in fundal height)
            a) Uterine cramping
        3) Extreme nausea
        4) Hyperthyroidism
        5) Preeclampsia
3. Diagnostic Testing
    a. Ultrasound
    b. Persistent, high, hCG levels
4. Collaborative Care
    a. Assess psyche
    b. Spontaneous expulsion
    c. Elective expulsion
        1) Curettage
        2) Induction not recommended
        3) RhoGAM post-expulsion if Rh-negative
        4) Post-expulsion
            a) Follow postpartum protocol.
            b) Continue to monitor hCG levels.
            c) Follow up to rule out choriocarcinoma.
            d) Discuss birth control.

D. Abortion: Expulsion of the fetus prior to viability

1. Types
    a. Spontaneous
        1) Occurs from natural causes
        2) Lay term: miscarriage
    b. Therapeutic
        1) Intentional abortion for health reasons

c. Elective

    1) Intentional abortion without health reasons

d. Others

    1) Complete/incomplete; missed; habitual; threatened; inevitable; septic

2. Collaborative Care

  a. Assess client's psychological reaction.

  b. Provide assessment as with postpartum care.

  c. Assess all vaginal discharge for products of conception, clots, amount.

3. Discharge Teaching

  a. Notify provider if signs of infection occur, bleeding increases, depression.

  b. Discuss future pregnancy plans, birth control.

  c. Provide follow-up exam.

E. Incompetent Cervix: Premature dilation of the cervix, usually in 2nd trimester

1. Contributing Factors

  a. Cervical trauma

  b. Previous spontaneous delivery in 2nd trimester

  c. Unknown

2. Manifestations

  a. Bleeding

  b. Fetal membranes visible

  c. Delivery of premature infant

3. Collaborative Care

  a. Emotional support

  b. If able to maintain pregnancy:

    1) Bed rest

    2) Monitor client and fetus

    3) Tocolytics

    4) Hydration

    5) Cerclage (purse string suture)

  c. Future pregnancies

F. Ectopic Pregnancy: Fertilized egg implants in pelvis or abdomen, often in fallopian tube

1. Contributing Factors

  a. Narrowing of fallopian tubes

  b. Previous STI or PID

  c. Malformation of tubes

  d. Constriction of tube from tumor, endometriosis, surgery, etc.

2. Manifestations

  a. Sharp abdominal pain

  b. Hemorrhage

  c. Shock

3. Collaborative Care

  a. Assess psyche.

  b. Surgery.

  c. Treat for shock.

  d. Provide postoperative care.

  e. Discuss concerns about future pregnancies.

SECTION 4
Labor and Delivery

Labor and Delivery

Labor and delivery include the period during which the baby and placenta are delivered and up to 1–2 hr after delivery.

A. Components of Labor—The Five P's are signifigant factors that affect the Labor and Delivery process.

1. Psyche—The mothers psychological response to labor

2. Powers—Uterine contractions

  a. Uterine contractions: Rhythmic tightening of the uterine muscle that act to dilate and efface the cervix resulting in the delivery of the fetus and placenta.

    1) Frequency—The amount of time from the beginning of one contraction to the beginning of the next contraction.

    2) Duration—The amount of time elapsed form the beginning of one contraction to the end of the contraction. Any duration greater than 90 seconds is considered hyperstimulation.

    3) Intensity—The strength of the uterine contraction. The only true measurement of this can be achieved with an Internal Uterine Pressure monitoring or IUPC.

    4) Regularity—The amount of regularity and consistency of frequency and intensity of contractions

  b. Effacement—Shortening and thinning of the cervix, the goal is 100% effacement

    1) Primigravida may complete effacement before dilation.

  c. Dilation—The opening of the cervix. The diameter of the cervix ranges from 0 cm (closed) to 10 cm (fully dilated).

3. Passenger—The fetus and placenta

  a. Lie—The relationship of the long axis or spine of fetus to the long axis or spine of the mother.

    1) Transverse—The long axis of the fetus is at a right angle to the mother's long axis. This is incompatible with a vaginal delivery if the fetus remains in a transverse lie.

2) Longitudinal—The fetus's long axis is parrellel to the mother's long axis or spine. The fetus is either in a breech or vertex presentation.

3) Oblique—when the fetus is lying at an angle. These fetus's will sometimes convert to a longitudinal lie, if they do not a vaginal delivery is not possible.

4. Presentation—the part of the fetus that enters the pelvic inlet first. The three primary presentations are cephalic, breech, and shoulder.

   a. Cephalic—head first

   b. Breech—buttocks or feet first

     1) Complete—sacrum and feet presenting are the presenting parts..

     2) Frank—Sacrum is the presenting part

     3) Footling—sacrum with a single or double leg extended.

     4) Shoulder—When the shoulder enters first, only seen in 1% of births.

5. Position—Relationship of presenting part (occiput, mentum, sacrum) to the maternal pelvic inlet. The fetal position is represented by a three letter abbreviation. The first letter refers to which side of the mothers pelvic inlet that the presenting part is facing, Left or Right. The second letter refers to the specific presenting part of the fetus (O—occiput, M—Mentum, S—for sacrum, Sc—for scapula or shoulder. The third letter stands for the relationship of the fetuses presenting part to maternal pelvis. A anterior, P posterior, or T transverse. Example LOA the occiput is located in the left anterior quadrant of the maternal pelvis.

   • Vertex—the presenting part is the occiput

   • Brow—forehead is the presenting part

   • Mentum—chin is the presenting part

   a. Attitude—The relationship of fetal body parts to one another. Degree of flexion

     1) Degree of flexion

   b. Station—The relationship of the presenting part to the maternal ischial spines that measures the degree of descent of the fetus.

     1) Negative stations are above ischial spines (–1, –2).

     2) Zero station is at the ischial spines, or engaged (0).

     3) Positive stations are below the ischial spines (+1, +2, +3).

6. Passageway—The birth canal or maternal pelvis. Composed of bony prominences of the pelvis, cervix, pelvic floor and vagina. The pelvic inlet is the upper portion of the pelvis. The pelvic cavity is the midpelvis, the pelvic outlet is the lower border of the pelvis.

   a. Cephalopelvic disproportion—When the fetus has a head size, shape or position that does not allow for passage through the pelvis. This can also occur secondary to maternal pelvic structure or associated problems.

B. Manifestations of False vs. True Labor

False vs. True Labor

Sign	False Labor	True Labor
Uterine contractions	Braxton Hicks, irregular, do not increase in frequency or intensity. Usually felt in the lower back or the abdomen above the umbilicus. Decrease in frequency intensity and duration with walking or position changes. Contractions often cease with sleep, comfort measures, oral hydration, and emptying of bladder..	My begin irregularly but become regular in frequency, become stronger and last longer, Walking can increase contraction intensity. Contractions continue despite comfort measures. Usually felt the lower back radiating to the abdomen.-.
Cervical dilation and effacement	No significant change in dilation or effacement. Cervix often stays in posterior position.	Cervical dilation and effacement steadily progress
Bloody show	Usually not present	Present as cervix dilates
Fetus	Presenting part not engaged in pelvis	Presenting part engages in pelvis

C. Medications Used in Labor and Delivery

Medications Used in Labor and Delivery

Medication	Use	NURSING INTERVENTIONS
Oxytocin (Pitocin)	Induces labor, stimulates labor, or contracts the uterus after delivery	Monitor uterine contractions, FHR, and maternal V/S. Must be given IV on pump through a secondary line. Stop immediately if any late decelerations or hyperstimulation occurs. May cause painful UC and postpartum edema. Assist with pain control. Given IV or IM.
Methylergonovine maleate (Methergine)	Contracts the uterus after delivery, used to treat/prevent postpartum hemorrhage	Monitor fundus for firmness and monitor bleeding.

Medication	Use	NURSING INTERVENTIONS
Calcium gluconate (generic only)	Antidote for magnesium sulfate toxicity	Monitor VS and DTRs. Monitor magnesium levels (therapeutic range is 4–8 mg/dL); Administer via infusion pump in diluted form; Use indwelling catheter to monitor urinary elimination. Administer calcium gluconate 10% available signs of toxicity.
Terbutaline (Brethine)	Beta-Adrenergic Agonists (Betamimetics). They relax smooth muscles. The uterus is a smooth muscle therefore they can be utilized as Tocolytics, in premature labor.	Assess VS, FHR, UC. Monitor for side effects: tremors, dizziness, headache, tachycardia, hypotension, anxiety. Given PO or SC. May give 0.25 mg every 20 minutes as needed. Maternal heart rate should be assessed prior to administration. Terbutaline should d be held for a HR greater than 120 beats per minute.
Indomethacin (Indocin)	Prostaglandin Synthetase Inhibitor (NSAIDS) Cn be utilized as as Tocolytic, in premature labor	Assess VS, FHR, UC. May cause maternal GI upset; other maternal side effects are rare. Fetus may develop cardiovascular problems and low UO. Given IV or PO.
Magnesium sulfate	Tocolytic, used in premature labor; CNS depressant; also used in management of preeclampsia	Assess VS, FHR, UC, DTRs, LOC, UO, magnesium plasma levels. Must be Given IV on pump through a secondary line. Stop Magnesium Sulfate immediately: if respirations are < 12, DTRs are absent, UO falls below protocol 25–30 ml/hr or less than 100/4 hrs, pulmonary edema, severe hypotension, chest pain, altered level of consciousness occurs or magnesium levels are above 10 mEq/L or 9 mg/dl. Calcium gluconate is the antidote given for magnesium toxicity.

Medication	Use	NURSING INTERVENTIONS
Magnesium sulfate (continued)		Magnesium Sulfate can cause decreased fetal movement and fetal breathing as well as decreased fetal heart rate variability. In the neonate you can see hypocalcemia, hypotonia, lethargy, and respiratory depression.
Naloxone HCl (Narcan)	Treats respiratory depression	May give per ET tube, IM, or IV. Monitor respiratory effort.
Betamethasone (Celestone)	Stimulates fetal lung maturation, used if premature delivery is expected	Assess VS, FHR, UC. 2 doses of 12 mg are given 24 hr apart. Given deep IM. Can cause a rise in maternal glucose and pulmonary edema. Maternal glucose and lung sounds should be monitored closely.
Prostaglandin E2 gel (Cervidil)	Softens and thins the cervix	Explain procedure to client. Assess VS, FHR; monitor effects.

D. Pain in Labor and Delivery

1. Non-pharmaceutical pain management: The concept is to decrease anxiety: answer questions, stay with client, assist partner. Teach and/or do: massage, guided imagery, relaxation techniques, positioning, sacral pressure, heat/cold applications, water therapy.

   a. Gate-control theory of pain is based on the concept that the sensory nerve pathways that pain sensations use to travel to the brain will only allow a limited number of sensations to travel at any given time. By sending alternate signals through these pathways, the pain signals can be blocked from ascending the neurological pathway and inhibit the brain's perception and sensation of pain. The gate-control theory of pain assists in the understanding of how non-pharmacological pain techniques can work to relieve pain.

   1) Childbirth preparation methods such as Lamaze, Bradley, Dick-Read methods and/or pattern breathing methods are used to promote relaxation and pain relief.

   2) Sensory stimulation strategies (based on the gate-control theory) to promote relaxation and pain relief:

   a) Aroma therapy

   b) Breathing techniques

c) Imagery

d) Music

e) Use of focal points

b. Cutaneous strategies (based on the gate-control theory) to promote relaxation and pain relief:

1) Back rubs and massage

2) Effleurage: Light, gentle circular stroking of the client's abdomen with the fingertips in rhythm with breathing during contractions

3) Sacral counterpressure: Consistent pressure is applied by the support person using the heel of the hand or fist against the client's sacral area to counteract pain in the lower back

c. Frequent maternal position changes to promote relaxation and pain relief

1) Semi-sitting

2) Squatting

3) Kneeling

4) Kneeling and rocking back and forth

5) Supine position only with the placement of a wedge under one of the client's hips to tilt the uterus and avoid supine hypotension syndrome

2. Pharmaceutical pain management: see Medications Used in Labor and Delivery table, page 129. Analgesics given early in labor (prior to 4–5 cm dilation) may slow or stop labor. Analgesics given late in labor remain in the fetal circulation and may cause newborn Complications such as respiratory depression.

a. **Regional blocks** are most commonly used and consist of the pudendal block, epidural block, spinal block, and paracervical nerve block.

b. **Pudendal block** consists of a local anesthetic transvaginally into the space in front of the pudendal nerve. It does provide local anesthesia to the perineum, vulva, and rectal areas during delivery. It is administered during the second stage of labor 10–20 min before delivery,.

c. **Epidural block** consists of a local anesthetic along with an analgesic morphine (Duramorph) or fentanyl (Sublimaze) injected into the epidural space at the level of the fourth or fifth vertebra. This eliminates all sensation from the level of the umbilicus to the thighs, relieving the discomfort of uterine contractions, fetal descent, and pressure and stretching of the perineum. It is administered when the client is in active labor and dilated to at least 4 cm. Continuous infusion or intermittent injections may be administered through an indwelling epidural catheter. Patient-controlled epidural analgesia is a new technique for labor analgesia and is becoming a favored method of acute pain relief management for labor and birth.

 1) **NURSING INTERVENTIONS**

a) Administer a bolus of IV fluids

b) Position and maintain the client into either a sitting or side-lying modified Sims' position.

c) Encourage the client to remain in the side-lying position after insertion of the epidural catheter.

d) Monitor the maternal bladder for distention and catheterize if necessary to assist with voiding.

e) Monitor for the return of sensation in the client's legs after delivery

f) Assist the client with standing and walking for the first time

E. Therapeutic Procedures in Labor and Delivery

1. Amniotomy: The artificial rupture of the amniotic membranes (AROM) by the primary care provider using an Amnihook or other sharp instrument. Labor typically begins within 12 hr after the membranes rupture. The client is at an increased risk for cord prolapse or infection.

a. Indications

1) Labor progression is too slow and augmentation or induction of labor is indicated.

2) An amnioinfusion is indicated for cord compression or meconium-stained amniotic fluid necessitating AROM.

 b. **NURSING INTERVENTIONS**

1) Explain the procedure to the client

2) Assure that the presenting part of the fetus is engaged prior to an amniotomy.

3) Monitor FHR prior to and following AROM to assess for cord prolapse as evidenced by variable or late decelerations.

4) Monitor and document time of rupture, characteristics of amniotic fluid including color, odor, and consistency.

5) Monitor maternal activity following AROM to reduce the risk of infection or malposition of the fetus.

6) Monitor temperature every 2 hr.

2. Amnioinfusion: An amnioinfusion of 0.9% sodium chloride or lactated Ringer's solution, as prescribed, is instilled into the amniotic cavity through a transcervical catheter introduced into the uterus to supplement the amount of amniotic fluid. The instillation will reduce the severity of variable decelerations caused by cord compression or dilute meconium-stained amniotic fluid.

a. Indications

1) Oligohydramnios caused by any of the following:

a) Uteroplacental insufficiency

b) Premature rupture of membranes

c) Postmaturity of the fetus

2) Fetal cord compression secondary to:

    a) Postmaturity of fetus (macrosomic, large body), which places the fetus at risk for variable deceleration from cord compression.

 b. **NURSING INTERVENTIONS**

    1) **Explain the procedure to the client**

    2) Assist with the amniotomy and insertion of IUPC if not already present

    3) Warm fluid using a blood warmer prior to infusion.

    4) Maintain comfort and dryness of the client.

        a) Monitor the client continuously to prevent uterine overdistention and increased uterine tone.

        b) Continually assess intensity and frequency of the client's uterine contractions.

        c) Continually monitor FHR.

F. Nursing Care During Labor and Delivery

1. Admission

2. Labor is considered "active" until it is ruled out.

3. Active labor is considered an emergency medical condition by the Emergency Medical Treatment and Active Labor Act (EMTALA).

4. Review prenatal history.

5. Review birth plan with woman and partner.

6. Monitor maternal and fetal status:

    a. Vital signs

    b. FHR

        1) Normal rate is 120–160 bpm

        2) Variability

        3) External: auscultation, ultrasound transducer

        4) Internal: spiral electrode

           a) Requires ruptured membranes

> **Note:** Any internal monitoring increases the risk of infection.

    c. Uterine contractions

        1) External: manual or tocotransducer

        2) Internal: intrauterine pressure catheter (IUPC)

    d. Vaginal discharge

    e. Cervix

        1) Cervical exams are done with sterile gloves.

        2) Limit exams especially if a vaginal infection is suspected.

> **Note:** Try to limit the frequency of vaginal exams secondary to the risk of infection

        3) If placenta previa is suspected, the nurse will not do a vaginal exam. Note: If the patient presents with any vaginal bleeding a vaginal exam should not be done.

G. Nursing Care: Stages of Labor

Stages of Labor

Stage	NURSING INTERVENTIONS
First Stage: Cervix dilates from 0 to 10 cm. Three phases: 1. **Latent Phase:** 0–3 cm. Irregular mild –moderate contractions. 2. **Frequency 5–30 min apart. Duration 30–45 sec.** 3. Client may be talkative and excited. 4. **Active Phase:** 47 cm. Contractions become more regular and stronger; 5. Frequency may increase to every 3–5 minutes. Duration increases to 40–70 seconds. 6. Client may become anxious. 7. **Transitional phase:** 8–10 cm. Contractions very strong; Frequency every 2–3 minutes. 8. **Frequency every 2–3 minutes, duration 45–90 seconds.** 9. Client may have nausea/vomiting and may become irritable.	1. Admission assessment. Good time to teach; review birth plan; determine pain goals. In all stages include maternal/fetal assessments; fluid intake; frequent urination. 2. Continue assessing maternal and fetal status. Assist partner with non-pharmaceutical pain management. Provide pharmaceutical analgesia if requested. 3. Continue assessing maternal and fetal status. Assist/assess partner. Provide comfort for client. Reinforce her efforts. Talk her through contractions. No pushing until fully dilated.
Second Stage: from complete dilation through delivery of baby. Client may become fatigued.	Continue assessment. Coach with pushing, breathing (prevent hyperventilation), comfort. Record delivery time, medications, episiotomy/tear, etc.
Third Stage: immediate time after delivery of baby until delivery of placenta. Contractions are usually mild; client is usually focused on her baby.	Immediate care of newborn; Assess client's VS, bleeding, fundus. Provide for bonding as soon as infant is stabilized.
Fourth Stage: 1–2 hr after delivery of the placenta.	Encourage breast-feeding for bonding and involution. Assess client every 15 min × 4; every 30 min × 2; and in 60 min. If no problem, continue assessments every 8 hr.

SECTION 5
Complications During Labor and Delivery

A. Preterm Labor: Uterine contractions and cervical changes that occur between 20 and 37 weeks of gestation

1. Contributing Factors

   a. Demographic factors

      1) Age less than 15 and greater than 35

      2) Low socioeconomic status

      3) Non-Caucasian ethnicity

      4) Single mother

      5) Level of education less than 12th grade

   b. Biophysical factors

      1) Previous preterm labor or birth

      2) Multifetal pregnancy

      3) Hydramnios

      4) Bleeding or acute or recurrent infection

      5) Placental problems

      6) Gestational hypertension

      7) Diabetes mellitus

   c. Behavioral factors

      1) Lack of prenatal care

      2) Poor nutrition

      3) Substance abuse

      4) Excessive exercise, physical or emotional stress

 2. **NURSING INTERVENTIONS**

   a. Provide modified bed rest with bathroom privileges.

   b. Encourage rest in the left-lateral position to increase blood flow to the uterus.

   c. Assess for vaginal drainage or discharge, noting color, consistency, and odor.

   d. Monitor the client's vital signs including temperature.

   e. Monitor FHR.

   f. Maintain adequate hydration in the client.

   g. Administer tocolytic medications as prescribed.

   h. Prepare the client for delivery if near term.

B. Premature Rupture of Membrane (PROM)

1. Contributing Factors

   a. Infection

   b. Trauma

 2. **NURSING INTERVENTIONS**

   a. Assess FHR.

   b. Assess the client for infection.

   c. Assess her for a prolapsed umbilical cord.

   d. Give the client ampicillin 4 g IV load, then 2 g every 4 hr.

C. Fetal Distress

1. Contributing Factors

   a. Uteroplacental insufficiency

      1) Acute uteroplacental insufficiency

         a) Excessive uterine activity associated with induction and use of oxytocin (Pitocin).

         b) Maternal hypotension: epidural, venacaval compression, supine position, internal hemorrhage.

         c) Placental separation: abruptio, placenta previa

      2) Chronic uteroplacental insufficiency

         a) Gestational hypertension

         b) Chronic hypertension

         c) Smoking or illicit drug use

         d) Diabetes mellitus

         e) Postmaturity

 2. **NURSING INTERVENTIONS**

   a. Stop oxytocin induction.

   b. Administer 8–10 L of oxygen/face mask.

   c. Turn the client onto her left side.

   d. Increase the client's IV fluids.

   e. Notify the provider.

D. Umbilical Cord Compression

1. Contributing Factors

   a. Prolapsed cord: Pressure on the umbilical cord during pregnancy, labor, or delivery that reduces blood flow from the placenta to the fetus.

      1) Causes: abnormal presentation, inadequate pelvis, presenting part at high station, multiple gestations, prematurity, premature rupture of membranes, and/or polyhydramnios

      2) Complications: fetal asphyxia

   b. Nuchal cord (cord around neck)

   c. Cord compression

 2. **NURSING INTERVENTIONS**

   a. Prolapsed cord

      1) Place the client in the Trendelenburg or knee-chest position.

      2) Perform a sterile vaginal exam to support the presenting part and relieve pressure on the cord.

      3) Administer 8–10 L of oxygen to the client via a face mask.

      4) Prepare the client for emergency Cesarean delivery.

   b. Cord compression

      1) Administer 8–10 L of oxygen to the client via a face mask.

      2) Prepare to assist with an amnioinfusion.

E. Uterine Hyperstimulation

1. Contributing Factors

   a. Often secondary to the use of oxytocin to induce or augment labor

2. Manifestations

   a. Uterine contractions lasting greater than 90 sec and occurring more frequently than every 2 min

   b. Uterine resting tone greater than 20 mm Hg

   c. Fetal responses
      1) Non-reassuring FHR and pattern
      2) Abnormal baseline (less than 110 or greater than 160)
      3) Absent variability
      4) Repeated late or prolonged decelerations

 3. **NURSING INTERVENTIONS**

   a. Turn off oxytocin infusion.

   b. Increase primary infusion rate.

   c. Initiate oxygen at 8–10 L by face mask.

   d. Place client in side-lying position.

   e. Notify health care provider.

   f. Continue to monitor FHR and uterine contraction patterns.

   g. Prepare to administer terbutaline (Brethine) 0.25 mg subcutaneously, to decrease uterine activity.

> **Note:** Decelerations
>
> | | | |
> |---|---|---|
> | **Variables** | = | **C**ord compression |
> | **Early** | = | **H**ead compression |
> | **Accelerations** | = | **O**ther/OK |
> | **Late** | = | **P**lacenta |

F. Emergency Childbirth

1. Contributing Factors

   a. Precipitous delivery

 2. **NURSING INTERVENTIONS**

   a. Encourage mother to pant, unless the fetus is in breech presentation.

   b. Support the perineum.

   c. Rupture the membranes if they have not yet ruptured.

   d. Feel for the cord around the neonate's neck, and gently slip it over his head.

   e. Clear out mucus and keep the neonate dry and warm.

   f. Do not cut the cord.

   g. Deliver the placenta. Expect a gush of blood and a lengthening of the cord.

   h. Save the placenta.

   i. Massage the client's uterus to shrink it. Place the neonate on the client's breast.

G. Amniotic Fluid Emboli: Occur when amniotic fluid, fetal cells, hair, or other debris enter the maternal circulation, triggering a complex series of events leading to life-threatening maternal symptoms.

1. Contributing Factors

   a. Fluid enters the maternal circulation as a result of an opening in the amniotic sac or maternal uterine veins accompanied by intrauterine pressure

2. Manifestations

   a. Respiratory distress

   b. Circulatory collapse

   c. Hemorrhage

   d. Seizure activity

 3. **NURSING INTERVENTIONS**

   a. Administer 10 L of oxygen to the client via a face mask.

   b. Prepare the client for intubation.

   c. Initiate and/or assist with CPR.

   d. Administer IV fluids.

   e. Administer blood or blood products.

   f. Prepare for an emergency birth.

   g. Provide emotional support.
      1) Happens at delivery
      2) Emergency situation and often fatal

H. Dystocia: prolonged, difficult labor

1. Contributing Factors

   a. Dysfunction of uterine contractions

   b. Abnormal position

   c. Cephalopelvic disproportion

   d. Maternal exhaustion

2. Manifestations

   a. Short stature, overweight status

   b. Age > 40 years

   c. Multifetal pregnancy

   d. Inappropriate timing of analgesia

 3. **NURSING INTERVENTIONS**

   a. Assess fetus and status of the client's labor.

   b. Assist with the application of a fetal scalp electrode.

   c. Encourage the client to void and ambulate regularly.

   d. Assist the client in positioning and coaching during contractions.

   e. Prepare the client for a possible forceps, vacuum-assisted, or cesarean birth.

I. **Assisted/Operative Obstetrics**

1. **Episiotomy**: An incision that is made into the perineum to enlarge the vaginal outlet during delivery

   a. Indications

      1) To spare muscles from overstretching/lacerations
      2) To avoid difficulty holding urine later in life

    b. **NURSING INTERVENTIONS**

      1) Monitor for pain, healing, infection, laceration of the anal sphincter (4th-degree tear), and hemorrhage.
      2) Encourage the client to perform Kegel exercises to improve and restore perineal muscle tone.
      3) Apply ice packs as indicted
      4) Educate client on perineal care

2. **Forceps**: Obstetric instrument used to aid in delivery of the fetal head.

   a. Indications

      1) Poor progress
      2) Fetal distress
      3) Persistent occiput posterior position
      4) Abnormal presentation

    b. **NURSING INTERVENTIONS**

      1) Assess the neonate for intracranial hemorrhage, facial bruising, and facial palsy.
      2) Assist with the delivery as needed.
      3) Check FHR before traction is applied.

   c. Complications

      1) Lacerations to cervix or vagina
      2) Bladder or urethral injury
      3) Urine retention
      4) Hematoma formation in the pelvic soft tissues

3. **Vacuum Extraction**: Attachment of a vacuum cup to the fetal head to assist in birth of the head

   a. Indications

      1) Similar to those of outlet forceps
      2) Preferred method when compared to forceps assistance

   b. **NURSING INTERVENTIONS**

      1) Encourage the client to push during contractions.
      2) Monitor the neonate for trauma at the application site.
      3) Monitor the neonate for cerebral trauma. (poor suck, listlessness)
      4) Inform the parents that caput will begin to disappear in a few hours.

4. **Cesarean Birth**: Birth of fetus through a transabdominal incision of the uterus.

   a. Types

      1) Low transverse: decrease chance of uterine rupture with future pregnancies; less bleeding after delivery
      2) Classical: good for emergency delivery; provides more room

   b. Indications

      1) Fetal distress
      2) Cephalopelvic disproportion
      3) Placenta previa, abruptio
      4) Uterine dysfunction (dysfunctional labor pattern)
      5) Prolapsed cord
      6) Multiple gestation
      7) Malpresentation such as breech or shoulder

   c. Medical risk factors

      1) Hypertensive disorders
      2) Active genital herpes
      3) Positive HIV status
      4) Diabetes mellitus

    d. **NURSING INTERVENTIONS**

      1) Perform preoperative assessment.
      2) Ensure that patient understands the procedure and associated risk and that and informed consent has been signed
      3) Administer pre-op medications
      4) Ensure that patient has a patent IV
      5) Perform postpartum and postoperative assessment.
      6) Monitor effects of anesthesia.
      7) Maintain patent airway.
      8) Monitorr and treat pain.
      9) Monitor vital signs.
      10) Monitor incisional dressing, fundus, and lochia.
      11) Monitor I&O.
      12) Encourage client to turn, cough, and take deep breathe.
      13) Facilitate maternal/newborn bonding and attachment.
      14) Initiate breast-feeding as soon as possible.

J. **Induction of Labor**: The process of chemically or mechanically initiating uterine contractions prior to their spontaneous onset

   1. Indications

      a. Maternal disease: cardiac, gestational hypertension, preeclampsia, diabetes mellitus, chorioamnionitis, severe Rh isoimmunization, chronic renal disease, chronic pulmonary disease
      b. Inadequate uterine contractions (Pitocin is utilized to augment existing contractions)
      c. Placental malfunctions (partial previa)
      d. Fetal conditions (anomaly, intrauterine growth restriction, death)
      e. Postmaturity
      f. PROM
      g. History of rapid birth combined with client living a considerable distance from a health care facility

2. Contraindications for induction with oxytocin
   a. CPD (cephalopelvic disportion)
   b. Non-reassuring FHR
   c. Placenta previa or vasa previa
   d. Prior classical uterine incision or uterine surgery
   e. Active genital herpes
   f. HIV
   g. Cervical cancer
3. Medications
   a. Chemical methods used to soften cervix
      1) Cervidil: placed in cervix then removed after 12 hr; start oxytocin 1 hr after removal
      2) Prostaglandin E (Cervidil): used before induction to soften and thin the cervix
   b. Medications used to initiate induction
      1) IV oxytocin (Pitocin): chemical
      2) Rupture of membranes; amniotomy: mechanical

 c. **NURSING INTERVENTIONS**
   1) Perform a vaginal exam for effacement, dilation, and station.
   2) Monitor the client's vital signs every 4 hr.
   3) Monitor the client's contraction pattern.
   4) Monitor the client's I&O.
   5) Monitor the client's level of maternal discomfort and provide pain management.
   6) Monitor the client's emotional responses and provide support.

SECTION 6

Postpartum Care

Postpartum: Time body requires to return to prepregnant state.

Puerperium: The period of about 6 weeks after childbirth during which the mother's reproductive organs return to their original nonpregnant condition.

A. Assess Physical Status

1. Vital signs, Hgb, Hct, CBC, estimated blood loss in delivery
2. Pain
   a. Monitor location, intensity of pain
   b. Examine location of pain.
   c. Implement non-pharmaceutical measures.
   d. Implement pharmaceutical measures.
      1) Consider safety of medications related to breast feeding:
         a) Hydrocodone/acetaminophen (Vicodin)
         b) Ibuprofen (Motrin, Advil)
         c) Acetaminophen/codeine (Tylenol #3)
         d) PCA such as morphine sulfate

3. Breasts
   a. Colostrum
      1) Produced until about 2 days after delivery
      2) High nutrition
   b. Milk production occurs about day 2–3
      1) Composition changes to meet needs of newborn.
      2) Sucking stimulates milk production.
      3) Supplementing with bottle may decrease production.
   c. Engorgement
      1) About 48 hr postpartum
      2) May cause slight rise in temperature
      3) Non-lactating clients
         a) Avoid nipple stimulation
         b) Cold compress
         c) Cabbage leaves
         d) Medication
         e) Supportive bra
      4) Lactating clients
         a) Manually express some milk to facilitate latch
         b) Frequent feeding or pumping
         c) Warm shower
         d) Breast massage
         e) Supportive bra
         f) Medicate prior to nursing

Note: For engorgement breast feed every 2–3 hours. Immediately prior to breast feeding encourage a warm shower. Immediately after and between feeding use cold compresses or preferably ice cold cabbage leaves to breast.

Note: Know the differences between mastitis and engorgement.

4. Uterus
   a. Involution
      1) Firm
      2) Fundus near umbilicus after delivery
      3) Descends approximately 1 cm/day
      4) Breast-feeding enhances
      5) Full bladder impedes involution
         a) Location
            (1) Midline
   b. Subinvolution
      1) Massage
      2) Frequent voiding
      3) Oxytocin
   c. Lochia
      1) Color
         a) Rubra postpartum day 1–4
         b) Serosa postpartum day 4–9
         c) Alba 10 days to 6 weeks postpartum
      2) Amount
      3) Clots
      4) Odor

5) Increase
6) Return of menstruation
   a) Ovulation occurs prior to mensturation
   b) Non-lactating client: 6–8 weeks postpartum
   c) Fully lactating client: may be up to 6 months
   d) Need for birth control

5. Perineum
   a. Assess tears, episiotomy, bruising, hematoma using REEDA:
      1) **R**edness
      2) **E**dema
      3) **E**cchymosis
      4) **D**rainage
      5) **A**pproximation
   b. Comfort and healing
      1) Cold compress first 24 hr
      2) Sitz bath
      3) Positioning
      4) Perineal hygiene
      5) Kegel exercises
      6) Medication
         a) Oral
         b) Topical
         c) Stool softener

6. Bladder
   a. Retention
      1) Assess intake and blood loss.
      2) Assist with frequent urination.
      3) Provide noninvasive measures to promote urination.
      4) Perform bladder scan.
      5) If retention persists, catheterize.

7. Bowel
   a. Bowels move in 1–2 days.
   b. Assess for hemorrhoids.
      1) Promote Fiber, activity, fluids
      2) Stool softener
      3) Hygiene
      4) Sitz
      5) Topical anesthetic

8. Edema
   a. Know prenatal amount.
   b. Oxytocin used during or after labor may increase edema.

9. Deep vein thrombosis
   a. Encourage early ambulation.
   b. Assess pain, redness.
   c. Homans are not recommended.
   d. Doppler study is recommended.

10. Infection
    a. Temperature normally elevated to 38° C (100.4° F) after delivery.
    b. WBCs normally elevated to 20,000–25,000/mm^3.
    c. Do not assume "normal."
    d. Assess possible sources of infection:
       1) Perineum
       2) Uterus
       3) Bladder
       4) Lungs
       5) Breasts
          a) Mastitis

B. Assess Emotional Status
1. Level of consciousness
   a. Change may be first sign of hemorrhage
2. Self-concept
3. Bonding
   a. Initial contact within 30–60 min after birth
   b. Client exploration of infant
      1) Fingertips, then palms
      2) Extremities, then trunk
      3) En face
   c. Paternal bonding: engrossment
   d. Collaborative Care
      1) Provide time immediately after birth for bonding.
      2) Minimize pain, fatigue, hunger to enhance bonding.
      3) Describe newborn behaviors.
4. Maternal role: Reva Rubin (see table)

Maternal Role

Phase of Maternal Adjustment	Characteristics	Collaborative Care
Taking in	24–48 hr after birth: dependent, passive; focuses on own needs; excited, talkative	Assist with cares; provide comfort, nutrition, hygiene; listen; review labor and delivery
Taking hold	2nd–10th day postpartum, or up to several weeks: focuses on maternal role and care of newborn; eager to learn; may develop blues	Provide teaching, written material, follow-up appointments, community resources; assess emotional status, discuss blues
Letting go	Focuses on family and individual roles	Assess progress; discuss community resources

5. Postpartum blues and depression (see table)

Postpartum Blues and Depression

	Postpartum Blues	Postpartum Depression
Contributing Factors	Fatigue, hormonal changes, role change, family tension, finances	History of depression*; poverty; single client; unwanted pregnancy; low support systems; newborn health problems
Occurrence	50–80% of postpartum clients	10–15% of postpartum clients
Onset	First 1–10 days postpartum	Up to 1 year or more after delivery; may persist for years
Signs/ Symptoms	Emotionally labile	Persistent depression; overwhelmed; anxious; hopeless; unable to care for self and/or infant; thoughts of suicide
Collaborative Care	Discuss with client and partner: sleep, accept help with newborn, simplify, nutrition, community resources	Discuss with client and partner: seek assistance from community resources. This is a serious problem and needs rapid intervention.

*Note: Medications used to treat depression, such as SSRIs, are frequently Category C or D drugs and may be discontinued during pregnancy. The nurse ensures that the medications are resumed as needed after delivery.

SECTION 7

At-Risk Postpartum Care

A. Hemorrhage: Blood loss of > 500 mL with vaginal delivery or > 1000 mL with C-section

  1. Contributing Factors

    a. Grand multigravida

    b. Macrosomia

    c. Prolonged labor

    d. Rapid labor

    e. Multiple gestation

    f. Forceps

    g. Retained placenta

  2. Manifestations

    a. Saturation of 1 pad or more per hour

    b. Large clots

    c. Formation of hematomas

    d. Boggy fundus

    e. Change in level of consciousness

 3. **NURSING INTERVENTIONS**

    a. Massage boggy fundus.

    b. Encourage frequent urination.

    c. Administer oxytocin.

    d. Remove retained placenta or repair laceration.

B. Rh Incompatibility (see RhoGAM table)

RhoGAM

Mother	Baby	Maternal Coombs	RhoGAM given?
Rh+	Rh+	Not checked	No
Rh+	Rh–	Not checked	No
Rh–	Rh+	Negative	Yes
Rh–	Rh+	Positive	No
Rh–	Rh–	Not checked	No

 1. **NURSING INTERVENTIONS**

    a. Observe newborn for hyperbilirubinemia.

    b. Teach mother about Rh, RhoGAM.

      1) Prevents, does not reverse, formation of antibodies

      2) Given prenatally with any invasive procedure, at 28 weeks, and after delivery

    c. Administer RhoGAM.

      1) Rho(D) immune globulin

      2) IM

      3) Given within 72 hr after delivery

    d. If client requires immunizations such as rubella, it is okay to give.

      1) Recommend follow–up titer.

C. Thromboembolic Disorder

  1. Contributing Factors

    a. Increased clotting factors postpartum

    b. Immobility

    c. Pelvic pressure during labor/delivery

    d. History of thrombosis, varicosities, heart disease

  2. Manifestations

    a. Pain, heat, redness in affected leg

 3. **NURSING INTERVENTIONS**

    a. Assess extremities including peripheral pulses, measuring and comparing circumferences of both legs.

    b. Homan's sign is not recommended.

    c. Venous Doppler if preferred to rule out DVTs. If DVT is suspected:

      1) Bed rest

      2) Elevation of affected extremity

      3) Anti-thrombolytic stocking to unaffected leg

      4) Anticoagulant

Newborn Care

The Newborn (neonatal) period begins at birth and ends after 28 days of life. The newborn adapts to life without the support of the placenta and amniotic fluid.

A. Initial Care: Immediately after birth

1. Airway, Breathing, Circulation

2. Thermoregulation

3. Umbilical Cord

   a. Inspect the newborn's umbilical cord for two arteries and one vein. Observe for any bleeding from the cord, and ensure that the cord is clamped securely to prevent hemorrhage.

4. Apgar

   a. Assess

Five categories	0	1	2
Heart rate	Absent	Slow < 100	> 100
Respiratory effort	Absent	Slow weak cry	Good cry
Muscle tone	Flaccid	Some flexion of extremities	Well flexed extremities
Reflex irritability	No response	Grimace	Cry
Color	Blue, pale	Centrally pink with blue extremities	Completely pink

   b. Ratings
      1) 7–10 is within normal limits with no need for resuscitation
      2) 4–6 is moderately distressed
      3) 0–3 is severely distressed

5. Vital signs

Assessment	Normal Findings	Normal variations	Deviations from normal	NURSING INTER–VENTIONS
Heart Rate	120–160 bpm	100 bpm sleeping 180 bpm when crying	Persistent Tachycardia ≥ 160 bpm Persistent Bradycardia ≤ 120 bpm	Assess apical pulse for a full minute. Assess all pulses bilaterally should be equal and strong
Respirations	40 breaths per minute		Bradypnea: less than 25/min Tachypnea: greater than 60/min	Assess rate, rhythm, and adventious breath sounds .Respirations will often be shallow and irregular in the newborn. Note any signs of distress. Nasal flaring grunting, intercostal retractions or see-saw breathing
Temperature	Axillary 37° C	36.5–37.2° C	Temperature not stabilized after 10 hours	Take measure to prevent heat loss. Keep dry, head covered, avoid placing infant near air vents. Place infant under radiant warmer or encourage skin to skin contact with mother
Blood Pressure	60–80/40–50	Variations occur with crying or sleeping	**Hypotension** = Potential sepsis or hypovolemic. **Hypertension** = Potential coarctation of aorta	Usually only checked if a problem is suspected. Check arm and leg- significant differences between the lower and upper extremities can be an indication of coarctation of the arteries

NOTE: Rectal temperatures are contraindicated.

6. Umbilical Cord

   a. Inspect the newborn's umbilical cord for two arteries and one vein. Observe for any bleeding from the cord, and ensure that the cord is clamped securely to prevent hemorrhage.

B. Newborn Physical Assessment

Newborn Physical Assessment

Assessment Area	Findings
Posture	General flexion Spontaneous movement
Head	Circumference 2–5 cm > chest circumference **Fontanels** • Posterior:Triangle shape, Closes 8–12 weeks • Anterior: Diamond shape, Closes at 18 weeks, Pulse visible • Observe for bulge or depression **Shape** • Molding • Caput succedaneum • Cephalhematoma
Eyes	Vision best within 12 inches Strabismus; pseudo strabismus Subconjunctival hemorrhage Congenital cataracts
Ears	Responds to voice and other sounds Assess for low-set ears
Nose	Patent nares Preferential nose breather
Skin	Pink Acrocyanosis Erythema Jaundice Hyperpigmentations Milia Café au lait spots; giraffe spots Nevus flammeus (port wine stains) Nevus flammeus nuchae (stork bite Vernix Lanugo
Mouth	Symmetry of lip movement Soft/hard palate intact Epstein pearls
Chest	Symmetrical chest movement Clavicles intact Nipples prominent, well prormed Nipple buds are sign of maturity
Abdomen	Umbilical cord Liver may be palpable
Musculo-skeletal	Evaluate joints for full range of motion Note presence of asymmetrical gluteal folds Spine straight and easily flexed
Genitalia	Female: prominent labia, pseudomenstruation Male: scrotum large, palpable testes on each side, meatus at tip of penis, foreskin
GI/GU	Voiding within 24 hours Meconium passed 24-48 hr after birth

Reflex	Expected Finding	Expected Age
Sucking and rooting reflex	• This reflex is elicited by stroking the newborn's cheek or edge of his mouth. When this is done, the newborn turns his head toward the side that is touched and starts to suck.	Birth to 4 months
Palmar grasp	• This reflex is elicited by placing an object in the newborn's palm. The newborn will grasp the object.	Birth to 6 months
Plantar grasp	• This reflex is elicited by touching the sole of the newborn's foot. The newborn responds by curling his toes downward.	Birth to 8 months
Moro reflex (startle)	• This reflex is elicited by striking a flat surface that the newborn is lying on, or allowing the head and trunk of the newborn in a semisitting position to fall backward to an angle of at least 30°. The newborn's arms and legs symmetrically extend and then abduct while his fingers spread to form a "C".	Birth to 4 months
Tonic neck reflex (fencer position)	• The newborn will extend his arm and leg on the side when his head is turned to that side with flexion of his arm and leg of the opposite side. • The newborn will turn his head to one side. The newborn will respond by extending his arm and leg on that side, and flex his arm and leg on the opposite side.	Birth to 3 to 4 months

1. Periods of Reactivity
   a. In the **first 6–8 hr** of life as the newborn's body systems stabilize and pass through periods of adjustment, observe for periods of reactivity in the newborn.
      1) **First period of reactivity**: The newborn is alert and exhibits exploring activity, makes sucking sounds, and has a rapid heartbeat and respiratory rate. Heart rate may be as high as 160–180/min, but will stabilize at a baseline of 100–120/min that lasts 15–30 min after birth.
      2) **Period of relative inactivity**: The newborn will become quiet and begin rest and sleep. The newborn's heart rate and respirations will decrease, and this period will last from 30 min to 2 hr after birth.
      3) **Second period of reactivity**: The newborn reawakens, becomes responsive again, and often gags and chokes on mucus that has accumulated in his mouth. This period usually occurs 2–8 hr after birth and may last 10 min to several hr.

C. Gestational Age Assessment

1. Contributing Factors: Early assessment allows early observations and interventions for premature and postmature newborns.
2. Manifestations
   a. Physical Components
      1) Skin
      2) Lanugo
      3) Plantar surfaces
      4) Breast
      5) Eye/ear
      6) Genitals
   b. Neuromuscular
      1) Posture
      2) Square window
      3) Arm recoil
      4) Popliteal angle
      5) Scarf sign
      6) Heel to ear
3. Medications of Newborn Care
   a. Eye prophylaxis
      1) Erythromycin or tetracycline
   b. Vitamin K (Aquamephyton) IM
   c. Hepatitis vaccine
4. Diagnostic and Therapeutic Procedures Following Birth
   a. Cord blood: ABO blood type and Rh-status if the mother's blood type is "O" or she is Rh-negative.
   b. CBC (anemia, polycythemia, infection, or clotting problems).
   c. Glucose level
   d. Serum bilirubin
   e. Newborn genetic screening
   f. PKU
   g. Newborn hearing screening
5. Collaborative Care

   a. **NURSING INTERVENTIONS**
      1) Monitor for signs and symptoms of respiratory complications.
      2) Promote patent airway
         a) Routine and prn suctioning of the mouth and nasal passages with a *bulb syringe*

Note: When using bulb syringe remember M before N

Note: Newborns delivered by cesarean birth are more susceptible to fluid remaining in the lungs than newborns who were delivered vaginally.

      3) The newborn's naal passages are suctioned one nostril at a time.
      4) If bulb suctioning is unsuccessful, mechanical suction may be needed.
   b. Promoting thermoregulation of the newborn
      1) Maintain abody temperature of 36.5°C (97.7°F) axillary.
      2) Prevent heat loss.
      3) Monitor glucose levels.

Note: Identify potential risks and prevent heat loss: by evaporation, conduction, convection, radiant.

   c. Nutrition
      1) Initiate feedings immediately after birth (Breasts or Formula)
         a) Maintain a fluid intake of 100–140 mL/kg/24 hr.
         b) Monitor for normal weight gain (both breast milk and formula provide 20 kcal/oz.)

   d. **NURSING INTERVENTIONS** to promote successful breast-feeding
      1) Explain breast-feeding techniques to the mother. Have the mother wash her hands, get comfortable, and have fluids to drink during breast-feeding.
      2) Offer the newborn the breast immediately after birth and frequently thereafter.
      3) Explain the let down reflex (stimulation of maternal nipple releases oxytocin that causes the letdown of milk).
      4) Reassure the mother that uterine cramps are normal during breast-feeding, resulting from oxytocin.
      5) Express a few drops of colostrum or milk and spread it over the nipple to lubricate the nipple and entice the newborn.

6) Show the mother the proper latch-on position. Have her support the breast in one hand with the thumb on top and four fingers underneath. With the newborn's mouth in front of the nipple, the newborn can be stimulated to his mouth by tickling his lower lip with the tip of the nipple. The mother pulls the newborn to the nipple with his mouth covering part of the areola as well as the nipple.

e. Formula-feeding
1) Feed every 3–4 hr.
2) **NURSING INTERVENTIONS** to promote successful formula feeding
   a) Always hold the bottle and never prop it.
   b) The newborn should not be placed in the supine position during bottle-feeding because of the danger of aspiration
   c) Show the parents how to cradle the newborn in their arms in a semi-upright position.
   d) Newborns who are formula-fed do best when held close and at a 45-degree angle.
   e) Teach the parents how to prepare formula, bottles, and nipples.
   f) Teach the parents about the different forms of formula (ready-to-feed, concentrated, and powder) and how to prepare each correctly.
   g) Teach the parents to check the flow of formula from the bottle to assure it is not coming out too slow or too fast.
   h) Instruct the mother how to place the nipple on top of the newborn's tongue.
   i) Keep the nipple filled with formula to prevent the newborn from swallowing air.
   j) Newborns should be burped several times during a feeding, usually after each ½ to 1 oz of formula or breast milk.
   k) Place the newborn in a supine position after feedings.
   l) Tell the parents to discard any unused formula remaining in the bottle when the newborn is finished feeding due to the possibility of bacterial contamination.

f. Closely monitor the newborn's elimination habits.
1) Document number of voids and stools.
2) Monitor and document the newborn's numer of voidings and stools
3) Keep the perineal area of the newborn clean and dry.
4) Prevent infection.
   a) Newborns should have their own bassinet equipped with a thermometer, diapers, T-shirts, and bathing supplies.
5) All personnel caring for a newborn should follow strict infection control policies

6) Cord care: Cleanse with neutral pH cleanser and sterile water. The cord should be kept clean and dry to prevent infection.

Note: Cleansing of the umbilical cord with a neutral pH cleanser and sterile water is the most current EBP according to AWHONN.

g. First bath
1) After temperature stabilizes

Note: Nurses should wear gloves handling baby until after the infants bath.

h. Bonding
1) Encourage mothers and family to hold the newborn in order to promote successful bonding ion.
i. Promote safety and security for the newborn and family
1) Verify that identification wristbands are correctly placed according to facilityprotocol.
2) Each time the newborn is taken to the parents, the identification band should be verified against the mother's identification band.
3) All facility staff who assist in caring for the newborn are required to wear identification badges.
j. Circumcision
1) Ensure consent form is signed
2) Monitor for complications
3) Promote healing
6. Client Education
a. Safety
1) Positioning and holding
2) Thermoregulation
3) Nutrtion and weight gain
4) Elimination
5) Cord care
6) Circumcision care
7) Newborn behaviors
8) Car seats
9) Oral and Nasal suctioning
10) Sudden infant death syndrome
11) Signs of illness to report
12) Newborn Follow up care and immunization schedule

Complications of Newborn Care

This section highlights the assessment and management of newborn complications. Assessment, risk factors, collaborative care, and desired client outcomes will be discussed. It is essential for a nurse to immediately identify complications and implement appropriate interventions. Ongoing emotional support to a client and significant other is also imperative to the plan of care. The following contributing factors will be detailed in this section:

- Neonatal substance withdrawal
- Hypoglycemia
- Respiratory distress syndrome (RDS)
- Asphyxia/meconium aspiration
- Preterm newborn
- Small for gestational age (SGA)
- Large for gestational age (LGA)/macrocosmic
- Post-term newborn
- Neonatal infection/sepsis (sepsis neonatorum)
- Birth trauma or injury
- Hyperbilirubinemia
- Congenital anomalies

A. Maternal substance abuse during pregnancy consists of any use of alcohol or drugs.

1. Contributing Factors

   a. Intrauterine drug exposure can cause anomalies, neurobehavioral changes, and signs of withdrawal in the neonate.

   b. These changes depend on a specific drug or combination of drugs used, dosage, route of administration, metabolism and excretion by the mother and her fetus, timing of drug exposure, and the length of drug exposure.

B. Fetal alcohol syndrome (FAS)

1. Contributing Factors

   a. Results from the chronic or periodic intake of alcohol during pregnancy.

   b. Alcohol is considered teratogenic, so the daily intake of alcohol increases the risk of FAS.

2. Manifestations associated with FAS

   a. Subjective data
      1) Feeding problems
      2) Central nervous system dysfunction (mental retardation, cerebral palsy)
      3) Behavioral difficulties such as hyperactivity
      4) Language abnormalities
      5) Delayed growth and development
      6) Poor maternal-newborn bonding

   b. Objective data: Monitor the neonate for signs and symptoms of abstinence syndrome (withdrawal) and increased wakefulness using the neonatal abstinence scoring system that assesses for and scores the following:
      1) CNS
         a) Increased wakefulness
         b) A high-pitched, shrill cry, incessant crying
         c) Irritability, tremors
         d) Hyperactive with an increased Moro reflex
         e) Increased deep-tendon reflexes, increased muscle tone
         f) Seizures
         g) Developmental delays and neurologic abnormalities
         h) Prenatal and postnatal growth retardation
         i) Sleep disturbances
      2) Skin
         a) Abrasions and/or excoriations on the face and knees
      3) Metabolic, vasomotor, and respiratory findings
         a) Nasal congestion with flaring
         b) Frequent yawning, skin mottling
         c) Tachypnea greater than 60/min
         d) Sweating and a temperature greater than 37.2° C (99° F)
      4) Gastrointestinal
         a) Poor feeding, regurgitation (projectile vomiting)
         b) Diarrhea, and excessive, uncoordinated, and constant sucking
      5) Facial anomalies
         a) Eyes with epicanthal folds, strabismus, and ptosis
         b) Mouth with a poor suck, small teeth, and cleft lip or palate
      6) Deafness
      7) Abnormal palmar creases and irregular hair
      8) Vital organ anomalies
         a) Such as heart defects, including atrial and ventricular septal defects, tetralogy of Fallot, and patent-ductus arteriosus

C. Tobacco

1. Contributing Factors

   a. Use of tobacco during pregnancy

2. Manifestations

   a. Prematurity, low birth weight

   b. Increased risk for sudden infant death syndrome

   c. Increased risk for bronchitis, pneumonia

   d. Developmental delays

3. Medications

    a. Phenobarbital (Solfoton): anticonvulsant

        1) It is prescribed to decrease CNS irritability and control seizures for neonates who have alcohol or opioid addiction.

4. Diagnostic Procedures

    a. Laboratory tests: Blood tests should be done to differentiate between neonatal drug withdrawal and central nervous system irritability.

        1) CBC

        2) Blood glucose

        3) Calcium

        4) Magnesium

        5) TSH, T_4, T_3

        6) Drug screen of urine or meconium to reveal the agent abused by the mother

        7) Hair analysis

    b. Diagnostic Procedures

        1) Chest x-ray for FAS to rule out congenital heart defects

5. Collaborative Care

     a. **NURSING INTERVENTIONS** for maternal substance abuse and neonatal effects or withdrawal include the following in addition to normal newborn care.

        1) Perform a neonatal abstinence scoring system assessment, as ordered by the provider.

        2) Elicit and assess the newborn's reflexes.

        3) Monitor the newborn's ability to feed and digest intake.

        4) Monitor the newborn's fluids and electrolytes such as skin turgor, mucous membranes, fontanels, and I&O.

        5) Observe the infant's behavior.

        6) Assess IV site frequently.

        7) Check for any medication incompatibilities.

        8) Reduce external stimuli.

        9) Swaddle the newborn to reduce self-stimulation and protect the skin from abrasions.

        10) Administer frequent, small feedings of high-calorie formula—may need gavage feedings. Elevate the infant's head during and following feedings, and burp the infant to reduce vomiting and aspiration.

        11) Try various nipples to compensate for a poor suck reflex.

        12) Have suction available to reduce the risk for aspiration.

        13) For newborns who are addicted to cocaine, avoid eye contact and use vertical rocking and a pacifier.

        14) Prevent infection.

        15) Initiate a consult with child protective services.

        16) Consult lactation services to evaluate if breastfeeding is contraindicated or desired.

D. Hypoglycemia: A serum glucose level of less than 40 mg/dL. Routine assessment of all newborns, especially newborns who are LGA and SGA, should include observing for symptoms of hypoglycemia.

1. Contributing Factors

    a. Maternal diabetes mellitus

    b. Preterm infant

    c. LGA or SGA

    d. Stress at birth, such as cold stress and asphyxia

    e. Maternal epidural anesthesia

2. Manifestations

    a. Objective data: physical assessment findings

        1) Poor feeding

        2) Jitteriness/tremors

        3) Hypothermia

        4) Diaphoresis

        5) Weak shrill cry

        6) Lethargy

        7) Flaccid muscle tone

        8) Seizures/coma

        9) Irregular respirations

        10) Cyanosis

        11) Apnea

3. Diagnostic Laboratory Tests and Diagnostic Procedures

    a. Two consecutive plasma glucose levels less than 40 mg/dL in a newborn who is term, and less than 25 mg/dL in a newborn who is preterm

4. Collaborative Care

     a. **NURSING INTERVENTIONS**

        1) Obtain blood per heel stick for glucose monitoring.

        2) Provide frequent oral and/or gavage feedings or continuous parenteral nutrition early after birth to treat hypoglycemia.

        3) Monitor the neonate's blood glucose level closely per facility protocol

        4) Monitor IV if the neonate is unable to orally feed.

E. Respiratory Distress Syndrome (RDS)/Asphyxia/ Meconium Aspiration: RDS occurs as a result of surfactant deficiency in the lungs and is characterized by poor gas exchange and ventilatory failure. Surfactant is a phospholipid that assists in alveoli expansion. Surfactant keeps alveoli from collapsing and allows gas exchange to occur.

1. Contributing Factors

    a. Preterm gestation

    b. Perinatal asphyxia (meconium staining, cord prolapse, and nuchal cord)

    c. Maternal diabetes mellitus

    d. Premature rupture of membranes

    e. Maternal use of barbiturates or narcotics close to birth

f. Maternal hypotension

g. Cesarean birth without labor

h. Hydrops fetalis (massive edema of the fetus caused by hyperbilirubinemia)

i. Maternal bleeding during the third trimester

2. Manifestations: Physical Assessment

   a. Objective data

     1) Tachypnea (respiratory rate greater than 60/min)

     2) Nasal flaring

     3) Expiratory grunting

     4) Intercostal and substernal retractions

     5) Labored breathing

     6) Fine rales on auscultation

     7) Cyanosis

     8) Unresponsiveness, flaccidity, and apnea with decreased breath sounds (signs and symptoms of worsened RDS)

3. Diagnostic Procedures and Laboratory Tests

   a. Culture and sensitivity of the blood, urine, and cerebrospinal fluid

   b. Blood glucose and serum calcium

   c. ABGs reveal hypercapnia (excess of carbon dioxide in the blood) and respiratory or mixed acidosis.

   d. Chest x-ray

F. Preterm Newborn: A preterm newborn's birth occurs after 20 weeks of gestation and before 37 weeks of gestation. This may occur once the cervix has dilated to 4 cm.

1. Contributing Factors

   a. Maternal gestational hypertension

   b. Multiple pregnancies

   c. Adolescent pregnancy

   d. Lack of prenatal care

   e. Substance abuse

   f. Smoking

   g. Previous history of preterm delivery

   h. Abnormalities of the uterus

   i. Cervical incompetence

   j. Premature rupture of the membranes

   k. Placenta previa

   l. Premature labor

   m. Premature rupture of membranes

2. Manifestations: Physical Assessment

   a. Objective data

     1) A Ballard assessment shows a physical and neurological assessment totaling less than 37 weeks of gestation.

     2) Periodic breathing consists of 5- to 10-second respiratory pauses, followed by 10- to 15-second compensatory rapid respirations.

     3) Signs of increased respiratory effort and/or respiratory distress include nasal flaring or retractions of the chest wall during inspirations, expiratory grunting, and tachypnea.

     4) Apnea is a pause in respirations longer than 10 to 15 sec.

     5) The newborn has a low birth weight.

     6) The newborn has minimal subcutaneous fat deposits.

     7) The newborn's head is large in comparison to his body.

     8) The newborn has wrinkled features.

     9) The newborn's skull and rib cage feel soft.

     10) The newborn's eyes are closed if he is born at 22 to 24 weeks of gestation.

     11) The newborn has a weak grasp reflex.

     12) The newborn has an inability to coordinate suck and swallow, and a weak or absent gag, suck, and cough reflex; weak swallow.

     13) The newborn has hypotonic muscles, decreased level of activity, and a weak cry for more than 24 hr.

     14) The newborn is lethargic, is experiencing tachycardia, and has poor weight gain.

G. Post-term Infant

1. Contributing Factors

   a. Postmature infant: gestational age of more than 42 weeks

2. Manifestations: Physical Assessment

   a. Dry, parchment-like skin

   b. Longer, harder nails

   c. Profuse scalp hair

   d. Absent vernix

   e. Hypoglycemia

3. Complications

   a. Progressive aging of placenta

   b. Difficult delivery

   c. High perinatal mortality

   d. Jaundice (hyperbilirubinemia)

H. Physiological Jaundice: Not observed in the newborn during the first 24 hr; usually appears by the third day

1. Contributing Factors

   a. Due to an immature liver

   b. Bruising

   c. ABO-incompatibility (mother is O, newborn is A, B, or AB)

   d. Rh-incompatibility (erythroblastosis fetalis)

     1) A mother who is Rh-negative and has a newborn who is Rh-positive

     2) Kernicterus (bilirubin encephalopathy) can lead to brain damage, anemia, and/or hepatosplenomegaly

2. Manifestations

  a. Yellowish tint to skin, sclera, and mucous membranes.

  b. To verify jaundice, press the infant's skin on the cheek or abdomen lightly with one finger. Then, release pressure and observe the infant's skin color for yellowish tint as the skin is blanched.

  c. Note the time of jaundice onset to distinguish between physiologic and pathologic jaundice.

  d. Assess the underlying cause by reviewing the maternal prenatal, family, and newborn history.

3. Diagnostic and Laboratory Procedures

  a. An elevated serum bilirubin level may occur (direct and indirect bilirubin).

  b. Monitor the infant's bilirubin levels every 4 hr until the level returns to normal.

  c. Assess maternal and newborn blood type to determine if there is a presence of ABO-incapability. This occurs if the newborn has blood type A, B, or AB, and the mother is type O.

  d. Review Hgb and Hct.

  e. A direct Coombs' test reveals the presence of antibody-coated (sensitized) Rh-positive RBCs in the newborn.

  f. Check electrolyte levels for dehydration from phototherapy.

  g. Transcutaneous bilirubin level is a noninvasive method to measure an infant's.

 4. **NURSING INTERVENTIONS**

  a. Phototherapy, sunlight, and/or exchange transfusion is administered to the newborn.

  b. Observe the infant's skin and mucous membranes for signs of jaundice.

  c. Monitor the infant's vital signs.

  d. Maintain an eye mask over the newborn's eyes for protection of corneas and retinas.

  e. Keep the newborn undressed with the exception of a male newborn. A surgical mask should be placed (make like a bikini) over the genitalia to prevent possible testicular damage from heat and light waves. Be sure to remove the metal strip from the mask to prevent burning.

  f. Avoid applying lotions or ointments to the infant because they absorb heat and can cause burns.

  g. Remove the newborn from phototherapy every 4 hr and unmask the newborn's eyes, checking for signs of inflammation or injury.

  h. Reposition the newborn every 2 hr to expose all of the body surfaces to the phototherapy lights and prevent pressure sores. Check the lamp energy with a photometer per unit protocol.

  i. Turn off the phototherapy lights before drawing blood for testing.

  j. Observe the newborn for side effects of phototherapy.

    1) Bronze discoloration: not a serious complication

    2) Maculopapular skin rash: not a serious complication

    3) Development of pressure areas

    4) Dehydration (poor skin turgor, dry mucous membranes, decreased urinary output)

    5) Elevated temperature

  k. Monitor elimination and daily weights, watching for signs of dehydration.

  l. Check the newborn's axillary temperature every 4 hr during phototherapy, because temperature may become elevated.

  m. Feed the newborn early and frequently—every 3 to 4 hr. This will promote bilirubin excretion in the stools.

  n. Continue to breast-feed the newborn. Supplementing with formula may be prescribed.

  o. Maintain adequate fluid intake to prevent dehydration.

  p. Reassure the parents that most newborns experience some degree of jaundice.

  q. Explain hyperbilirubinemia, its causes, diagnostic tests, and treatment to parents.

  r. Explain that the newborn's stool contains some bile that will be loose and green. Administer an exchange transfusion for infants who are at risk for kernicterus.

SECTION 10
Reproductive Health Nursing

A. Contraception: refers to strategies or devices used to reduce the risk of fertilization or implantation in an attempt to prevent pregnancy

1. A nurse should assess a client's need/desire for contraception. In addition, a thorough discussion of benefits, risks, and alternatives of each method should be discussed.

2. A client's preference for contraception should be considered. The decision may be individual. Methods of contraception include natural-family planning, barrier, hormonal, and intrauterine methods, as well as surgical procedures.

3. Sexual partners often make a joint decision regarding a desired preference (vasectomy or tubal ligation). Postpartum discharge instructions should include thediscussion of future contraceptive plans.

4. Expected outcomes for family planning methods consist of preventing pregnancy until a desired time.

5. Nurses should support clients in making the decision that is best for their individualized situations.

6. Refer to tables in Pharmacology: Contraception-Forms of Contraception (see tables).

B. Infertility: An inability to conceive despite engaging in unprotected sexual intercourse for a period of at least 12 months

1. Contributing Factors

   a. Decreased sperm production

   b. Endometriosis

   c. Ovulation disorders

   d. Tubal occlusions

2. Factors Associated with Physical Inability to Conceive

   a. Expense

   b. Impact on the couple's relationship

   c. Lack of family support

3. Diagnostic Procedures

   a. Infertility procedures

   1) **Semen collection:** A procedure in which semen is collected from the man in a sterile collection device and evaluated and analyzed

      a) In 40% of couples who are infertile, inability to conceive is due to male infertility. Therefore, this infertility test is a preferred starting point in evaluating a couple. It costs less and is less invasive compared to female infertility testing. More than one sample may need to be provided.

   2) **Pelvic examination:** Monitor for uterine or vaginal anomalies. The nurse should position a client on the exam table and have equipment and supplies prepared for the primary care provider.

   3) **Ultrasonography:** A transvaginal or abdominal ultrasound procedure performed to visualize female reproductive organs.

   4) **Hysterosalpingography:** Radiological procedure that is outpatient where dye is used to assess the patency of the fallopian tubes. The nurse should obtain the client's history of allergies to iodine and seafood.

   5) **Hysteroscopy:** A radiographic procedure where the uterus is examined for signs of defect, distortion, or scar tissue that may impair successful impregnation.

   6) **Laparoscopy:** A procedure where gas insufflation is used to observe internal organs. This procedure may cause post-procedural pain. General anesthesia is required for this procedure.

4. Collaborative Care

   a. Perform Infertility Assessment

    b. **NURSING INTERVENTIONS** for Infertility

   1) Encourage couples to express and discuss their feelings.

   2) Monitor for side effects associated with medications to treat female and male infertility.

3) Advise that the use of medications to treat female infertility may increase the risk of multiple births by more than 25%.

4) Provide information regarding assisted reproductive therapies

c. Referrals to Support Groups

   1) Genetic counseling

C. Vaginal Infections

1. **Candidiasis (thrush):** A fungal infection of any of the Candida species of which *Candida albicans* is the most common. Encompasses infections that range from superficial, such as oral thrush and vaginitis, to systemic and potentially life-threatening diseases.

   a. Contributing Factors

   1) Use of oral contraceptives, frequent use of antibiotics, and frequent douching; diabetes mellitus and immunosuppression

   b. Manifestations

   1) A cheese-like discharge, itching, and discomfort; discomfort on urination and during intercourse

   c. Collaborative Care and **NURSING INTERVENTIONS**

   1) Administer miconazole (Monistat) or fluconazole (Diflucan).

   2) Discuss the importance of cleanliness and perineal care with the client.

   3) Ensure that both partners are treated.

2. **Trichomoniasis:** An infection caused by the single-celled protozoan parasite, *Trichomonas vaginalis.* The vagina is the most common site of infection in women, and the urethra is the most common site of infection in men.

   a. Contributing Factors

   1) The parasite is transmitted sexually through penis-to-vagina intercourse or vulva-to-vulva contact with an infected partner.

   2) Women can acquire the disease from infected men or women, but men usually contract it only from infected women.

   b. Manifestations

   1) Yellow, green, or gray discharge; discomfort with urination and intercourse; irritation and itching

   c. Collaborative Care and **NURSING INTERVENTIONS**

   1) Administer metronidazole (Flagyl) unless the client is in her first trimester of pregnancy.

   2) Treat both sexual partners and instruct them to abstain from sexual intercourse during treatment.

3. **Condyloma:** Genital warts, also known as vene-real warts

    a. Contributing Factors

       1) Condyloma is one of the most common types of STDs. Genital warts affect the moist tissues of the genital area. The virus that causes genital warts is the human papillomavirus, which has also been associated with cervical cancer.

    b. Manifestations

       1) Small, flesh-colored or gray swellings in the genital area; warts can clump together and take on a cauliflower shape; itching or discomfort in the genital area; bleeding may occur with intercourse

c. Collaborative Care and **NURSING INTERVENTIONS**

    1) Provide education related to risk factors, such as having unprotected sex with multiple partners, having had another STD, and/or becoming sexually active at a young age.

    2) Administer medications such as indicated (Aldara) and podophyllin (Condylox).

Sexually Transmitted Diseases

STD	Symptoms in Women	Symptoms in Men	Complications	Treatments
Chlamydia: Symptoms may appear 7–28 days after infection.	• Vaginal discharge • Vaginal bleeding • Painful/frequent urination • Abdominal pain • Fever/nausea	• White, watery penile discharge • Painful/frequent urination • Swollen/tender testicles	• Can pass to sexual partners and to neonate during childbirth • Damage to reproductive organs • Can lead to infertility in women and sterility in men	Caused by bacteria and can usually be cured with medication
Genital herpes: Symptoms may appear anytime after infection.	• Some have no symptoms • Blisters on mouth or genital region • Blisters last 7 to 21 days • Blisters can reoccur	• Some have no symptoms • Blisters on mouth or genital region • Blisters last 7–21 days • Blisters can reoccur	• There is no cure for herpes • Treatment is available • Can pass to sexual partners and to neonate during childbirth	• Caused by a virus • Antiviral medications are available to suppress herpes outbreaks
Gonorrhea: Symptoms may appear 2–21 days after infection.	• Yellow/gray vaginal discharge • Painful urination/bowel movement • Vaginal bleeding • Stomach cramps	• Yellow/green penile discharge • Painful urination/bowel movement • Frequent urination • Swollen/tender testicles	• Transmitted to sexual partner and to the neonate in uterus/during childbirth • Damage to reproductive organs • Can lead to infertility in women and sterility in men • Can cause heart problems, arthritis, and/or blindness	• Caused by bacteria and can usually be cured with medication • A health care professional can provide antibiotics to treat gonorrhea
HIV: Symptoms can appear months to several years after infection.	• Can be infected for several years without symptoms • Weight loss/fatigue • Recurring vaginal yeast infections • Diarrhea/flu-like symptoms • Oral thrush	• Can be infected for several years without symptoms • Weight loss/fatigue • Diarrhea/flu-like symptoms • Oral thrush	• There is no cure for HIV, but treatment is available • Can be passed by sex, sharing needles, to the fetus in uterus during childbirth, or during breast-feeding • Can cause several illnesses and can lead to death	• HIV is a virus and there is no cure • Medication is available to slow down the progression of HIV

(continues)

Sexually Transmitted Diseases (continued)

STD	Symptoms in Women	Symptoms in Men	Complications	Treatments
Human papillomavirus (HPV): There are more than 100 strains of HPV; some may cause genital warts and others have been linked to cancer (cervical, anal). Symptom appearance time varies.	• Genital warts: • Warts can reoccur • Itching/burning around the genitalia • Abnormal pap smear	• Genital warts – Warts can recur • Itching/burning around the genitalia	• There is no cure for HPV, but treatment is available • Can pass to sexual partners and neonate during childbirth • Warts can spread • Certain strains of HPV may lead to cancer	• HPV is a virus and there is no cure • Depending on the strain of HPV different treatment options are available

Pelvic inflammatory disease (PID): Several different bacteria can cause PID, and many cases have been related to chlamydia and gonorrhea. When pushed from the vagina and cervix higher into the female reproductive tract, bacteria can cause PID.	• Lower abdominal pain
	• Vaginal discharge
	• May have unpleasant odor
	• Painful intercourse/ urination
	• Vaginal bleeding
		• PID does not occur in males	• Can cause ectopic pregnancy (pregnancy in the fallopian tubes)
			• Can cause damage to the reproductive organs
			• May require surgery to treat
			• Can lead to infertility
			• May cause chronic pain in abdominal area
				• Depending on the severity of PID, the following may be used for treatment
				  – Antibiotics
				  – Hospitalization/bed rest
				  – Outpatient intensive treatment

Syphilis: There are three stages of syphilis. Stage 1 symptoms can appear 1 week to 3 months after infection.	• Stage 1
	  – Sore(s) on genitalia or mouth
	  – The sore(s) can last 2 to 6 weeks
	• Stage 2
	  – Rash on body
	  – Flu-like symptoms
	• Tertiary (last) Stage
	  – Neurological/ cardiovascular complications
		• Stage 1
		  – Sore(s) on genitalia or mouth
		  – The sore(s) can last 2–6 weeks
		• Stage 2
		  – Rash on body
		  – Flu-like symptoms
		• Tertiary (last) Stage
		  – Neurological/ cardiovascular complications
			• Can pass to sexual partners and to the neonate during pregnancy
			• May cause miscarriage in women
			• May cause heart disease, blindness, and/or brain damage
			• Can lead to death
				• Syphilis is caused by bacteria and may be cured
				• A health care professional may provide penicillin for syphilis
				• Other antibiotics may be available for individuals allergic to penicillin

Trichomoniasis (Trich): Symptoms can appear 3 days to 2 weeks after infection.	• Often no symptoms • Vaginal itching or • burning • Yellow/green/gray • vaginal discharge	• Often no symptoms • White, watery penile discharge • Painful/frequent urination	• Can pass to sexual partners • Continuation of unpleasant symptoms • Can lead to prostate infection in men	• Trich is caused by a parasite and may be cured • A health care professional may provide medication for trich

D. Cancer

1. **Cervical Cancer:** Forms in the tissue of the cervix

   a. Contributing Factors

     1) Human papillomavirus is responsible for most cervical cancer, and half of cervical cancer cases occur between the ages 35 and 55. A history of STDs, becoming sexually active at a young age, immunosuppression, and cigarette smoking are contributing factors.

     2) Many partners with initial sex before age 18

     3) History of STDs

     4) Immunosuppression

     5) Cigarette smoking

   b. Manifestations

     1) Abnormal bleeding

     2) Pelvic pain or pain during intercourse

   c. Diagnostic Screening

     1) Annual Pap smear

     2) HPV, DNA test

   d. Collaborative Care/Treatment

     1) Conization, laser surgery, loop electrocautery excision procedure, cryosurgery, hysterectomy, radiation, and/or chemotherapy

     2) Prevention

       a) Delay initial intercourse.

       b) Avoid smoking.

       c) Have fewer sexual partners.

       d) Gardasil (human papillomavirus quadrivalent) is a vaccine for ages 12–26 that is given as three injections over a 6-month period.

2. Endometrial Cancer: Originates in the cells of the endometrium and is often detected at an early stage, as it produces early vaginal bleeding between menstrual cycles or after menopause.

  a. Contributing Factors

    1) Obesity increases the risk three-fold for women who are 21 to 50 lb overweight

    2) Nulliparity

    3) Late menopause

  b. Manifestations

    1) Postmenopausal bleeding

    2) Abnormal bleeding

  c. Diagnostic Screening

    1) There is no specific diagnostic test.

    2) At the time of menopause, all women should be informed about the risks and symptoms of endometrial cancer.

    3) Report any unusual bleeding to the provider.

  d. Collaborative Care

    1) Radium

    2) X-ray therapy

    3) Hysterectomy

 e. **NURSING INTERVENTIONS**

    1) Assess the client for grieving.

    2) Provide preoperative teaching.

    3) Provide postoperative care.

    4) Assess the client's psychosexual needs.

3. Ovarian Cancer: Cancerous growth originating from different parts of the ovary.

  a. Contributing Factors

    1) Contributing factors are unknown.

    2) There is a high incidence with family history.

      a) Ovarian cancer is the fifth leading cause of cancer death after lung, breast, colorectal, and pancreatic.

      b) Mortality rates are greater in Caucasian women.

  b. Risk factors

    1) Age 50 and older

    2) One or more relatives has a history (mother, daughter, sister)

  c. Manifestations

    1) Early symptoms are not obvious.

    2) Later symptoms may include:

      a) Pressure or pain in the abdomen, pelvis, back, or legs

      b) A swollen or bloated abdomen, nausea and indigestion, constipation or diarrhea, fatigue, shortness of breath, frequent urination, and/or vaginal bleeding

  d. Diagnostic Screening

    1) CA 125 blood test: more than 35 u/mL is considered abnormal

    2) Intravaginal ultrasound

    3) Pelvic exam

  e. Collaborative Treatment

    1) Chemotherapy

    2) Radiation, surgery

4. Breast Cancer: Abnormal growth of breast tissue

  a. Contributing Factors

    1) Initial menses before age 12, initial menopause after age 51

      a) First pregnancy after age 35

      b) Did not breast-feed

      c) Never been pregnant

      d) Family history of breast cancer

      e) Overweight and sedentary lifestyle

      f) Long-term use of hormone replacement therapy

      g) Use of oral contraceptives

      h) Alcohol use greater than one drink per day

  b. Manifestations

    1) Lump in breast or armpit

    2) Thickening, dimpling, redness, pain, or asymmetry in breasts

    3) Pulling, discharge, or pain in nipple area

  c. Diagnostic Screening

    1) Mammogram: Women 40 and older should get a mammogram every 1–2 years.

    2) Clinical breast exam: Women should receive this exam annually.

    3) Breast self-exam: Women should perform this monthly, 1 week after menses.

  d. Treatment

    1) Surgery

    2) Chemotherapy

    3) Radiation

    4) Hormone therapy

E. Uterine Disorders

1. Myomas (uterine fibroids): Benign fibroid tumors of the uterine muscle

  a. Contributing Factors

    1) African Americans older than age 30 who have never been pregnant

  b. Manifestations

    1) Pelvic pain or pressure

    2) Hypermenorrhea

  c. Collaborative Treatment

    1) Medication

    2) Surgery

2. **Endometriosis:** Endometrial tissue located outside of the uterus.

   a. Contributing Factors

      1) May involve retrograde menstruation

      2) Hereditary factors

      3) Impaired immune function

   b. Manifestations

      1) Severe dysmenorrhea

      2) Lower abdominal pain, pain during intercourse, back and rectal pain

      3) Abnormal bleeding

   c. Collaborative Treatment

      1) Oral contraceptives (hormone therapy), surgery, or pregnancy

3. **Pelvic Inflammatory Disease:** An infection of the female reproductive organs, which usually occurs when sexually transmitted bacteria spread from the vagina to the upper genital tract

   a. Contributing Factors

      1) Infections

      2) Venereal disease

   b. Manifestations

      1) Vaginal discharge that is foul smelling, purulent

      2) Pain in abdomen, and/or the lower back

      3) Elevated temperature, nausea, and/or vomiting

      4) Complications

         a) Ectopic pregnancy

         b) Infertility

         c) Chronic pelvic pain.

   c. Treatment

      1) Antibiotics

      2) Treating all sexual partners

      3) Avoiding sexual intercourse until treatment is completed

       4) **NURSING INTERVENTIONS**

         a) Administer antibiotic therapy.

         b) Educate the client.

F. Menopause: Complete cessation of menstruation for 1 year

   1. Manifestations

      a. Hot flashes

      b. Palpitations

      c. Diaphoresis

      d. Osteoporosis

   2. Collaborative Care and **NURSING INTERVENTIONS**

      a. Assess the client's psychosocial response.

      b. Discuss the merits of estrogen therapy, including prevention of osteoporosis and heart disease.

      c. Use alternative therapies (diet, exercise, and/or calcium supplements).

UNIT SIX

Nursing Care of Children

SECTION 1

Foundations of Nursing Care of Children: Family-Centered Care

A. Family

1. Family is defined as what an individual considers it to be

2. Families are groups that should remain constant in children's lives

3. Positive family relationships are characterized by parent–child interactions that show mutual warmth and respect

B. Manifestations of Positive Family-Centered Care

1. Respecting cultural diversity and incorporating cultural views in the plan of care

2. Understanding growth and developmental needs of children and their families

3. Treating children and their families as clients

4. Working with all types of families

5. Collaborating with families regarding hospitalization, home, and community resources

6. Allowing families to serve as experts regarding their children's health conditions, usual behaviors in different situations, and routine needs

C. Manifestations of Positive Parental Influences

1. Parents have positive mental health.

2. Structure and routine is maintained in the household.

3. Parents engage in activities with the child.

4. There is communication that validates the child's feelings.

5. The child is monitored for safety with special consideration for his developmental needs.

D. Collaborative Care

 1. **NURSING INTERVENTIONS**

   a. Nurses should perform comprehensive family assessments to identify strengths and weaknesses of families.

   b. Nurses should pay close attention when family members state that a child "isn't acting right" or have other concerns.

   c. Children's opinions should be considered when providing care.

2. Client Education and Referral

   a. Referral to social services for any signs of unhealthy or dysfunctional family manifestations

Family Composition

Type	Members
Nuclear family	Two parents and their children (biologic, adoptive, step, foster)
Tradit ional nuclear family	Married couple and their biologic children (only full brothers and sisters)
Single-parent family	One parent and one or more children
Blended family (also called reconstituted)	At least one stepparent, stepsibling, or half sibling
Extended family	At least one parent, one or more children, and other individuals either related or not related
Gay/Lesbian family	Two members of the same sex that have a common-law ie and mayor may not have children
Foster family	A child or children that have been placed in an approved living environment away from the family of origin -usually with one or two parents
Binuclear family	Parents that have terminated spousal roles but continue their parenting roles
Communal family	Individuals that share common ownership of property and goods and exchange services without monetary consideration

Parenting Styles

Type	Description	Example
Dictatorial or authoritarian	Parents or caregivers try to control the child's behaviors and attitudes through unquestioned rules and expectations.	The child may not watch television on school nights.
Permissive or laissez-faire	Parents or caregivers exert little or no control over the child's behaviors.	The child may watch television whenever he wants to watch it.
Democratic or authoritative	Parents or caregivers direct the child's behavior by setting rules and explaining the reason for each rule setting. The privilege is taken away but may be reinstated based on new guidelines.	Parents negatively reinforce deviations from the rules. The children may watch television for an hour if her homework is completed.

Physical Assessment Findings

A. Vital Sign Guidelines

1. Temperature

Age	Temperature (°C)	Temperature (°F)
Birth to 1 year (axillary)	36.5–37.2° C	97.7–98.9° F
1–12 years (oral)	36.7–37.7° C	98.1–99.9° F
12 years and older (oral)	36.6–36.7° C	97.8–98.0° F

2. Pulse

Age	Pulse
Birth to 1 week	100–160/min with brief fluctuations above and below this range, depending on activity level (crying, sleeping)
1 week to 3 months	100–220/min
3 months to 2 years	80–150/min
2 to 12 years	70–110/min
12 years and older	50–90/min

3. Respirations

Age	Respirations
Newborn	30–60/min with short periods of apnea (less than 15 seconds)
Newborn to 1 year	30/min
1 to 2 years	25–30/min
2 to 6 years	21–24/min
6 to 12 years	19–21/min
12 years and older	16–18/min

4. Blood Pressure

   a. Age, height, and gender all influence blood pressure readings. The following chart provides examples of expected ranges of blood pressure by age and gender.

Vital Sign Summary

Age	Girls		Boys	
	Systolic (mm Hg)	Diastolic (mm Hg)	Systolic (mm Hg)	Diastolic (mm Hg)
1 year	97–107	53–60	94–106	50–59
3 years	100–110	61–68	100–113	59–67
6 years	104–114	67–75	105–117	67–76
10 years	112–122	73–80	110–123	73–82
16 years	122–132	79–86	125–138	79–87

B. Physical Characteristics

1. General Appearance

   a. Appears undistressed

   b. Appears clean and well kept

   c. Muscle tone

      1) Limp posture with extension of the extremities is expected.

      2) Erect head posture is expected in infants after 4 months of age.

   d. Has no body odors

   e. Makes eye contact when addressed (except infants)

   f. Follows simple commands as age appropriate

   g. Uses speech, language, and motor skills spontaneously

2. Growth: Growth can be evaluated using weight, height, body mass index (BMI), and head circumference. Growth charts are tools that can be used to assess the overall health of a child. To see growth charts by age and gender, visit the website for the Centers for Disease Control and Prevention (CDC) (http://www.cdc.gov).

3. Skin, Hair, and Nails

   a. Skin

      1) Skin color may show normal variations based on race and ethnicity.

      2) Temperature should be warm or slightly cool to the touch.

      3) Skin turgor should demonstrate brisk elasticity with adequate hydration.

      4) Skin texture should be smooth and slightly dry.

      5) Lesions are not normal findings.

      6) Skin folds should be symmetric.

   b. Hair

      1) Hair should be evenly distributed, smooth, and strong.

      2) Children approaching adolescence should be assessed for the presence of secondary hair growth.

   c. Nails

      1) Pink over the nail bed and white at the tips

      2) Smooth and firm (but slightly flexible in infants)

      3) No clubbing

4. Head and Neck

   a. Head

      1) The shape of the head should be symmetric.

      2) Fontanels should be flat. The posterior fontanel usually closes between 2 and 3 months of age, and the anterior fontanel usually closes between 12 and 18 months of age.

   b. Face

      1) Symmetric appearance and movement

      2) Proportional features

c. Neck
  1) Short in infants
  2) No palpable masses
     a) Lymph nodes should be nonpalpable, but lymph nodes that are small, palpable, non-tender, and mobile in children may still be considered normal
  3) Midline trachea
  4) Full range of motion present whether assessed actively or passively

5. Eyes
  a. **Visual acuity** may be difficult to assess in children under 3 years of age. Visual acuity in infants can be assessed by holding an object in front of the eyes and checking to see if the infant is able to fix on the object and follow it. Older children should be tested using a Snellen chart or symbol chart.
  b. **Color vision** should be assessed using the Ishihara color test. The child should be able to correctly identify shapes.
  c. **Peripheral visual** fields should be:
     1) Upward 50°
     2) Downward 70°
     3) Nasally 60°
     4) Temporally 90°
  d. **Extraocular movements** may not be symmetric in newborns
     1) Corneal light reflex should be symmetric
     2) Cover/uncover test should demonstrate equal movement of the eyes. The presence of strabismus should be further evaluated in children between 4 and 6 years of age.
     3) Six cardinal fields of gaze should demonstrate no nystagmus
  e. **Eyebrows** should be symmetric and evenly distributed from the inner to the outer canthus.
  f. **Eyelids** should close completely and open to allow the lower border and most of the upper portion of the iris to be seen.
  g. **Eyelashes** should curve outward and be evenly distributed with no inflammation around any of the hair follicles.
  h. **Conjunctiva**
     1) Palpebral is pink.
     2) Bulbar is transparent.
  i. **Lacrimal apparatus** is without excessive tearing, redness, or discharge.
  j. **Sclera** should be white.
  k. **Corneas** should be clear.
  l. **Pupils** should be:
     1) Equal in size
     2) Round
     3) Reactive to light
     4) Accommodating (can be tested in older children)

m. **Irises** should be round with the permanent color manifesting around 6 to 12 months of age.
n. **Internal exam**
  1) Red reflex should be present in infants.

6. Ears
  a. Alignment
     1) The top of the auricles should meet in an imaginary horizontal line that extends from the outer canthus of the eye.
  b. External ear
     1) The external ear should be free of lesions and nontender.
     2) The ear canal should be free of foreign bodies or discharge.
     3) Cerumen is an expected finding.
  c. Internal ear
     1) In infants, pull the pinna down and back to visualize the tympanic membrane.
     2) In children older than 3 years of age, pull the pinna up and back to visualize.
     3) The tympanic membrane should be pearly gray.
     4) The light reflex should be visible.
     5) The ear canal should be pink with fine hairs.

7. Hearing
  a. Newborns should have intact acoustic blink reflexes to sudden sounds.
  b. Infants should turn toward sounds.
  c. Older children can be screened by whispering a word from behind to see if they can identify the word.

8. Nose
  a. The position should be midline.
  b. Patency should be present for each nostril without excessive flaring.
  c. Internal structures.
     1) The septum is midline and intact.
     2) The mucosa is deep pink and moist with no discharge.
  d. Smell can be assessed in older children.

9. Mouth and Throat
  a. Lips
     1) Darker pigmented than facial skin
     2) Smooth, soft, and moist
  b. Gums
     1) Coral pink
     2) Tight against the teeth
  c. Mucous membranes
     1) Without lesions
     2) Moist and pink
  d. Tongue
     1) Infants may have white coatings on their tongues from milk that can be easily removed. Oral candidiasis coating is not easily removed.

2) Children and adolescents should have pink, symmetric tongues that they are able to move beyond their lips.

e. Teeth

    1) Infants should have 6 to 8 teeth by 1 year of age.

    2) Children and adolescents should have teeth that are white and smooth, with 20 deciduous and 32 permanent teeth.

f. Dentition

    1) Drools at 4 months

    2) Six primary teeth by 1 year (age of child in months minus 6 equals number of teeth)

    3) Collaborative Care

      a) **NURSING INTERVENTIONS**

        (1) Avoid phenytoin (Dilantin) because it causes gingivitis and gingival hyperplasia. Also, avoid medications that may stain the infant's teeth (tetracycline, iron).

        (2) Teach the parents to monitor for increased drooling, finger sucking, and biting on objects, which are all indicators of teething.

        (3) Reinforce to the parents that cool or cold items such as teething rings are soothing.

        (4) Use acetaminophen (Tylenol) for continued irritability.

      b) Client Education and Referral

        (1) Educate the parents that once dentition occurs to avoid giving the infant a nighttime bottle that contains juice or formula, because it increases the incidence of dental caries (bottle mouth caries).

g. Hard and soft palates

    1) Intact, firm, and concave

h. Uvula

    1) Intact and moves with vocalization

i. Tonsils

    1) Infants (may not be able to visualize)

    2) Children (barely visible to prominent, same color as surrounding mucosa, deep crevices that hold food particles)

j. Speech

    1) Infants (strong cry)

    2) Children and adolescents (clear and articulate)

10. Thorax and Lungs

a. Chest shape

    1) Infants: Shape is almost circular with anteroposterior diameter equaling the transverse or lateral diameter.

    2) Children and adolescents: The transverse diameter to anteroposterior diameter changes to 2:1.

b. Ribs and sternum: More soft and flexible in infants, symmetric, and smooth with no protrusions or bulges

    1) Movement: Symmetric, no retractions

      a) Infants: Irregular rhythms are common.

      b) Children younger than 7 years: More abdominal movement is seen during respirations.

    2) Breath sounds

      a) Infants: Harsher and easier to hear than in adults; harder to differentiate between upper versus lower respiratory sounds

      b) Children and adolescents: Vesicular sounds heard over the lung fields

    3) Breasts

      a) Newborns: Breasts may be enlarged during the first several months.

      b) Children and adolescents: Nipples and areolas are darker pigmented and symmetric.

      c) Females: Breasts typically develop between 10 and 14 years of age. The breasts should appear asymmetric, have no masses, and be palpable.

      d) Males may develop a firm, approximately 2-cm area of breast tissue or gynecomastia.

11. Circulatory System

a. Heart sounds: S1 and S2 heart sounds should be clear and crisp. S1 is louder at the apex of the heart. S2 is louder near the base of the heart. Sinus arrhythmias that are associated with respirations are common. Physiologic splitting of S2 and S3 heart sounds are expected findings in children.

b. Pulses

    1) Infants: Brachial, temporal, and femoral pulses should be palpable, full, and localized.

    2) Children and adolescents: Pulse locations and expected findings are the same as those in adults.

12. Abdomen

a. Without tenderness, no guarding. Peristaltic waves may be visible in thinner children.

b. Shape: Symmetric and without protrusions around the umbilicus

    1) Infants and toddlers have rounded abdomens.

    2) Children and adolescents should have flat abdomens.

c. Bowel sounds should be heard every 5 to 30 seconds.

d. Descending colon: Cylindrical mass that is possibly palpable in the lower left quadrant due to the presence of stool

13. Musculoskeletal System

a. Length, position, and size are symmetric.

b. Joints: Stable and symmetric with full range of motion and no crepitus or redness

c. Spine
  1) Infants: Spines should be without dimples or tufts of hair. They should be midline with an overall C-shaped lateral curve.
  2) Toddlers appear squat with short legs and protuberant abdomens.
  3) Preschoolers appear more erect than toddlers.
  4) Children should develop the cervical, thoracic, and lumbar curvatures like that of adults.
  5) Adolescents should remain midline (no scoliosis noted).

d. Gait
  1) Toddlers and young children: A bowlegged or knock-knee appearance is a common finding. Feet should face forward while walking.
  2) Older children and adolescents: A steady gait should be noted with even wear on the soles of shoes.

14. Neurological System

  a. Height: Increases by 50% in first year

  b. Weight: Birth weight doubles by 6 months; birth weight triples by 1 year

  c. Head: 70% of adult size at birth; 80% of adult size by end of first year
    1) Posterior fontanel: Closes by 2 months of age
    2) Anterior fontanel: Closes between 12 to 18 months of age
    3) Bulging: Classic sign of increased intracranial pressure
    4) Sunken: Classic sign of dehydration

  d. Deep tendon reflexes should demonstrate the following:
    1) Partial flexion of the lower arm at the biceps tendon
    2) Partial extension of the lower arm at the triceps tendon
    3) Partial extension of the lower leg at the patellar tendon
    4) Plantar flexion of the foot at the Achilles tendon

  e. Cerebellar function (children and adolescents)
    1) Finger to nose test: Rapid coordinated movements
    2) Heel to shin test: Able to run the heel of one foot down the shin of the other leg while standing
    3) Romberg test: Able to stand with slight swaying while eyes are closed

  f. Language, cognition, and fine and gross motor development can be screened using a standardized tool such as the *Denver Developmental Screening Test*, Revised (Denver II). Referrals for further evaluation should not be based solely on results of one tool, but on a combination of data collected from psychosocial and medical histories and a physical examination.

15. Genitalia
  a. Male
    1) Hair distribution is diamond shaped after puberty in adolescent males. No pubic hair is noted in infants and small children.
    2) Penis
      a) Penis should appear straight.
      b) Urethral meatus should be at the tip of the penis.
      c) Foreskin may not be retractable in infants and small children.
      d) Enlargement of the penis occurs during adolescence.
    3) Scrotum
      a) The scrotum hangs separately from the penis.
      b) The skin on the scrotum has a rugated appearance and is loose.
      c) The left testicle hangs slighter lower than the right.
      d) The inguinal canal should be absent of swelling.
      e) During puberty, the testes and scrotum enlarge with darker scrotal skin.
  b. Female
    1) Hair distribution over the mons pubis should be documented in terms of amount and location during puberty. Hair should appear in an inverted triangle. No pubic hair should be noted in infants or small children.
    2) Labia: Symmetric, without lesions, moist on the inner aspects
    3) Clitoris: Small, without bruising or edema
    4) Urethral meatus: Slit-like in appearance with no discharge
    5) Vaginal orifice: The hymen may be absent, or it may completely or partially cover the vaginal opening prior to sexual intercourse
    6) Anus: Surrounding skin should be intact with sphincter tightening noted if the anus is touched. Routine rectal exams are not done with the pediatric population.

Expected Growth and Development

A. Infant (first year of life)

1. Physical Development

  a. The infant's posterior fontanel closes by 2 to 3 months of age.

  b. The infant's anterior fontanel closes by 12 to 18 months of age.

  c. Weight, height, and head circumference measurements are used to track the size of infants.
    1) Weight: Infants gain approximately 150–210 g (about 5–7 oz) per week the first 6 months of age. Infants triple their birth weights by the end of the first year of life.

2) Height: Infants grow approximately 2.5 cm (1 in) per month the first 6 months of age, and then approximately 1.25 cm (0.5 in) per month for the next 6 months.

3) Head circumference: The circumference of infants' heads increases approximately 1.5 cm (0.6 in) per month for the first 6 months of life, and then approximately 0.5 cm (0.2 in) between 6 and 12 months of age.

4) Dentition: Six to eight teeth should erupt in infants' mouths by the end of the first year of age.

   a) Teething pain can be eased using cold teething rings, over-the-counter teething gels, or acetaminophen (Tylenol) and/or ibuprofen (Advil). Ibuprofen should be used only in infants over the age of 6 months.

   b) Clean infants' teeth using cool, wet washcloths.

   c) Bottles should not be given to infants when they are falling asleep. This will help to avoid prolonged exposure to milk or juice that can cause dental caries (bottle mouth syndrome)

Motor Skill Development of the Infant

Age	Gross Motor Skills	Fine Motor Skills
1 month	Demonstrates head lag	• Has a grasp reflex
2 months	Lifts head off mattress	• Holds hands in an open position
3 months	Raises head and shoulders off mattress	• No longer has a grasp reflex • Keeps hands loosely open
4 months	Rolls from back to side	• Places objects in mouth
5 months	Rolls from front to back	• Uses palmar grasp dominantly
6 months	Rolls from back to front	• Holds bottle
7 months	Bears full weight on feet	• Moves objects from hand to hand
8 months	Sits unsupported	• Begins using pincer grasp
9 months	Pulls to a standing position	• Has a crude pincer grasp
10 months	Changes from a prone to a sitting position	• Grasps rattle by its handle
11 months	Walks while holding on to something	• Places objects into a container
12 months	Sits down from a standing position without assistance	• Tries to build a two-block tower without success

2. Cognitive Development

   a. Piaget: Sensorimotor stage (birth to 24 months)

      1) There are three things that occur during this time: separation, object permanence, and mental representation.

         a) Separation is when infants learn to separate themselves from other objects in the environment.

         b) Object permanence is the process by which infants know that an object still exists when it is hidden from view. This occurs at approximately 9 months of age.

         c) Mental representation is the recognition of symbols.

   b. Language

      1) Vocalizes with cooing noises

      2) Responds to noises

      3) Turns head to the sound of a rattle

      4) Laughs and squeals

      5) Pronounces single-syllable words

      6) Begins speaking two-word phrases and progresses to speaking three-word phrases

3. Psychosocial Development

   a. The stage of psychosocial development for infants, according to Erikson, is **trust versus mistrust**.

   b. The infants trust that their feeding, comfort, stimulation, and caring needs will be met. Social development is initially influenced by infants' reflexive behaviors and includes attachment, separation, recognition/anxiety, and stranger fear.

      1) Attachment is seen when infants begin to bond with their parents. This development is seen within the first month, but it actually begins before birth. The process is enhanced when infants and parents are in good health, have positive feeding experiences, and receive adequate rest.

      2) Separation recognition occurs during the first year as infants learn physical boundaries from other people. Learning how to respond to people in their environments is the next phase of development. Positive interactions with parents, siblings, and other caregivers help to establish trust.

      3) Separation anxiety develops between 4 and 8 months of age. Infants will protest loudly when separated from parents, which can cause considerable anxiety for parents.

      4) Stranger fear becomes evident between 6 and 8 months of age, when infants are less likely to accept strangers.

4. Self-Concept Development

   a. By the end of the first year, infants will be able to distinguish themselves as being separate from their parents.

5. Body Image Changes

    a. Infants will discover that their mouths are pleasure producers.

    b. **Hands and feet are seen as objects of play.**

    c. Infants discover that smiling causes others to react.

6. Age-Appropriate Activities

    a. Infants will have short attention spans and will not interact with other children during play (solitary play). Appropriate toys and activities that stimulate the senses and encourage development include:

        1) Rattles

        2) Mobiles

        3) Teething toys

        4) Nesting toys

        5) Playing pat-a-cake

        6) Playing with balls

        7) Having books read to them

7. Health Promotion for Infants

    a. Immunizations

> **Note:** Always refer to the CDC website (http://www.cdc.gov) for the latest immunization requirements and schedules.

    b. Nutrition

        1) Feeding alternatives

           a) Breast-feeding provides a complete diet for infants during the first 6 months of life and is recommended by health care providers.

           b) Iron-fortified formula is an acceptable alternative to breast milk. **Cows' milk is not recommended during the first year of life.**

           c) Solids can be introduced between 4 and 6 months of age.

           d) Iron-fortified rice cereal should be offered first.

           e) New foods should be introduced one at a time, over a 5- to 7-day period to observe for signs of allergy or intolerance, which may include fussiness, rash, vomiting, diarrhea, and constipation. Vegetables or fruits are first started between 6 and 8 months of age. After both have been introduced, meats may be added.

           f) Milk, eggs, wheat, citrus fruits, peanuts, peanut butter, and honey should be delayed until after the first year of life.

           g) Breast milk/formula should be decreased as intake of solid foods increases.

           h) Table foods that are cooked, chopped, and unseasoned are appropriate by 9 months of age.

           i) Appropriate finger foods include ripe bananas; toast strips; graham crackers; cheese cubes; noodles; and peeled chunks of apples, pears, or peaches.

           j) Parents should be encouraged to use iron-enriched foods after infants are 6 months of age.

        2) Health promotion of the infant (birth to 1 year)

           a) **Weaning** can be accomplished when infants are able to drink from cups with handles (sometime after 6 months).

               (1) One feeding may be replaced with breast milk or formula in a cup with handles.

               (2) Bedtime feedings are the last to be replaced.

    c. Injury Prevention

        1) Aspiration of foreign objects

           a) Small objects that can become lodged in the throat (e.g., grapes, coins, candy) should be avoided.

           b) Age-appropriate toys should be provided.

           c) Clothing should be checked for safety hazards (e.g., loose buttons).

        2) Bodily harm

           a) Sharp objects should be kept out of reach.

           b) Infants should be kept away from heavy objects that they can pull down onto themselves.

           c) Infants should not be left unattended with any animals present.

           d) Infant should be monitored for shaken baby syndrome.

        3) Burns

           a) The temperature of bath water should be checked.

           b) Thermostats on hot water heaters should be turned down.

           c) Working smoke detectors should be kept in the home.

           d) Handles of pots and pans should be kept turned to the back of stoves.

           e) Sunscreen should be used when infants will be exposed to the sun.

           f) Electrical outlets should be covered.

        4) Drowning

           a) Infants should not be left unattended in bathtubs.

        5) Falls

           a) Crib mattresses should be kept in the lowest position possible with the rails all the way up.

           b) Restraints should be used in infant seats.

           c) Infant seats should be placed on the ground or floor if used outside of the car, and they should not be left unattended or on elevated surfaces.

           d) Safety gates should be used across stairs.

        6) Poisoning

           a) Exposure to lead paint should be avoided.

           b) Toxins and plants should be kept out of reach.

c) Safety locks should be kept on cabinets with cleaners and other household chemicals.

d) The phone number for a poison control center should be kept near the phone.

e) Medications should be kept in childproof containers, away from the reach of infants.

f) A working carbon monoxide detector should be kept in the home.

7) Motor vehicle injuries

a) Infants should be placed in approved rear-facing car seats in the backseat, preferably in the middle (away from air bags and side impact). Infants should be in rear-facing car seats until 2 years of age and until they weigh 20 lb (9.1 kg).

b) A five-point harness or T-shield should be part of a convertible restraint.

8) Suffocation

a) Plastic bags should be avoided.

b) Balloons should be kept away from infants.

c) Crib mattresses should fit snugly.

d) Crib slats should be no farther apart than 6 cm (2.4 in).

e) Crib mobiles or crib gyms should be removed by 4 to 5 months of age.

f) Pillows should be kept out of the crib.

g) Infants should be placed on their backs for sleep.

h) Toys with small parts should be kept out of reach.

i) Drawstrings should be removed from jackets and other clothing.

9) Sudden infant death syndrome (SIDS)

a) Contributing Factors (Cause of SIDS is unknown, but multiple theories exist.)

(1) Mostly boys who are ages 2 to 4 months

(2) Preterm infants who have apnea problems

(3) Multiple births

(4) Occurs during sleep, usually in winter months

b) Client (Parent) Education and Referral

(1) The infant should sleep in a supine or side-lying position, not prone.

(2) Provide a firm mattress with no pillows, comforters, or stuffed animals. Avoid overheating the infant during sleep.

(3) There is a lower incidence of SIDS if the infant is breast-fed.

d. Health Promotion Client (Parent) Education Guidelines

1) Childproof the environment.

2) Constantly supervise the infant.

3) Provide anticipatory guidance.

4) Provide an appropriate car seat restraint.

5) Assess the temperature of the infant's bath water, formula, and food.

6) Do not prop the bottle during the infant's feedings or at bed time.

7) Supervise the infant during bath time, changing table, and play time.

8) Select age-appropriate toys for the infant.

9) Turn handles of pots/pans away from the infant's reach.

10) Keep side rails of the infant's crib up during bed time.

B. Toddler (1 to 3 years)

1. Physical Development

a. Anterior fontanels close by 18 months of age.

b. Weight: At 30 months of age, toddlers should weigh four times their birth weights.

c. Height: Toddlers grow about 7.5 cm (3 in) per year.

Motor Skill Development of the Toddler

Age	Gross Motor Skills	Fine Motor Skills
15 months	• Walks without help • Uses a cup well	• Creeps up stairs • Builds a tower of two blocks
18 months	• Assumes a standing position	• Manages a spoon without rotation • Turns pages in a book, two or three at a time
2 years	• Walks up and down stairs	• Builds a tower of six or seven blocks
2.5 years	• Jumps in place with both feet • Stands on one foot momentarily	• Draws circles • Has good hand-finger coordination

2. Cognitive Development

a. Piaget: The sensorimotor stage transitions to the preoperational stage

1) The concept of object permanence is fully developed.

2) Toddlers have and demonstrate memories of events that relate to them.

3) Domestic mimicry (e.g., playing house) is evident.

4) Preoperational thought does not allow for toddlers to understand other viewpoints, but it does allow them to symbolize objects and people to imitate previously seen activities.

b. Language

1) Language increases to about 400 words, with toddlers speaking in two- to three-word phrases.

3. Psychosocial Development

a. The stage of psychosocial development for toddlers, according to Erikson, is **autonomy versus shame and doubt**.

b. Independence is paramount for toddlers, who are attempting to do everything for themselves.

c. Separation anxiety continues to occur when parents leave toddlers.

4. Moral Development

a. Moral development is closely associated with cognitive development.

b. Egocentric: Toddlers are unable to see things from the perspectives of others; they can only view things from their personal points of view.

c. Punishment and obedience orientation begin with a sense that good behavior is rewarded and bad behavior is punished.

5. Self-Concept Development

a. Toddlers progressively see themselves as separate from their parents and increase their explorations away from them.

6. Body Image Changes

a. Toddlers appreciate the usefulness of various body parts.

b. Toddlers will develop gender identity by 3 years of age.

7. Age-Appropriate Activities

a. Solitary play evolves into parallel play, in which toddlers observe other children and then may engage in activities nearby.

1) Filling and emptying containers
2) Playing with blocks
3) Looking at books
4) Playing with toys that can be pushed and pulled
5) Tossing balls
6) Temper tantrums result when toddlers are frustrated with restrictions on independence. Providing consistent, age-appropriate expectations helps toddlers to work through frustration.

b. Toilet training can begin when it is recognized that toddlers have the sensation of needing to urinate or defecate. Parents should demonstrate patience and consistency in toilet training. Nighttime control may develop last of all.

c. Discipline should be consistent with well-defined boundaries that are established to develop appropriate social behavior.

8. Health Promotion for the Toddler

a. Immunizations: See preceding immunization chart.

b. Nutrition

1) Toddlers are generally picky eaters who will repeatedly request their favorite foods.
2) Toddlers should consume 24–30 oz of milk per day, and they may switch from drinking whole milk to drinking low-fat milk (2% fat) at 2 years of age.
3) Juice consumption should be limited to 4–6 oz per day.

4) Food serving size should be 1 tbsp for each year of age.
5) Exposure to a new food may need to occur 8 to 15 times before toddlers develop an acceptance of it.
6) If there is a family history of allergy, then cows' milk, chocolate, citrus fruits, egg whites, seafood, and nut butters may be gradually introduced while monitoring for reactions.
7) Toddlers generally prefer finger foods because of increasing autonomy.
8) Regular meal times and nutritious snacks best meet nutrient needs.
9) Snacks or desserts that are high in sugar, fat, or sodium should be avoided.
10) Foods that are potential choking hazards (nuts, grapes, hot dogs, peanut butter, raw carrots, tough meats, popcorn) should be avoided.
11) Adult supervision should always be provided during snack and mealtimes.
12) Foods should be cut into small, bite-size pieces to make them easier to swallow and to prevent choking.
13) Toddlers should not be allowed to engage in drinking or eating during play activities or while lying down.
14) Parents should follow dietary recommendations outlined by the United States Department of Agriculture (http://www.mypyramid.gov).

c. Injury Prevention

1) Aspiration of foreign objects—small objects (e.g., grapes, coins, candy) that can become lodged in the airway
   a) Toys that have small parts should be kept out of reach.
   b) Age-appropriate toys should be provided.
   c) Clothing should be checked for safety hazards (e.g., loose buttons).
   d) Balloons should be kept away from toddlers
2) Bodily harm
   a) Sharp objects should be kept out of reach.
   b) Firearms should be kept in locked boxes or cabinets.
   c) Toddlers should not be left unattended with any animals present.
   d) Toddlers should be taught stranger safety.
3) Burns
   a) The temperature of bath water should be checked.
   b) Thermostats on hot water heaters should be turned down.
   c) Working smoke detectors should be kept in the home.
   d) Pot handles should be turned toward the back of the stove.

e) Electrical outlets should be covered.

f) Toddler should wear sunscreen when outside.

4) Drowning

a) Toddlers should not be left unattended in bathtubs.

b) Toilet lids should be kept closed.

c) Toddlers should be closely supervised when near pools or any other body of water.

d) Toddlers should be taught to swim.

5) Falls

a) Doors and windows should be kept locked.

b) Crib mattresses should be kept in the lowest position with the rails all the way up.

c) Safety gates should be used across stairs both at the top and bottom of stairs.

6) Motor vehicles injuries

a) Approved car seats should be used in the backseats of cars (away from air bags).

b) Toddlers should be in approved rear-facing car seats in the backseat until they weigh 20 lb (9.1 kg). Toddlers may then sit in approved forward-facing car seats in the backseat. Toddlers may usually remain in car seats until 4 years of age and/or 40 lb (18.1 kg).

7) Poisoning

a) Exposure to lead paint should be avoided.

b) Safety locks should be placed on cabinets that contain cleaners and other chemicals.

c) The phone number for a poison control center should be kept near the phone.

d) Medications should be kept in childproof containers, away from the reach of toddlers.

e) A working carbon monoxide detector should be placed in the home.

8) Suffocation

a) Plastic bags should be avoided.

b) Crib mattresses should fit tightly.

c) Crib slats should be no farther apart than 6 cm (2.4 in).

d) Pillows should be kept out of cribs.

e) Drawstrings should be removed from jackets and other clothing.

C. Preschooler (3 to 6 years)

1. Physical Development

a. Weight: Preschoolers should gain about 2–3 kg (4.5–6.5 lb) per year.

b. Height: Preschoolers should grow about 6.2–7.5 cm (2.5–3 inches) per year.

c. Preschoolers' bodies evolve away from the characteristically unsteady wide stances and protruding abdomens of toddlers, into a more graceful, posturally erect, and sturdy physicality.

d. Fine and gross motor skills

1) Preschoolers should show improvement in fine motor skills, which will be displayed by activities like copying figures on paper and dressing independently.

Motor Skills of the Preschooler

Age	Gross Motor Skills
3 years	• Rides a tricycle • Jumps off bottom step • Stands on one foot for a few seconds
4 years	• Skips and hops on one foot • Throws a ball overhead
5 years	• Jumps rope • Walks backward with heel to toe • Moves up and down stairs easily

2. Cognitive Development

a. Piaget: Preschoolers are still in the preoperational phase of cognitive development. They participate in preconceptual thought (from 2 to 4 years of age) and intuitive thought (from 4 to 7 years of age).

b. Preconceptual thought: Preschoolers make judgments based on visual appearances. Misconceptions in thinking during this stage include:

1) Artificialism: Everything is made by humans.

2) Animism: Inanimate objects are alive.

3) Imminent justice: A universal code exists that determines law and order.

4) Intuitive thought: Preschoolers can classify information, and they become aware of cause-and-effect relationships.

5) Time: Preschoolers begin to understand the concepts of the past, present, and future. By the end of the preschool years, children may comprehend days of the week

6) Language: The vocabulary of preschoolers continues to increase. Preschoolers can speak in sentences and identify colors, and they enjoy talking.

3. Psychosocial Development

a. The stage of psychosocial development for preschoolers, according to Erikson, is **initiative versus guilt**.

b. Preschoolers may take on many new experiences, despite not having all of the physical abilities necessary to be successful at everything. Guilt may occur when preschoolers are unable to accomplish a task and believe they have misbehaved. Guiding preschoolers to attempt activities within their capabilities while setting limits is appropriate.

4. Moral Development

a. Preschoolers continue in the good–bad orientation of the toddler years, but they begin to understand behaviors in terms of what is socially acceptable.

5. Self-Concept Development
   a. Preschoolers feel good about themselves with regard to mastering skills that allow independence (e.g., dressing, feeding). During stress, insecurity, or illness, preschoolers may regress to previous immature behaviors or develop habits (e.g., nose picking, bedwetting, thumb sucking).

6. Body Image Changes
   a. Mistaken perceptions of reality coupled with misconceptions in thinking lead to active fantasies and fears. The greatest fear is that of bodily harm, resulting in fear of the dark or animals.
   b. Sex-role identification is occurring.

7. Social Development
   a. Preschoolers generally do not exhibit stranger anxiety and have less separation anxiety. However, prolonged separation, such as during hospitalization, can provoke anxiety. Favorite toys and appropriate play should be used to help ease preschoolers' fears.
   b. Pretend play is healthy and allows preschoolers to determine the difference between reality and fantasy.
   c. Sleep disturbances frequently occur during early childhood, and problems range from difficulties going to bed to night tremors.
   d. Advise parents to assess whether or not the bedtime is too early if preschoolers are still taking naps (on average, preschoolers need about 12 hr of sleep per day). Some still require a daytime nap.
   e. Keep a consistent bedtime routine.
   f. Use a night-light.
   g. Reassure preschoolers who have been frightened, but avoid allowing preschoolers to sleep with their parents.

8. Age-Appropriate Activities
   a. Parallel play shifts to associative play during the preschool years. Play is not highly organized, but cooperation does exist between children. Appropriate activities include:
      1) Playing ball
      2) Putting puzzles together
      3) Riding tricycles
      4) Playing pretend and dress-up activities
      5) Role playing
      6) Painting
      7) Sewing cards and beads
      8) Reading books

9. Health Promotion for the Preschooler
   a. Immunizations: See preceding immunization chart.
   b. Health screenings
      1) Vision screening is routinely done in the preschool population as part of the prekindergarten physical exam. Visual impairments such as myopia and amblyopia can be detected and treated before poor visual acuity impairs learning.

c. Nutrition
   1) Preschoolers consume about half the amount of energy that adults do (1,800 kcal).
   2) Picky eating may remain a behavior in preschoolers, but often by 5 years of age they become more willing to sample different foods.
   3) Preschoolers need 13 to 19 g/day of complete protein in addition to adequate calcium, iron, folate, and vitamins A and C.
   4) Parents need to ensure that preschoolers are receiving a balance of nutrients.
   5) Healthy food recommendations are posted by the United States Department of Agriculture (http://www.mypyramid.gov).

d. Injury Prevention
   1) Bodily harm
      a) Firearms should be kept in locked cabinets or containers.
      b) Preschoolers should be taught stranger safety.
      c) Preschoolers should be taught to wear protective equipment (e.g., helmet, pads).
   2) Burns
      a) Thermostats should be turned down on hot water heaters.
      b) Working smoke detectors should be kept in the home.
      c) Preschoolers should have sunscreen applied when outside.
   3) Drowning
      a) Preschoolers should not be left unattended in bathtubs.
      b) Preschoolers should be closely supervised when near the pool or any other body of water.
      c) Preschoolers should be taught to swim.
   4) Motor vehicle injuries
      a) Preschoolers should sit in approved forward-facing car seats in the backseat away from air bags. Usually preschoolers may remain in car seats until 4 years of age and/or 40 lb (18.1 kg). When preschoolers have outgrown car seats, booster seats in the backseat should be used. Children should be restrained in car seats or booster chairs until adult seat belts fit correctly. Laws may vary from state to state, and requirements may be up to a weight of 80 lb (36.3 kg) and a height of 4 feet 9 inches, which is when adult seat belts will most likely fit correctly.
   5) Poisoning
      a) Exposure to lead paint should be avoided.
      b) Plants should be kept out of reach.
      c) Safety locks should be placed on cabinets with cleaners and other chemicals.
      d) The phone number for a poison control center should be kept near the phone.
      e) Medications should be kept in childproof containers, out of reach of preschoolers.
      f) A working carbon monoxide detector should be placed in the home.

D. School-Age Child (6 to 12 Years)

1. Physical Development

   a. Weight: School-age children will gain about 2–4 kg (4.4–8.8 lb) per year.
      1) Weight gain typically occurs between 9 and 12 years of age (girls from 9 to 12 and boys from 10 to 12 years of age).

   b. Height: School-age children will grow about 5 cm (2 inches) per year. Changes in height usually occur after 10 to 12 years of age for girls and 12 to 14 years of age for boys (after the period of weight gain).

   c. Changes related to puberty begin to appear in females.
      1) Budding of breasts
      2) Appearance of pubic hair
      3) Onset of menarche

   d. Changes related to puberty begin to appear in males.
      1) Enlargement of testicles with changes in the scrotum (increased looseness)
      2) Appearance of pubic hair

   e. Permanent teeth erupt.

   f. Visual acuity improves to 20/20.

   g. Auditory acuity and sense of touch is fully developed.

   h. Fine and gross motor development: During the school-age years, coordination continues to improve.

2. Cognitive Development

   a. Piaget: Concrete operations
      1) Sees weight and volume as unchanging
      2) Understands simple analogies
      3) Understands time (days, seasons)
      4) Classifies more complex information
      5) Understands various emotions
      6) Becomes self-motivated
      7) Is able to solve problems

   b. Language
      1) Defines many words and understands rules of grammar
      2) Understands that a word may have multiple meanings

3. Psychosocial Development

   a. The stage of psychosocial development for school-age children, according to Erikson, is **industry versus inferiority**.
      1) A sense of industry is achieved through advancements in learning.
      2) School-age children are motivated by tasks that increase self-worth.
      3) Fears of ridicule by peers and teachers over school-related issues are common.
      4) Some children manifest nervous behaviors (nail biting) to deal with the stress.

4. Moral Development

   a. Early on, school-age children may not understand the reasoning behind many rules and may try to find ways around them. Instrumental exchange ("I'll help you if you help me") is in place. Children want to make the best deal, and they do not really consider elements of loyalty, gratitude, or justice as they make decisions.

   b. In the latter part of the school-age years, children move into a law-and-order orientation with more emphasis placed on justice being administered.

5. Self-Concept Development

   a. School-age children strive to develop a healthy self-respect by finding out in what areas they excel.

   b. School-age children need parents to encourage them regarding educational or extracurricular successes.

6. Body Image Changes

   a. This is the age at which solidification of body image occurs.

   b. Curiosity about sexuality should be addressed with education regarding sexual development and the reproductive process.

   c. School-age children are more modest than pre-schoolers and place more emphasis on privacy issues.

7. Social Development

   a. Peer groups play an important part in social development. Peer pressure begins to take effect.

   b. Friendships begin to form between same-gender peers. This is the time period when clubs and best friends are popular.

   c. Children prefer the company of same-gender companions.

   d. Most relationships come from school associations.

   e. Children may rival same-gender parents.

   f. Conformity becomes evident.

8. Age-Appropriate Activities

   a. Competitive and cooperative play is predominant

   b. Children from 6 to 9 years of age
      1) Play simple board and number games
      2) Play hopscotch
      3) Jump rope
      4) Collect rocks, stamps, cards, coins, or stuffed animals
      5) Ride bicycles
      6) Build simple models
      7) Join organized sports (for skill building)
      8) Make crafts
      9) Build models
      10) Collect things/engage in hobbies
      11) Solve jigsaw puzzles
      12) Play board and card games
      13) Join organized competitive sports

9. Health Promotion for School-Aged Children

a. Immunizations

1) 2010 CDC immunization recommendations for healthy school-age children 6 to 12 years of age (http://www.cdc.gov) include:

a) If not given between 4 and 5 years of age, **children should receive the following vaccines by 6 years of age**:

(1) Diphtheria and tetanus toxoids and pertussis (DTaP)

(2) Inactivated poliovirus (IPV)

(3) Measles, mumps, and rubella (MMR)

(4) Varicella

b) Yearly seasonal influenza vaccine: Trivalent inactivated influenza vaccine (TIV) or live, attenuated influenza vaccine (LAIV) by nasal spray

c) 11 to 12 years

(1) Tetanus

(2) Diphtheria toxoids and pertussis vaccine (Tdap)

(3) Human papillomavirus vaccine (HPV2) in three doses (for females), and HPV4 (for males)

b. Health Screenings

1) Scoliosis: School-age children should be screened for scoliosis by examining for a lateral curvature of the spine before and during growth spurts. Screening may take place at schools or at a health care facilities.

c. Nutrition

1) By the end of the school-age years, children should be eating adult proportions of food. They need quality nutritious snacks.

2) Obesity is an increasing concern of this age group that predisposes children to low self-esteem, diabetes, heart disease, and high blood pressure.

a) Advise parents to:

(1) Avoid using food as a reward.

(2) Emphasize physical activity.

(3) Ensure that a balanced diet is consumed. Recommendations posted by the United States Department of Agriculture may be found at http://www.mypyramid.gov.

(4) Teach children to make healthy food selections for meals and snacks.

(5) Avoid eating fast food frequently.

(6) Avoid skipping meals.

d. Dental health

1) Brush daily.

2) Floss daily.

3) Have regular checkups.

4) Have regular fluoride treatments.

e. Injury Prevention

1) Bodily harm

a) Firearms should be kept in locked cabinets or boxes.

b) Children should not be allowed to use trampolines.

c) Safe play areas should be identified.

d) Stranger safety should be taught.

e) Children should be taught to wear helmets and/or pads when rollerblading, skateboarding, bicycling, riding scooters, skiing, and snowboarding.

2) Burns

a) Children should be taught fire safety and potential burn hazards.

b) Working smoke detectors should be kept in the home.

c) Children should use sunscreen when outside

3) Drowning

a) Children should be supervised when swimming or when near a body of water.

b) Children should be taught to swim.

4) Motor vehicle injuries

a) Children should be restrained in car seats or booster chairs until adult seat belts fit correctly. Laws may vary from state to state and requirements may be up to a weight of 80 lb (36.3 kg) and a height of 4 feet 9 inches, which is when adult seat belts will most likely fit correctly. Properly fitting adult seat belts should have the lap belt lying across the upper thighs and the shoulder belt fitting across the chest. Children less than 13 years of age are safest in the backseat.

5) Poisoning and substance abuse

a) Cleaners or chemicals should be kept in locked cabinets or out of reach of younger children.

b) Children should be taught to say "no" to illegal drugs and alcohol.

E. Adolescent (12 to 20 years)

1. Physical Development

a. The final 20–25% of height is achieved during puberty.

b. Acne may appear during adolescence.

c. Girls may cease to grow at about 2–2.5 years after the onset of menarche. They will grow 5–20 cm (2–8 in) and gain 7–25 kg (15.5–55 lb).

d. Boys tend to stop growing at around 18 to 20 years of age. They will grow 10–30 cm (4–12 inches) and gain 7–30 kg (15.5–66 lb).

e. In girls, sexual maturation occurs in the following order:
1) Appearance of breast buds
2) Growth of pubic hair (although some girls may have hair growth prior to breast bud development)
3) Onset of menstruation

f. In males, sexual maturation occurs in the following order:
1) Increase in the size of the testes and scrotum
2) Appearance of pubic hair
3) Rapid growth of genitalia
4) Growth of axillary hair
5) Appearance of downy hair on upper lip
6) Change in voice

g. Sleep habits change with puberty due to increased metabolism and rapid growth during the adolescent years. Changes are characterized by staying up late, sleeping in later in the morning, and perhaps sleeping longer than was done during the school-age years.

2. Cognitive Development

a. Piaget: Formal operations
1) Capable of thinking at an adult level
2) Able to think abstractly and deal with principles
3) Capable of evaluating the quality of their own thinking
4) Able to maintain attention for longer periods of time
5) Highly imaginative and idealistic
6) Capable of making decisions through logical operations
7) Future oriented
8) Capable of using deductive reasoning
9) Able to understand how the actions of an individual influence others

b. Language
1) Adolescents develop jargon within their peer groups. They are able to communicate one way with peer groups and another way with adults or teachers.
2) Development of communication skills is essential for adolescents.

3. Psychosocial Development

a. The psychosocial development stage of adolescents, according to Erikson, is **identity versus role confusion**.

b. Adolescents develop a sense of personal identity that is influenced by expectations of their families.

c. Group identity: Adolescents may become part of a peer group that greatly influences behavior.

d. Vocationally: Adolescents solidify work habits and plan for future college and careers.

e. Sexually: There is increased interest in the opposite gender.

f. Health perceptions: Adolescents may view themselves as invincible to bad outcomes of risky behaviors.

4. Moral Development

a. Conventional law and order: Rules are not seen as absolutes. Each situation needs to be looked at, and perhaps the rules will need to be adjusted. Not all adolescents attain this level of moral development during these years.

5. Self-Concept Development

a. A healthy self-concept is developed by having healthy relationships with peers, family, and teachers. Identifying a skill or talent helps maintain a healthy self-concept. Participation in sports, hobbies, or the community can have a positive outcome.

6. Body Image Changes

a. Adolescents seem particularly concerned with the body images portrayed by the media. Changes that occur during puberty result in comparisons between individual adolescents and their surrounding peer groups. Parents also give their input as to hair styles, dress, and activities. Adolescents may require help if depression or eating disorders result due to poor body image.

7. Social Development

a. Peer relationships develop. These relationships act as a support system for adolescents.

b. Best-friend relationships are more stable and longer lasting than they were in previous years.

c. Parent–child relationships change to allow a greater sense of independence.

8. Age-Appropriate Activities

a. Nonviolent video games
b. Nonviolent music
c. Sports
d. Caring for a pet
e. Career training programs
f. Reading
g. Social events (going to the movies, school dances)

9. Health Promotion for Adolescents

a. Immunizations: See the preceding immunization chart

b. Health Screenings
1) Scoliosis: Screenings for scoliosis should continue during the adolescent years. These screenings should include an examination for a lateral curvature of the spine before and during growth spurts. Screenings may take place at school or at a health care facility.

c. Nutrition
1) Rapid growth and high metabolism require increases in quality nutrients. Nutrients that tend to be deficient during this stage of life are iron, calcium, and vitamins A and C.

2) Eating disorders commonly develop during adolescence (more prevalent in girls than in boys) due to a fear of being overweight, fad diets, and/or the desire to maintain control over some aspect of life. Eating disorders include anorexia nervosa, bulimia nervosa, and obesity.

    a) Advise parents to:

        (1) Avoid using food as a reward.

        (2) Emphasize physical activity.

        (3) Ensure that a balanced diet is consumed. Healthy food recommendations are posted by the United States Department of Agriculture (http://www.mypyramid.gov).

    b) Teach children to make healthy food selections for meals and snacks.

d. Dental health

    1) Brush daily.

    2) Floss daily.

    3) Have regular checkups.

    4) Have regular fluoride treatments.

e. Injury Prevention

    1) Three leading causes of death in adolescents are homicide, suicide, and motor vehicle accidents.

    2) Sources of accidental injury

        a) Keep firearms in a locked cabinet or box.

        b) Teach proper use of sporting equipment prior to use.

          (1) Insist on helmet use and/or pads when rollerblading, skateboarding, bicycling, riding scooters, skiing, and snowboarding.

          (2) Avoid trampolines.

    3) Be aware of changes in mood. Monitor for self-harm in adolescents who are at risk. Watch for:

        a) Poor school performance

        b) Lack of interest in things that were of interest to the adolescent in the past

        c) Social isolation

        d) Disturbances in sleep or appetite

        e) Expression of suicidal thoughts

    4) Burns

        a) Teach fire safety.

        b) Teach to apply sunscreen when outside.

    5) Drowning

        a) Teach adolescents to swim.

        b) Teach adolescents not to swim alone.

    6) Motor vehicle injuries

        a) Encourage attendance at drivers' education courses. Emphasize the need for adherence to seat belt use.

        b) Insist on helmet use with bicycles, motorcycles, skateboards, roller blades, and snowboards.

        c) Discourage use of cell phones while driving and enforce laws regarding use.

        d) Teach the dangers of combining substance abuse with driving.

        e) Role model desired behavior.

    7) Substance abuse

        a) Monitor for signs of substance abuse in adolescents who are at risk.

        b) Teach adolescents to say "no" to illegal drugs and alcohol.

        c) Present a no-tolerance attitude.

    8) Sexually transmitted diseases (STDs)

        a) Provide education and resources for treatment.

    9) Pregnancy prevention

        a) Provide education.

SECTION 3

Nursing Care of Children: The Hospitalized Child

A. Stress of Hospitalization: The stress that may be experienced by families and children related to hospitalization. The nurse should be alert to signs of stress and intervene as appropriate. The family should be considered as clients when a child is hospitalized or ill.

B. Separation anxiety during hospitalization manifests in three behavioral responses:

  1. Protest (screaming)

  2. Despair (developmental regression)

  3. Detachment (lack of interaction with unfamiliar people)

C. Contributing Factors

  1. Family structure and response to illness

  2. Chronological age

  3. Developmental stage

  4. Cognitive ability

D. Impact of Hospitalization Based on Development Stage of Child

E. Family Responses

  1. Fear and guilt regarding not bringing the child in for care earlier

  2. Frustration due to the perceived inability to care for the child

  3. Altered family roles

  4. Worry regarding finances if work is missed

  5. Worry regarding care of other children within the household

  6. Fear related to lack of knowledge regarding illness or treatments

Impact of Hospitalization on Children

Age	Level of Understanding	Impact of Hospitalization
Infant	• Inability to describe symptoms and follow directions • Lack of understanding for the need of therapeutic procedures	• Experiences stranger anxiety between 6 to 18 months of age • Displays physical behaviors as expressions of discomfort due to inability to verbalize • May experience sleep deprivation due to strange noises, monitoring devices, and procedures
Toddler	• Limited ability to describe symptoms • Poorly developed sense of body image and boundaries • Limited understanding for the need for therapeutic procedures • Limited ability to follow directions	• Experiences separation anxiety • May exhibit an intense reaction to any type of procedure due to the intrusion of boundaries
Preschooler	• Limited understanding of the cause of illness but knows what illness feels like • Limited ability to describe symptoms • Fears related to magical thinking • Ability to understand cause and effect inhibited by concrete thinking	• May experience separation anxiety • May harbor fears of bodily harm • May believe illness and hospitalization are a punishment
School-age child	• Beginning awareness of body functioning • Ability to describe pain symptoms • Increasing ability to understand cause and effect	• Fears loss of control • Seeks information as a way to maintain a sense of control • May sense when not being told the truth • May experience stress related to separation from peers and regular routine
Adolescent	• Increasing ability to understand cause and effect • Perceptions of illness severity are based on the degree of body image changes	• Develops body image disturbance • Attempts to maintain composure but is embarrassed about losing control • Experiences feelings of isolation from peers • Worries about outcome and impact on school/activities • May not adhere to treatments/medication regimen due to peer influence

F. Assessment of Family

1. Child's and family's understanding of the illness or the reason for hospitalization
2. Stressors unique to the child and family (needs of other children in the family, socioeconomic situation, health of other extended family members)
3. Past experiences with hospitalization and illness
4. Developmental level and needs of child/family
5. Parenting role and the family's perception of role changes
6. Support available to the child/family

G. NURSING INTERVENTIONS

1. Teach the child and family what to expect during hospitalization.
2. Encourage parents or family members to stay with the child during the hospital experience to reduce the stress.
3. Attempt to maintain routine as much as possible.
4. See table below for age-related nursing interventions.

Age-Related Interventions

Age	Interventions
Infant	• Place infants whose parents are not in attendance close to nursing stations so that their needs may be quickly met.
Toddler	• Provide consistency in assigning caregivers. • Encourage parents to provide routine care for the child, such as changing diapers and feeding the child. • Encourage the child's autonomy by giving the child appropriate choices. • Provide consistency in assigning caregivers.
Preschooler	• Explain all procedures using simple, clear language. Avoid medical jargon and terms that can be misinterpreted by the child. • Encourage the child's independence by letting the child provide selfcare. • Encourage the child to express feelings. • Validate the child's fears and concerns. • Provide toys that allow for emotional expression, such as a pounding board to release feelings of protest.

(continues)

Age-Related Interventions (continued)

Age	Interventions
Preschooler *(continued)*	• Provide consistency in assigning caregivers. • Give choices when possible, such as "Do you want your medicine in a cup or a spoon?" • Allow younger children to handle equipment if it is safe.
School-age	• Provide factual information. • Encourage the child to express feelings. • Try to maintain a normal routine for long hospitalizations, including time for school work. • Encourage contact with peer group.
Adolescent	• Provide factual information. • Include the adolescent in the planning of care to relieve feelings of powerlessness and lack of control. • Encourage contact with peer group.

H. Play

1. Overview
   a. Play allows children to express feelings and fears.
   b. Play facilitates mastery of developmental stages and assists in the development of problem-solving abilities.
   c. Play allows children to learn socially acceptable behaviors.
   d. Play activities should be specific to each child's stage of development.
   e. Play can be used to teach children.
   f. Play is a means of protection from everyday stressors.

2. Content of Play
   a. Social affective: Taking pleasure in relationship
   b. Sense-pleasure: Objects in the environment catching the child's attention
   c. Skill: Demonstrating new abilities
   d. Unoccupied behavior: Focusing attention on something of interest
   e. Dramatic; Pretending and fantasizing
   f. Games: Imitative, formal, or competitive

3. Social Character of Play
   a. Onlooker: The child observing others
   b. Solitary: The child playing alone
   c. Parallel: Children playing independently but among other children, which is characteristic of toddlers
   d. Associative: Children playing together without organization, which is characteristic of preschoolers
   e. Cooperative play: Organized playing in groups, which is characteristic of school-age children

4. Functions of Play
   a. Play helps in the development of the following types of skills:
      1) Intellectual
      2) Sensorimotor
      3) Social
         a) Self-awareness
         b) Creativity
         c) Therapeutic and moral values

5. Play Activities Related to Age
   a. Infants
      1) Birth to 3 months: Visual and auditory stimuli
      2) 3 to 6 months: Noise-making objects and soft toys
      3) 6 to 9 months: Teething toys and social interaction
      4) 9 to 12 months: Large blocks, toys that pop apart, and push-and-pull toys
   b. Toddler
      1) Cloth books
      2) Large crayons and paper
      3) Push-and-pull toys
      4) Tricycles
      5) Balls
      6) Puzzles with large pieces
      7) Educational television
      8) Videos for children
   c. Preschoolers
      1) Associative, imitative, and imaginative play
      2) Drawing, painting, riding a tricycle, swimming, jumping, and running
      3) Educational television and videos
   d. School-age children
      1) Games that can be played alone or with another person
      2) Team sports
      3) Musical instruments
      4) Arts and crafts
      5) Collections
   e. Adolescents
      1) Team sports
      2) School activities
      3) Reading and listening to music
      4) Peer interactions

6. Therapeutic Play
   a. Makes use of dolls and/or stuffed animals
   b. Encourages the acting out of feelings of fear, anger, hostility, and sadness
   c. Enables the child to learn coping strategies in a safe environment
   d. Assists in gaining cooperation for medical treatment

7. Assessment Regarding Play

   a. Developmental level of the child

   b. Motor skills

   c. Level of activity tolerance

   d. Child's preferences

 8. **NURSING INTERVENTIONS** Regarding Play

   a. Select activities that enhance development.

   b. Observe the child's play for clues to the child's fears or anxieties.

   c. Encourage parents to bring one favorite toy from home.

   d. Use dolls and/or stuffed animals to demonstrate a procedure before it is done.

   e. Provide play opportunities that meet the child's level of activity tolerance.

   f. Allow the child to go to the play room if able.

   g. Encourage the adolescent's peers to visit.

I. Collaborative Care

1. Consult child life specialist.

2. Consult social services if needed.

3. Consult resource management as needed.

SECTION 4

Nursing Care of Children: Pain Management

A. Overview

1. Assessment of pain in children is complex and challenging.

2. Children have a right to adequate assessment and management of pain. The nurse's role is to advocate for the child and family and educate about proper pain management.

3. Pain is whatever the child says it is, and it exists whenever the child says it does. The child's report of pain is the most reliable diagnostic measurement of pain. Behavioral measures are also used to evaluate pain.

4. The type of pain children experience includes procedure-related pain, operative and trauma-associated pain, and/or acute and chronic pain from illness or injury.

5. Pain assessments should be performed and recorded frequently by the nurse, and pain may be considered the fifth vital sign.

6. The effectiveness of treatment should be evaluated in a timely manner (15 min after IV pain medication administration, 30 min after IM pain medication, 30–60 min after oral medication administration and non-pharmacologic therapies).

   a. Assessment is more difficult to determine in infants and young children because they lack the verbal skills to state how severe the pain is. Older children and adolescents are able to self-report information about what they are experiencing.

   b. Behaviors in a child with pain can vary from immobility and stillness to restlessness and constant mobility.

   c. Changes in blood pressure, pulse, and respiratory rate are temporary physiologic changes associated with the pain. Initially, elevated vital signs will return to normal despite the persistence of pain.

   d. Children from 3 to 7 years of age may comprehend how to use a pain rating scale, and self-report using pain scales may be useful with children over 7 years of age. However, each child's ability should be assessed. Verification with parents will validate assessment. Often, parents may indicate that the child is experiencing pain, and the nurse should be attuned to this report.

   e. Proper pain management includes the use of pharmacologic and non-pharmacologic pain management therapies, such as guided imagery.

   f. Children receiving opioid medications need to be monitored closely for respiratory depression.

B. Contributing Factors

1. Age can influence how pain is perceived and how it can be communicated.

2. Fatigue, anxiety, and fear can increase sensitivity to pain.

3. Genetic sensitivity can increase or decrease the amount of pain tolerated.

4. Cognitive impairment may impact a child's ability to report pain or report it accurately.

5. Prior experiences can increase or decrease sensitivity depending on whether or not adequate relief was obtained, especially in older children and adolescents.

6. Family and friends may decrease sensitivity to pain by staying with the child.

7. Culture may influence how a child expresses pain or the meaning given to it.

C. Manifestations

1. Behaviors complement self-report and assist in pain assessment of children who are unable to verbalize their feelings.

   a. Facial expressions (grimace, wrinkled forehead) and body movements (restlessness, pacing, guarding)

   b. Moaning and crying

   c. Decreased attention span

2. Physiologic measures of blood pressure, pulse, and respiratory rate will be temporarily increased by acute pain. Eventually, increased vital signs will return to normal despite the persistence of pain. Therefore, physiologic indicators may not be an accurate measure of pain over time.

3. Common pain scales (see table below)

Tools Used in Pain Assessment

Pain Assessment Tool	Form of Evaluation	Age of Child

CRIES Neonatal Postoperative Scale	• Pain rated on a scale of 0 to 10
	• Behavior indicators
	  – Crying
	  – Changes in vital signs
	  – Changes in expression
	  – Altered sleeping patterns
		32 weeks of gestation to 20 weeks of life

Faces, Legs, Activity, Cry, and Consolability (FLACC) Postoperative Pain Tool	• Behavior indicators • Facial expressions • Position of legs • Activity • Crying • Ability to be consoled	2 months to 7 years
FACES Pain Rating Scale	• Rating scale uses drawings of happy and sad faces to depict levels of pain.	3 years and older
Visual Analog Scale (VAS)	• Pain is rated on a scale of 0 to 10. • Child points to the number that best describes the pain he is experiencing	7 years and older (may be effective with children as young as 4.5 years)

Noncommunicating Children's Pain Checklist	• Pain is rated on a scale of 0 to 18.
	• Behavior indicators
	  – Vocalization
	  – Socialization
	  – Facial expressions
	  – Activity level
	  – Movement of extremities
	  – Physiologic changes
		3 to 18 years of age (for children with or without cognitive impairments)

D. Collaborative Care

 1. **NURSING INTERVENTIONS**

a. Interventions should be determined in conjunction with the family and child. Severity of the pain will also guide the choice of treatment.

b. Medications

1) Administer medications routinely versus PRN (as needed) to manage pain that is expected to last for an extended period of time.

2) Use caution when administering medications to newborns less than 2 to 3 months of age because of immature liver function.

3) Combine adjuvant medications (steroids, antidepressants, sedatives, antianxiety medications, muscle relaxants, anticonvulsants) with other analgesics.

4) Use non-opioid and opioid medications.

  a) Acetaminophen (Tylenol) and NSAIDs are acceptable for mild to moderate pain.

  b) Opioids are acceptable for moderate to severe pain. Medications used include morphine sulfate, oxycodone (OxyContin), and fentanyl (Duragesic).

  c) Combining a non-opioid and an opioid medication treats pain peripherally and centrally. This offers greater analgesia with less adverse effects (respiratory depression, constipation, nausea).

5) Appropriate Routes (See table below)

c. Non-pharmacologic Measures

1) Positioning

2) Teaching breathing and relaxation techniques

3) Splinting

4) Maintaining a calm environment (low noise, reduced lighting)

5) Providing ice to swollen or injured area

6) Offering warm blankets

7) Assisting with guided imagery

8) Offering distractions (video games, cartoons, videos)

9) Providing comfort with physical contact (holding, rocking)

10) Administering sucrose pacifiers for infants during procedures.

Routes of Medication Administration

Route	Nursing Implications
Oral	• The oral medication route is preferred due to its convenience, cost, and ability to maintain steady blood levels. • Oral medications take 1 to 2 hr to reach peak analgesic effects. Therefore, these medications are not suited for children experiencing pain that requires rapid relief or pain that is fluctuating in nature.

Topical/transdermal	• One type of topical/transdermal medication is a eutectic mixture of local anesthetics (EMLA), which contains equal quantities of lidocaine and prilocaine in the form of a cream or disk.
	  – Use EMLA for any procedure in which the skin will be punctured (IV insertion, biopsy) 60 min prior to a superficial puncture and 2 hr prior to a deep puncture.
	  – Place an occlusive dressing over the cream after application.
	  – Prior to the procedure, remove the dressing or disk and clean the skin. An indication of an adequate response is reddened or blanched skin.
	  – Demonstrate to the child that the skin is not sensitive by tapping or scratching lightly.
	  – Instruct parents to apply EMLA at home prior to coming to a health care facility for the procedure.
	• Fentanyl
	  – Use for children older than 12 years of age.
	  – Use to provide continuous pain control. It has an onset of 12 to 24 hr and a duration of 72 hr.
	  – Use an immediate-release opioid for breakthrough pain.
	  – Treat respiratory depression with naloxone (Narcan).

Continuous intravenous (IV)	• Use continuous intravenous (IV) medication administration to provide stable blood levels.
Patient-controlled analgesia (PCA)	• Use a PCA to control pain from injury and chronic conditions. • Administer morphine, fentanyl, and hydromorphone (Dilaudid) via PCA. • Allow child to control PCA if appropriate. • Designate one family member or one nurse to control PCA.

SECTION 5

Nursing Care of Children: Safe Medication Administration

A. Overview

1. Organ system immaturity affects drug sensitivity in infants and children.

2. Variations

   a. Newborns and young infants may have intense and prolonged responses to medications.

   b. In comparison to adults, medications administered by IM injection are absorbed more slowly in newborns, but faster in infants.

   c. A limited protein-binding capacity may lead to high concentrations of free drugs.

   d. Newborns are highly sensitive to medications that affect the CNS and are metabolized by the liver.

   e. Newborns have limited renal excretion abilities. Therefore, they must have reduced dosages of medications that are eliminated by the renal system.

   f. Starting at 1 year of age, children's pharmacokinetic responses to medication will start to be similar to those of adults, with the exception of faster metabolism until age 12.

3. Pediatric dosages are based on body weight, body surface area (BSA), and maturation of body organs.

4. Nurses should be particularly alert when administering medications to children due to the high risk for medication error.

   a. Adult medication forms and concentrations may require dilution, calculation, preparation, and administration of very small doses. Certain medications should be double-checked by another nurse. Nurses should be aware of those medications and follow facility policies on administration.

B. Pediatric-Specific Considerations of Safe Medication Administration

1. **Right client**: Verify the client's identification each time a medication is administered.

   a. Infants and young children cannot be relied upon to identify themselves.

   b. Young children may answer to any name that is called. A parent or guardian can be asked to identify an infant or young child.

2. **Right dose**: Calculate the correct medication dose; many pediatric medication doses will be weight based. Check medication reference to ensure the dose is within the safe and therapeutic range. Have a second nurse check if unsure or if facility policy requires it.

3. **Right route**: If administering an oral medication, the nurse should use a pediatric-approved medication administration device. The nurse should also educate parents not to use household measuring devices for medication administration.

C. Contributing Factors Influencing Medication Administration

1. Organ system immaturity is the greatest factor that affects medication response in children.
2. Psychosocial variables affecting medication responses in children:
   a. Health/illness beliefs of the child and family
   b. Previous experiences with medications
   c. Developmental stage

D. Nursing Assessments

1. Medication dose appropriate for child's weight
2. Child's ability to cooperate with medication administration

E. Collaborative Care

1. **NURSING INTERVENTIONS**
   a. Oral Medication Administration
      1) Consider the oral route as the preferred route for children and milliliters (mL) as the preferred measurement (5 mL = 1 tsp, 30 mL = 1 oz).
      2) Use plastic, needleless syringes for measurement and administration of small doses of medications.
      3) To ensure that the total dose is given, use only a small amount of liquid or soft food when mixing medications.
      4) Strategies for administering oral medications to infants
         a) Do not mix a medication with formula because the infant may not take all of the formula, which will result in the infant not receiving the full dose of medication. This may also alter the taste of the formula, which may cause the infant to refuse to drink it in the future.
         b) Hold the infant in a semi-upright or semi-Fowler's position to prevent aspiration.
         c) Use a medicine cup once the infant is able to drink from a cup.
         d) Place the medication into nipples from which the infant can suck.
   b. Other Medication Administration Routes
      1) Optic, otic, and nasal administration
         a) Procedures for these routes are similar to adult administration.
         b) Pull the auricle down and back when instilling otic solutions for children up to 3 years of age. Pull the auricle up and back for older children.
      2) Use strategies to gain the child's cooperation.
      3) Allow the parent to be present. The parent may also hold the child.
      4) Warm otic solutions to room temperature before instilling.
      5) Hyperextend the child's neck for nasal medication administration to prevent the medication from sliding down into the child's throat.
      6) Subcutaneous (SQ) and Intradermal Medication Administration
         a) Strategies to decrease pain
            (1) Apply a eutectic mixture of local anesthetics (EMLA) in the form of a cream or disk 60 min prior to injection.
            (2) Ensure that the amount of medication injected is appropriate for the child's muscle size (approximately 0.5 mL in infants and 2.0 mL in children).
      7) Intramuscular (IM) Medication Administration
         a) Strategies to decrease pain
            (1) Apply a eutectic mixture of local anesthetics (EMLA) in the form of a cream or disk a minimum of 60 min, preferably 2 to 2.5 hr, prior to injection.
            (2) Ability to obtain proper positioning of the child
      8) Intravenous (IV) Medication Administration
         a) A child who requires short-term therapy may be discharged with a peripheral line that is maintained by a home health care nurse.
         b) Central venous access devices (VADs)
            (1) If a child is to go home with a VAD, discharge instructions should include how to prepare and inject medication, flush the line, and perform dressing changes.
         c) Peripherally inserted central catheters (PICCs)
            (1) PICC lines are used for short- to moderate-length therapy.
            (2) PICCs are the least costly and have the fewest incidences of complications.

SECTION 6

Nursing Care of Children: Death and Dying

A. Overview

1. The death of a child may be traumatic and devastating for a family.
2. Parental grief may last a lifetime, place stress on marital relations, and impact a parent's ability to assist siblings in dealing with their grief.
3. Children, regardless of age, will experience grief and loss, which is expressed sporadically through behavior and play and is present for a long period of time. Grief in children is expressed and dealt with in an individual manner. Children who have sustained the loss of siblings may experience physical symptoms (sleep disturbances, depression) or may display behaviors like trying to be perfect or acting out for attention.

4. Dysfunctional grief is a type of complicated grief that persists for more than a year after the loss. This type of grief presents with the following characteristics: intense and prolonged feelings of loneliness, emptiness, and yearnings; distractive thoughts; an inability to sleep; lowered self-esteem; and loss of interest in daily activities.

5. Family-centered care is required to meet the needs of each individual family member who is experiencing grief.

Palliative Care (End-of-Life Care)

Palliative care is a multidisciplinary approach that focuses on the process of dying rather than prolonging life in cases in which cures are no longer possible.

A. Factors Influencing Loss, Grief, and Coping Ability

1. Interpersonal relationships and social support networks

2. Type and significance of loss

3. Culture and ethnicity

4. Spiritual and religious beliefs and practices

5. Prior experience with loss

6. Socioeconomic status

7. Current stage of development

Children's Response to Death/Dying

Age	Relevant Factors
Infants/Toddlers (birth to 3 years)	• Have little to no concept of death • Have egocentric thinking that prevents them from understanding death (toddlers) • Mirror parental emotions (sadness, anger, depression, anxiety) • React in response to the changes brought about by being in the hospital (change of routine, painful procedures, immobilization, less independence, separation from family) • May regress to an earlier stage of behavior
Preschool children (3 to 6 years)	• Have egocentric thinking • Have magical thinking that allows them to believe that their thoughts can cause an event such as death (As a result, they may feel guilty and shameful.) • Interpret separation from parents as punishment for bad behavior • View dying as temporary because they have no concept of time and because the dead person may still have attributes of the living (sleeping, eating, breathing)
School-age children (6 to 12 years)	• Start to respond to logical or factual explanations • Begin to have an adult concept of death (inevitable, irreversible, universal), which generally applies to school-age children who are older (9 to 12 years)

Age	Relevant Factors
School-age children (6 to 12 years) *(continued)*	• Experience fear of the disease process, the death process, the unknown , and loss of control – Fear is often displayed through un cooperative behavior. • May be curious about funeral services and what happens to the body after death
Adolescents (12 to 20 years)	• May have an adult-like concept of death • May have difficulty accepting death because they are discovering who they are, establishing an identity, and dealing with issues of puberty • Rely more on their peers rather than the influence of their parents, which may cause the reality of a serious illness to cause adolescents to feel isolated. • May be unable to relate to peers and communicate with their parents • May become more stressed by changes in physical appearance from the medications or illness than the prospect of death • May experience guilt and shame

B. Contributing factors that may increase the family's potential for dysfunctional grieving following the death of a child include:

1. Lack of a support system

2. Presence of poor coping skills

3. Association of violence or suicide with the death of the child

4. Sudden and unexpected death of the child

5. Lack of hope or presence of preexisting mental health issues

C. Assessment

1. Knowledge regarding diagnosis, prognosis, and care

2. Perceptions and desires regarding diagnosis, prognosis, and care

3. Nutritional status, as well as growth and development patterns

4. Activity and energy level of the child

5. Parents' wishes regarding the child's end-of-life care

6. Presence of a do-not-resuscitate (DNR) order

7. Family coping and available support

8. The stage of grief the child and family are experiencing

9. Symptoms of normal grief, which may include:

   a. Feelings of sadness, denial, anxiety, and/or yearning

   b. Feelings of guilt and/or anger toward the deceased

   c. Somatic reports of chest pain, palpitations, headaches, nausea, changes in sleep patterns, or fatigue

   d. Experience of hearing the deceased person's voice

D. Collaborative Care

 1. **NURSING INTERVENTIONS**: Terminally Ill Children

Care for Terminally Ill Children

Care	Focus
Hospital care	• The child cannot be managed at home (the family does not want or is not able to provide necessary care, the child requires intensive nursing care).
Home care	• A home care agency nurse provid es assessments, treatments, medications, supplies, and equipment under the direction of the health care provider.
Hospice care	• The psychological, spiritual, physical, and social needs of the child and family will be managed. • Family members providing most of the care with support from the hospice team. • Priority is given to pain and symptom control. • Support to the family will continue post death. Family needs will be addressed after death occurs.

a. Allow an opportunity for anticipatory grieving, which impacts the way a family will cope with the death of a child.

b. Offer primary nursing.

c. Offer strategies specific to developmental level.

Strategies for Caring for Terminally Ill Children

Age Group	Developmental Approach
Infants and toddlers	• Encourage parents to stay with the child. • Attempt to maintain a normal environment.
Preschoolers	• Encourage parents to stay with the child. • Communicate with the child in honest, simple terms. • Be aware of medical jargon that may frighten the child.
School-age children	• Encourage parents to stay with the child. • Use language that is dear regarding the disease, medications, procedures, and expectations. • Encourage self-care to promote independence and self-esteem. • Allow participation in plans for funeral services.
Adolescents	• Be honest and respectful when co mmuni cating. • Encourage self-care to prom ote independence and self-esteem • Allow participation in plans for funeral services • Encourage parents or other family members to stay with the adolescent.

 2. **NURSING INTERVENTIONS**: Palliative Care

a. Consider the child, siblings, and parents as the units of care.

b. Provide an environment that is as close to being like home as possible.

c. Consult with the child and family for desired measures.

d. Respect the family's cultural and religious preferences and rituals.

e. Provide and clarify information and explanations.

f. Encourage physical contact; address feelings; and show concern, empathy, and support.

g. Provide comfort measures (warmth, quiet, noise control, dry linens).

h. Provide adequate nutrition and hydration.

i. Control pain.
   1) Give medications on a regular schedule.
   2) Treat breakthrough pain.
   3) Increase doses as necessary to control pain.
   4) Encourage use of relaxation, imagery, and distraction to help manage pain.

 3. **NURSING INTERVENTIONS**: End-of-Life Care for the Terminally Ill Client

a. Provide information to the child and family about the disease, medications, procedures, and expected events.

b. Encourage and support parents to participate in caring for the child.

c. Encourage parents to remain near the child as much as possible.

d. Encourage the child's independence and control as developmentally and physically appropriate.

e. Allow for visitation of family and friends as desired.

f. Emphasize open, honest communication among the child, family, and health care team.

g. Provide support to the child and family with decision making.

h. Provide opportunities for the child and family to ask questions.

i. Assist the child with completion of unfinished tasks.

j. Assist parents to cope with their feelings and help them to understand the child's behaviors.

k. Use books, movies, art, music, and play therapy to stimulate discussions and provide an outlet for emotions.

l. Provide and encourage professional support and guidance from a trusted member of the health care team.

m. Remain neutral and accepting.

n. Give reassurance that the child is not in pain and that all efforts are being made to maintain comfort and support of the child's life.

o. Recognize and support the individual differences of grieving. Advise families that each member may react differently on any given day.

p. Give families privacy, unlimited time, and opportunities for any cultural or religious rituals. Respect the family's decisions regarding care of the child.

q. Encourage discussion of special memories and people, reading of favorite books, providing favorite toys/objects, physical contact, sibling visits, and continued verbal communication, even if the child seems unconscious.

r. After death, validate the loss.
   1) The nurse should express his own feelings of loss and sadness to someone who can offer support.

s. Issues and decisions to be addressed at the time of death include the following:
   1) Organ and/or tissue donation if applicable
   2) Autopsy
   3) Viewing of the body
   4) Sibling's attendance at the funeral

SECTION 7

Nursing Care of the Child with a Congenital Anomaly

A. Congenital Heart Disease (CHD): Anatomic defects of the heart prevent normal blood flow to the pulmonary and/or systemic system. Many defects will spontaneously close, but some will require surgical repair. Most children with CHD will be diagnosed in the first year of life, but certain children may not exhibit manifestations until later. Children with CHD have an increased incidence of other anatomic defects, which may impact their care.

1. Contributing Factors
   a. Cardiac development occurs very early in fetal life, making it difficult to identify the cause of defects.
      1) Maternal factors
         a) Rubella in early pregnancy
         b) Alcohol and/or other substance abuse during pregnancy
         c) Diabetes mellitus
      2) Genetic factors
         a) History of congenital heart disease in other family members
         b) Trisomy 21 (Down syndrome)
         c) Presence of other congenital anomalies or syndromes

B. Heart failure (HF): Impaired myocardial function.

1. Contributing factors
   a. Structural anomalies such as septal defects
   b. Increased blood volume and pressure within the heart
   c. Decreased contractility of the heart
   d. Excessive demands on the cardiac muscle such as sepsis, and severe anemia
   e. Pulmonary congestion

2. Manifestations—can be divided into three categories. See table below.

Impaired Myocardial Function	Pulmonary Congestion	Systemic Venous Congestion
Tachycardia	Tachypnea	Weight gain
Excessive diaphoresis	Dyspnea	Hepatomegaly
Decreased output	Flaring nares	Peripheral edema
Fatigue	Intercostal retractions (infants)	Periorbital edema
Weakness	Activity intolerance	Ascites
Restlessness	Cough	Clubbing
Poor appetite	Hoarseness	Polycythemia
Pale cool extremities	Cyanosis	Jugular Vein Distention (JVD) seen only in children, not seen in infants).
Weak peripheral pulses	Wheezing	
Decreased B/P	Grunting	**Hypercyanotic spells (blue, or Tet, spells) are manifested as acute cyanosis**
Cardiomegaly	Orthopnea	
Gallop heart rhythm		

3. Diagnostic Procedures
   a. Laboratory Tests
      1) Hemoglobin (Hgb)
      2) Hematocrit (Hct)
      3) Serum electrolytes
   b. ECG monitoring

4. Collaborative Care
    a. **NURSING INTERVENTIONS**
      1) Assist with the application of electrodes.
      2) Assist with maintaining the child in a quiet position.
   b. Client Education
      1) Tell the child that the test will not be painful.
   c. Radiography (chest x-ray)
   d. Echocardiography

5. Therapeutic Measures
   a. Cardiac catheterization
    1) **NURSING INTERVENTIONS**
      Pre catherization
      a) Perform a nursing history and physical exam. Signs and symptoms of infections, such as a severe diaper rash, may necessitate canceling the procedure if femoral access is required.
      b) Check for allergies to iodine and shellfish.
      c) Provide age-appropriate teaching.
      d) Provide for NPO status 4–6 hr prior to the procedure.
      e) Obtain baseline vital signs including oxygen saturation.
      f) Locate and mark the dorsalis pedis and posterior tibial pulses on both extremities.
      g) Administer presedation.

2) **NURSING INTERVENTIONS**
    Post catherization
    a) Provide for continuous cardiac monitoring and oxygen saturation.
    b) Assess pulses for equality and symmetry.
    c) Assess temperature and color. A cool extremity with skin that blanches may indicate arterial obstruction.
    d) Assess insertion site (femoral or antecubital area) for bleeding and/or hematoma.
    e) Maintain clean dressing.
    f) Monitor I&O.
    g) Monitor for hypoglycemia.
    h) Prevent bleeding by maintaining the affected extremity in a straight position for 4–8 hr.
    i) Encourage oral intake, starting with clear liquids.
    j) Encourage the child to void to promote excretion of the contrast medium.

6. Collaborative Care

 a. **NURSING INTERVENTIONS**
    1) Conserve the child's energy by providing frequent rest periods; clustering care; providing small, frequent meals; bathing PRN; and keeping crying to a minimum in cyanotic children.
    2) Perform daily weight and I&O.
    3) Monitor heart rate, blood pressure, serum electrolytes, and renal function.
    4) Allow the child to sleep with several pillows.
    5) Allow the infant to rest during feedings, taking approximately 30 minutes to complete the feeding.
    6) Gavage feed the infant if he is unable to consume enough formula or breast milk.
    7) Monitor oxygen saturation every 2–4 hr.
  b. Medications
    1) Digoxin (Lanoxin): improves myocardial contractility

> **Note:** If an *infant's pulse is less than 90/min*, the medication should be withheld. In children, the medication should be withheld if the pulse is less than 70/min.

    2) Captopril (Capoten) or enalapril (Vasotec)
    3) Furosemide (Lasix) or chlorothiazide (Diuril)
  c. Client Education and Referrals
    1) Dieticians should be consulted to assist the family with appropriate food choices.

Review of Acyanotic Congenital Heart Defects

Anomaly	Hemodynamics	Manifestations	Treatment
Patent ductus arteriosus • A vascular channel between the left main pulmonary artery and the descending aorta, as a result of failure of the fetal ductus arteriosus to dose	• Shunt of oxygentated blood from the aorta into the pulmonary artery • Increased left ventricular output and work load	• Usually asymptomatic, but frequent impairment of growth or heart failure • "Machinery murmur" • Wide pulse pressure	• Medical: adminstration of indomethacin (Indocin) (prostaglandin inhibitor) is effective in some newborns and premature newborns • Surgical: ligation of patent ductus (in infancy)
Ventricular septal defect • In membranous muscular portion of the ventricular septum; may vary from small to large defect	• Shunt of oxygenated blood from left to right ventricle • Leads to right ventricular hypertrophy • Needs surgical repair • Bidirectional shunting may occur with very large defect (Eisenmenger's complex)	• May be asymptomatic • Heart murmur is heard in first week of life (systolic) • Growth failure, feeding problems during the first year of life; failure to thrive; frequent respiratory infections • Heart failure	• Some small defects may close spontaneously • Open heart: direct closure suturing with plastic prosthesis (usually preschooler; may be done earlier in infancy for large defects)
Atrial septal defect • Malfunctioning foramen ovale; or abnormal opening between the atria	• Shunting of oxygenated blood from the left to right atrium • Increased right ventricular output and work load • May develop pulmonary hypertension in adulthood (if not surgically treated in childhood)	• Acyanotic; asymptomatic • Soft blowing, systolic murmur • Thin and asthenic • Frequent episodes of pulmonary inflammatory diseases • Poor exercise intolerance	• Open heart with direct closure or suturing with plastic prosthesis (usually preschooler)
Coarctation of aorta • Preductal constriction of the aorta between subclavian artery and ductus arteriosus • Postductal constriction of aorta directly beyond the ductus	• Obstructions of the flow of blood through the constricted segments • Increased left ventricular pressure and work load • Extensive collateral circulation bypasses coarctated area to supply lower extremities with blood	• Hypertension in upper extremities with decreased blood pressure in lower extremities • Weak or absent pulsations in lower extremities • Heart failure • May be asymptomatic; occasionally fatigue, headaches, leg cramps, epistaxis	• Surgical resection of coarctate area with direct anastomosis or use of a graft • Correction usually done by 2 years of age to prevent permanent hypertension

Review of Cyanotic Congenital Heart Anomalies

Anomaly	Hemodynamics	Manifestations	Treatment

• Tetralogy of Fallot—combination of four defects
  – Pulmonary stenosis
  – ventricular septal defect (vSd)
  – Overriding aorta
  – hypertrophy of right ventricle
	• Obstruction to outflow of blood from the right ventricle into pulmonary circuit and increased pressure in the right ventricle leads to right to left shunting of oxygenated blood through the vSd directly into the aorta
	• Severity of defect depends on degree of pulmonary stenosis and size of vSd
		• Acute cyanosis at birth
		• Cyanosis developing during early months that increases with physical exertion
		• Clubbing of fingers and toes
		• Systolic murmur
		• Acute episodes of cyanosis and hypoxia called "tet spells" or hypercyanotic episodes occur if oxygen supply cannot meet demand (crying, exertion, exercise, feeding)
		• Squatting
		• Growth retardation
			• Surgical—blalock-taussig procedures; provides blood flow to pulmonary arteries from the left to right subdavian artery
			• Repair—open heart closure of vSd and resection of stenosis. Usually performed in the first 2 years of life.

• Transposition of great vessels (TGV)
  – the aorta originates from the right ventricle and the pulmonary artery from the left ventricle
	• Two separate circulations without mixture of oxygenated and unoxygenated blood except through shunts
	• Mixture of blood may occur through one or more septal defects
	  – ventricular septal defect (vSd)
	  – Atrial septal defect (ASd)
	  – Patent ductus arteriosus (PdA)
		• Usually deep cyanosis shortly after birth or after closing of ductus
		• Early clubbing of toes and fingers
		• Poor growth and development, failure to thrive
		• Rapid respirations; fatigue
		• Heart failure
			• Prostaglandin medications are given to keep ductus arteriosus open until surgery. Prostaglandin inhibitors are given to close duct.
			• Repair—arterial switch treatment of choice; must be done within the first few days of life; great vessels reimplanted under complete circulatory arrest
			• Several other types of repair are all multiple stage approaches

C. Club Foot: Congenital clubfoot is a complex deformity of the ankle and foot. Description of the deformity will be dependent upon the position of the ankle and foot. The most common deformity is talipes equinovarus (inward and downward position), and it may be bilateral. Congenital clubfoot occurs as an isolated defect or is diagnosed in association with other disorders, including cerebral palsy and spina bifida. Variations of the deformity and manifestations may be present in one or both feet. The etiology is not known, but it may be related to abnormal embryonic development.

1. Contributing Factors
   a. Positional (intrauterine crowding)
   b. Syndromic (associated with other deformities).
   c. Congenital anomalies
2. Manifestations

Manifestations of Clubfoot

Deformity Name	Manifestation
Talipes equinovarus (most common)	Plantar flexion with feet bending inward
Talipes calcaneus	Dorsiflexion of feet with toes higher than heels

Deformity Name	Manifestation
Talipes equinus	Plantar flexion of feet with toes lower than heels
Talipes varus	Inversion of feet (toes pointing toward midline)
Talipes valgus	Eversion of feet (toes pointing laterally)

3. Diagnostic Procedures
   a. Prenatal ultrasound: used to identify the deformity
   b. Radiograph: used to determine bone placement and tissue involvement for clubfoot
4. Collaborative Care
    a. **NURSING INTERVENTIONS**
      1) Encourage parents to hold and cuddle the child.
      2) Encourage parents to meet the developmental needs of the child.
      3) Assess and maintain the cast or harness used to treat clubfoot.
      4) Perform neurovascular and skin integrity checks after cast or harness placement.

b. Therapeutic Measures

   1) Management of clubfoot will depend upon the severity of the deformity.

   2) Passive exercise should be performed for a minor deformity.

   3) Serial casting is begun after birth before the newborn is discharged home. Weekly casting to stretch the skin and other structures of the foot is done until maximum correction is accomplished.

   4) Surgical intervention should occur if maximum correction is not achieved by 3 months of age.

c. Client Education

   1) Educate the family about how to perform gentle stretching of the foot as prescribed.

   2) Educate the family about the importance of serial casting, cast care, and follow-up appointments.

D. Developmental Dysplasia of the Hip (DDH): A broad term that is used to describe a variety of disorders resulting in abnormal development of the hip structures. **DDH** may be identified during prenatal or postnatal periods or early in childhood.

1. Contributing Factors

  a. DDH may be affected by family history, gender, birth order, intrauterine position, and/or laxity of a joint.

  b. Predisposing factors include intrauterine placement, mechanical situations (e.g., size of infant, multiple births, breech presentation), and genetic factors.

2. Manifestations

  a. Asymmetrical gluteal and thigh folds

  b. Limited abduction of hips. One knee that appears shorter when the infant is supine with thighs flexed at 90° toward the abdomen (Allis sign)

  c. For infants from birth to 3 months of age, the provider performs the Barlow and Ortolani tests

    1) Barlow test: The hips are taken through adduction (the thighs are brought toward the midline) and abduction, and an audible click or clunk is heard from the head of the femur on the affected hip, which can be moved from the socket.

    2) Ortolani test: The affected hip is then reduced back into the socket by manipulation of the joint.

  d. For children able to walk, observe postural gait

    1) Trendelenburg sign: Abnormal downward tilting of pelvis on the unaffected side when bearing weight on the affected side

    2) Waddling gait or abnormal lordosis of spine if bilateral dislocation

3. Diagnostic Procedures

  a. Ultrasound: An ultrasound should be performed at 2 weeks of age to determine the cartilaginous head of the femur.

  b. X-ray: An x-ray can diagnose DDH in infants older than 4 months of age.

4. Collaborative Care

 a. **NURSING INTERVENTIONS**

   1) Assess and maintain the cast or harness used to treat clubfoot or DDH.

   2) Perform neurovascular and skin integrity checks after cast or harness placement.

   3) Ensure proper positioning of Pavlik harness at all times.

   4) Assess and maintain the hip spica cast.

   5) Perform range of motion with the unaffected extremities.

   6) Assess for pain control using an age-appropriate pain tool.

   7) Evaluate hydration status frequently.

   8) Assess elimination status daily.

b. Therapeutic Measures

   1) A Pavlik harness can be used from birth up to 5 or 6 months of age. Until the hip is determined, by radiograph, to be stable. Frequent follow-up will be needed for strap adjustment.

   2) Hip spica cast can be used for infants older than 6 months of age. It can also be used in children whose hips were not stabilized by use of the Pavlik harness. A short course of traction is sometimes used prior to the application of a hip spica cast.

c. Client Education and Referrals

   1) Instruct the family to keep the Pavlik harness on continuously, except during bathing, if prescribed.

   2) Instruct the family to return for follow-up visits weekly at the start of therapy and then as needed.

   3) Teach and reinforce skin care.

   4) Encourage application of a cotton shirt and cotton socks under the Pavlik harness to prevent irritation and the avoidance of powders and lotions.

   5) Position casts on pillows.

   6) Reinforce to parents the importance of monitoring color and temperature of toes on casted extremity.

   7) Encourage parents to hold and cuddle the child.

   8) Encourage parents to meet the developmental needs of the child.

   9) Educate regarding care after discharge with emphasis on using appropriate equipment (stroller, wagon, car seat) for maintaining mobility.

E. Scoliosis: A complex deformity of the spine that also affects the ribs. Scoliosis is characterized by a lateral curvature of the spine and spinal rotation that causes rib asymmetry. Not all curvatures of the spine are scoliosis. A curve of less than 10° may be a postural variation.

1. Contributing Factors

    a. Idiopathic or structural scoliosis is the most common form of scoliosis and can be seen in isolation or associated with other conditions.

2. Manifestations

    a. Asymmetry in scapula, ribs, flanks, shoulders, and hips

    b. Improperly fitting clothing (one leg shorter than the other)

3. Diagnostic Procedures

    a. Screen during preadolescence for boys and girls.

    1) Observe the child, who should be wearing only underwear, from the back.

    2) Have the child bend over at the waist with arms hanging down and observe for asymmetry of ribs and flank.

    3) Diagnosis is made using x-rays of the child in a standing position from the neck to the groin and determining the angle of curvature using the Cobb technique with a scoliometer.

4. Collaborative Care

     a. **NURSING INTERVENTIONS**

    1) Monitor for signs of skin breakdown in the child wearing a brace.

    2) Monitor adherence to therapy.

    3) Postoperatively, monitor pain using an age-appropriate pain tool.

    4) Administer analgesia using a patient-controlled analgesic pump as prescribed.

    5) Turn the adolescent frequently by log rolling to prevent damage to the spinal fusion.

    6) Assess skin for pressure areas, especially if a brace has been prescribed.

    7) Prevent rubbing and pressure from brace.

    8) Provide skin care by keeping skin clean and dry.

    9) Monitor surgical and drain sites for signs of infection. Provide wound care as prescribed.

    10) Assess bowel sounds and monitor, observing for paralytic ileus.

    11) Monitor for decreases in Hgb and Hct. Observe for signs of bleeding.

    12) Administer blood transfusion as prescribed. The adolescent may have self-donated blood available for transfusion.

    13) Encourage mobility as soon as tolerated.

    b. Medications

    1) Administer analgesia using a patient-controlled analgesic pump as prescribed.

    c. Therapeutic Measures

    1) Surgery is generally needed for curves greater than 40°. A type of internal fixation system (Harrington, Dwyer, Zielke) may be used to straighten and realign the spine along with a bony fusion to stabilize the correction.

    2) Repair is performed from either an anterior and/or posterior approach. The type of instrumentation selected is based on surgeon preference and client needs.

    3) The goal of repair is to achieve maximal correction and maximal mobility with minimal complications.

    d. Client Education

    1) Suggest that the family arrange the environment to facilitate the adolescent's ability to be as independent as possible (keep favorite items within reach).

    2) Emphasize the necessity of follow-up care.

F. Hydrocephalus: An imbalance in either absorption or production of cerebrospinal fluid within the intracranial cavity. Classification is either congenital or acquired. Usually diagnosed at birth or within 2 to 4 months of life. Often associated with other neural tube defect (myelomeningocele).

1. Contributing Factors

    a. Impaired absorption of cerebrospinal fluid (CSF) within the subarachnoid space

    b. Obstruction to the flow of CSF through the ventricular system

    c. Developmental malformations: neoplasm, infection, and trauma

2. Manifestations (categorized by age)

    a. Infant: increased head circumference, tense bulging anterior fontanel, distended scalp veins, high-pitched cry, irritability, feeding problems, discomfort when held

    b. Older child: headache, vomiting (especially in the morning), diplopia, blurred vision, behavioral changes, decreased motor function, decreased level of consciousness, seizures

3. Diagnostic Procedure

    a. May be detected on prenatal sonogram

    b. Clinical signs

    1) Increased intracranial pressure

    2) Increased head circumference

    c. Computed tomography or magnetic resonance imaging scan confirms diagnosis by showing excessive fluid in ventricles

4. Collaborative Care

 a. **NURSING INTERVENTIONS**

1) **Preoperatively**: Measure head circumference by obtaining occipitofrontal measurement.

2) **Postoperatively**

a) Perform frequent neurological assessment by measuring head circumference daily.

b) Position on nonoperative site; check anterior fontanel to determine positioning of the head; do not pump shunt without order.

c) Monitor for signs and symptoms of shunt failure: lethargy, vomiting, and irritability.

d) Institute seizure precautions.

e) Decrease shunt infection:

(1) Monitor for elevated vital signs, decreased level of consciousness, vomiting, and feeding problems.

(2) Assess the incision site frequently for manifestations of inflammation or leakage.

(3) Implement care to meet physiologic and developmental needs.

b. Medications

1) Administer IV antibiotics

2) Assist Health Care Provider with intraventricular instillation of antibiotics

c. Therapeutic Measures

1) Surgical placement of a Ventriculoperitoneal (VP) shunt

2) Endoscopic third ventriculostomy-only used for children with a non-communicating hydrocephalus.

d. Client Education and Referrals

1) Instruct primary care givers on how to recognize signs and symptoms of shunt malfunction.

2) Instruct care givers on how to recognize signs and symptoms of infection as well as how to prevent infection.

3) Instruct care givers on of safe transportation and positioning of child.

4) Instruct care givers on how to pump shunt when necessary.

5) Refer families to Home Health when indicated.

6) Refer families to The National Hydrocephalus Foundation and The Hydrocephalus Foundation

Note: Arbitrary pumping of the VP shunt is contraindicated unless ordered by the neurosurgeon. Arbitrary pumping can cause obstruction of the VP shunt.

Note: Shunts will need to be routinely replaced as the child grows.

G. Neural Tube Defects

1. Types

a. Myelomeningocele (Spina Bifida): A spinal defect, in which a fissure in spinal column is open, leaving meninges and A spinal cord exposed; the sac also includes spinal fluid and nerves. The level of impairment depends on the level of the neural tube defect on the spine.

b. Meningocele: A spinal defect and sac-like protrusion are present, but only spinal fluid and meninges are present in the sac. After the sac is repaired, no further symptoms are usually seen because spinal nerves are not damaged.

2. Contributing Factors (etiology unknown)

a. Failure of posterior laminae to fuse with herniation of saclike cyst of meninges, cerebrospinal fluid, spinal nerves

b. Usually associated with other neurological defects (hydrocephalus)

c. May be prevented by folic acid supplementation for women of childbearing age prior to conception and through first trimester

d. Assess family history of neural tube defects

3. Manifestations

a. Partial to complete paralysis determined by location of defect (usually lumbosacral)

b. Musculoskeletal problems such as clubfoot, scoliosis, congenital hip dysplasia

c. Varying degrees of sensory disturbances

d. Parallel motor dysfunction

e. Bowel and bladder problems including constipation, incontinence, and neurogenic bladder

4. Diagnostic Procedure

a. An elevated Maternal Serum Alpha Fetal Protein is a screening tool for neural tube defects

b. Amniocentesis: 98% accurate; elevated amniotic alpha-fetoprotein, confirmed by prenatal sonogram

c. Apparent at birth: visible sac

d. MRI, Ultrasound, and CT are used to determine the degree and causative factors of NTDs.

e. Early closure of myelomeningocele when possible.

5. Collaborative Care

 a. **NURSING INTERVENTIONS**

1) Prevent infection.

2) **Preoperatively**: Priority of care is to preserve integrity of sac.

a) Keep infant in prone position.

b) Cover sac with 4 × 4 gauze moistened with sterile saline.

c) Check sac frequently for tears or cracks.

d) Do not cover sac with clothing or diapers because that places too much pressure on the sac.

e) Perform perineal care to prevent contamination of sac.

f) Monitor for manifestations of meningitis such as irritability, anorexia, fever, and seizures.

3) **Postoperatively**: Priority of care is to promote healing and preserve neurological integrity.

a) Place the infant in a prone position with head slightly lower than body.

b) Place a protective barrier across the incision to prevent contamination.

c) Be aware of long-term problems of infection related to urinary retention, reflux, and chronic urinary tract infections.

d) Monitor for manifestations of increased intracranial pressure.

e) Perform neurological checks by measuring head circumference daily.

f) Promote effective parental and familial coping strategies.

b. Therapeutic Measures

1) Pressure is relieved by surgically inserting a VP shunting device for associated hydrocephalus.

2) Early treatment is necessary to prevent progressive mental retardation.

3) Decision to correct the defect or not is difficult as well as controversial.

4) Early surgical closure is advocated to preserve neural function, reduce risk of infection, and control hydrocephalus.

c. Client Education and Referrals

1) Teach parents the *Credé maneuver*.

2) Encourage independent intermittent self-catheterization, which can be performed as early as 5 to 6 years of age.

3) Stress hydration and early recognition of urinary tract infections.

4) Explain to parents that urinary diversion procedures are often required.

5) Refer to appropriate disciplines for optimal outcomes

a) Orthopedics

b) Physical therapy

c) Neurosurgery

d) Pediatrics

e) Urology

f) Physical therapy

g) Rehabilitation services

h) Social services

! POINT TO REMEMBER: Increased risk for latex allergy—recognize that children with neural tube defects are at increased risk for latex allergy to common medical (or other) products containing latex. Vinyl gloves and balloons should be avoided.

H. Cerebral Palsy: Group of permanent disorders of movement and posture causing activity limitation and disturbances of sensation, perception, communication, cognition, and behavior. CP is categorized into 3 main categories. See the table below for manifestations of each type. The Pathways Awareness Foundation for Parents encourages parents to report any early manifestations of CP early.

1. Contributing Factors

a. Causes undetermined; may be related to prenatal, perinatal, or postnatal factors

b. Birth asphyxia

c. Prenatal brain abnormalities

2. Manifestations (Early): Parents should be instructed to report any of these symptoms immediately.

a. Persistent primitive reflexes

b. Hyper- or hypotonicity (stiff or floppy arms and legs)

c. Poor hand control and body control

d. Feeding difficulties

e. Irritability

f. Delayed attainment of developmental milestones

Manifestations of Cerebral Palsy

Spastic	Dyskinetic	Ataxic
Hypertonicity	Involuntary movements of face and extremities	Lack of coordination and equilibrium
Hyperreflexive DTRs + Clonus	Involuntary movements increase with stress	Gait instability
Difficulty with both gross and fine motor skills	Involuntary movements do not occur during sleep	Orthopedic problems are rare
Contractures of knee and heel cord	DTR's are normal	Decreased reflexes and muscle tone
Gait in crouched with scissoring and toes pointe inward	Rarely have contractures	Speech is often slurred , sporadic or explosive
Elbows, wrist, and fingers are usually in a flexed position with thumbs in an adducted		Nystagmus are often present
Flexor and adductor muscles more affected than extension and abductor muscles		Inability to judge distance speed or strength of movements

3. Diagnostic Procedures

a. Classified by nature and distribution of neuromuscular dysfunction

b. May not be diagnosed until child is several months old

c. Confirmed by physical evaluation or supplemental tests (electroencephalogram test, tomography, or metabolic screening)

4. Collaborative Care

   a. **NURSING INTERVENTIONS**
      1) Institute seizure precautions if appropriate.
      2) Encourage physical safety techniques such as aspiration precautions and adequate rest.
      3) Encourage self-care activities to foster independence and confidence.
      4) Modify the environment, and introduce devices to enhance development, enhance safety, and increase functional abilities.

   b. Medications
      1) Administer anticonvulsants if ordered
      2) Administer antibiotics and analgesics as ordered pre- and postoperatively

   c. Therapeutic Measures
      1) Treatment (based on degree of disability)
      2) Physical therapy (active and passive)
      3) Occupational Therapy
      4) Potentially speech therapy
      5) Modified toys or equipment to enhance development
      6) Modify the environment to enhance safety
      7) Surgery to correct contractures or spastic deformities

   d. Client Education and Referrals
      1) Refer to occupational and speech therapy for evaluation and development of verbal and nonverbal communication skills.
      2) Teach parents alternative communication methods to facilitate positive adjustments of child and family.

I. Gastrointestinal Structural Disorders

   1. Types of Disorders

      a. **Gastroesophageal reflux (GER)** occurs when the gastric contents reflux back up into the esophagus, making esophageal mucosa vulnerable to injury from gastric acid and resulting in gastroesophageal reflux disease (GERD). GER in infants is usually self-limiting and resolves by the end of the first year of life. It may result in failure to thrive, bleeding, and difficulty with swallowing.

      b. **Hypertrophic pyloric stenosis** is the thickening of the pyloric sphincter, which creates an obstruction.

      c. **Hirschsprung's disease, or congenital aganglionic megacolon** is a structural anomaly of the gastrointestinal (GI) tract that is caused by lack of ganglionic cells in segments of the colon and results in mechanical obstruction. Stool accumulates due to lack of peristalsis in the non-innervated area of the bowel (usually rectosigmoid), causing the bowel to dilate. Hirschsprung's disease is usually diagnosed in infants, but chronic milder symptoms may occur in late childhood.

      d. **Meckel's diverticulum** is a complication resulting from failure of the omphalomesenteric duct to fuse during embryonic development. The diverticulum may be up to 4 inches in length and is found in the small intestine.

      e. **Intussusception** is the telescoping of the intestine over itself. This usually occurs in infants and young children up to 5 years of age, but it is most common between 5 and 9 months of age.

      f. **Cleft lip (CL)** results from the incomplete fusion of the maxillary processes during intrauterine life. May be unilateral or bilateral.

      g. **Cleft palate (CP)** results from the incomplete fusion of the palatine plates during intrauterine life.

SECTION 8

Nursing Care of the Child with an Acute Illness

A. Fever: Classified as temperature in excess of **38° C (100.4° F).**

   1. Contributing Factors
      a. Not always related to severity of illness; varies from child to child
      b. Always consider age of the child (below 6 months is a more serious concern)
      c. Child who is immunosuppressed or receiving chemotherapy
      d. Most fevers in children are viral and self-limiting; may play a role in recovery from infection

   2. Manifestations
      a. May vary secondary to the source of fever

   3. Diagnostic Procedures
      a. Feeling a child's skin for warmth is not an accurate indicator.
      b. Always investigate family epidemiology and take a careful history for exposure to communicable diseases.
      c. Remember that diet, activity level, and behavioral changes are subtle diagnostic clues.
      d. Laboratory tests may include:
         1) CBC, urinalysis, chest film, and blood cultures; a "septic workup" includes all of the above with the addition of a lumbar puncture and urine culture.

Gastrointestinal Disorders

Types of Disorders	Contributing Factors	Manifestations	Diagnostic Procedures
Gastroesophageal reflux (GERD)	**GER(D)** is more likely to occur in premature infants and infants born with congenital defects (neurological disorders, esophageal disorders, hiatal hernia, cystic fibrosis, cerebral palsy).	**Infant** Excessive spitting up or forceful vomiting, irritability, excessive crying, blood in stool or vomitus, arching of back and stiffening Apnea or apparent life-threatening event **Older child** Reports of heartburn, abdominal pain, difficulty swallowing, chronic cough, and Sandifer syndrome (in which there is repetitive stretching and arching of head and neck that may mimic seizure activity)	a) Upper GI series to detect GI structural abnormalities b) 24-hr intraesophageal pH monitoring study to measure the amount of gastric acid reflux into the esophagus c) Endoscopy with biopsy to detect esophagitis and strictures d) Scintigraphy to identify cause of gastric content aspiration
Hypertrophic pyloric stenosis	**Hypertrophic pyloric stenosis** has a genetic component.	**Vomiting** that often occurs 30 to 60 min after a meal and becomes projectile as obstruction worsens **Constant hunger** **Olive-shaped mass** in the right upper quadrant of the abdomen and possible peristaltic wave that moves from left to right when lying supine **Failure to gain weight and signs of dehydration**, such as skin that is dry and/or pale, cool lips, dry mucous membranes, decreased skin turgor, diminished urinary output, concentrated urine, thirst, rapid pulse, sunken eyes, and decreased blood pressure	Ultrasound of the abdomen. An ultrasound will reveal an elongated, sausage-shaped mass and an elongated pyloric area.
Hirschsprung's disease, or congenital aganglionic megacolon	**Hirschsprung's disease** may be either an acute or chronic disorder.	**Newborn** Failure to pass meconium within 24 to 48 hr, refusal to eat, episodes of vomiting bile, and abdominal distention **Infant** Failure to thrive, constipation, abdominal distention, episodes of vomiting and diarrhea **Older child** Constipation, abdominal distention, visible peristalsis, ribbon-like stool, palpable fecal mass, and a malnourished appearance	a) Rectal biopsy b) Full-thickness biopsies to reveal the absence of ganglion cells
Meckel's diverticulum		Abdominal pain, bloody stools without pain, bright red mucus in infant stools	a) Radionucleotide scan to show the presence of gastric mucosa
Intussusception	**Intussusception** occurs with cystic fibrosis.	Normal comfort interrupted by periods of sudden and acute pain Palpable, sausage-shaped mass in the right upper quadrant of the abdomen and/or a tender, distended abdomen Stools that are mixed with blood and mucus that resemble the consistency of red currant jelly	a) Ultrasound, barium enema
Cleft lip (CL) and Cleft palate (CP)	**Multifactorial**, but there are strong indicators of genetic or environmental factors **Cleft palate** is more common in males; **Cleft lip** is more common in females and may or may not be accompanied by cleft palate **Heredity** (as the incidence of cleft palate is higher in relatives of people with the defect) **Teratogens** (especially maternal intake of phenytoin [Dilantin]), maternal smoking, and family tendency)	Cleft lip is visible. Cleft palate alone may only be visible when examining the mouth. Individuals are prone to ear, nose, and throat infection. Long-term problems include speech, hearing, and dentition problems.	Cleft lip visible Cleft palate—palates are palpated during the newborn assessment.

Collaborative Care of GI Disorders

Types of Disorders	🩺 NURSING INTERVENTIONS	Medications	Therapeutic Measures	Client Education and Referrals
Gastroesophageal reflux	a) Position the child on her side or with her head elevated when vomiting to prevent aspiration. b) Document the amount and characteristics of vomitus, and describe vomiting behavior to aid in diagnosis of etiology. c) Monitor fluid and electrolyte balance to assess for deficits. d) Provide oral care after the child vomits to prevent damage to teeth from hydrochloric acid contact. e) Offer small, frequent feedings of thickened formula for infants with GERD. f) Position the child with GERD with the head elevated at 30° after she has eaten. g) Place infants in a prone position for sleep, which can prevent aspiration of stomach contents. This is only recommended for infants with severe GERD.	a) Proton pump inhibitors (Prilosec) b) H$_2$ receptor antagonist (Zantac) c) Antibiotics as ordered	Surgical manipulation or Nissen fundoplicaton (wraps the fundus of the stomach around the distal esophagus to decrease the chance of reflux)	a) Teach the parents signs and symptoms of dehydration. b) Teach the parents to assess the incision and monitor for signs of infection. c) Demonstrate proper hand hygiene techniques. d) Encourage the parents to be active in the care of the child. e) Teach the parents of a child who has a temporary colostomy for Hirschsprung's disease how to perform colostomy care before discharge.
Hypertrophic pyloric stenosis	a) Position the child on her side or with her head elevated when vomiting to prevent aspiration. b) Document the amount and characteristics of vomitus, and describe vomiting behavior to aid in diagnosis of etiology. c) Monitor fluid and electrolyte balance to assess for deficits. d) Provide oral care after the child vomits to prevent damage to teeth from hydrochloric acid contact.	a) Proton pump inhibitors (Prilosec) b) H$_2$ receptor antagonist (Zantac) c) Antibiotics as ordered	Surgical incision into the pyloric sphincter (pylorotomy)	a) Teach the parents signs and symptoms of dehydration. b) Teach the parents to assess the incision and monitor for signs of infection. c) Demonstrate proper hand hygiene techniques. d) Encourage the parents to be active in the care of the child. e) Teach the parents of a child who has a temporary colostomy for Hirschsprung's disease how to perform colostomy care before discharge.
Hirschsprung's disease, or congenital aganglionic megacolon	a) Position the child on her side or with her head elevated when vomiting to prevent aspiration. b) Document the amount and characteristics of vomitus, and describe vomiting behavior to aid in diagnosis of etiology. c) Monitor fluid and electrolyte balance to assess for deficits. d) Provide oral care after the child vomits to prevent damage to teeth from hydrochloric acid contact.	a) Proton pump inhibitors (Prilosec) b) H$_2$ receptor antagonist (Zantac) c) Antibiotics as ordered	Surgical removal of the aganglionic section (may require temporary colostomy)	a) Teach the parents signs and symptoms of dehydration. b) Teach the parents to assess the incision and monitor for signs of infection. c) Demonstrate proper hand hygiene techniques. d) Encourage the parents to be active in the care of the child. e) Teach the parents of a child who has a temporary colostomy for Hirschsprung's disease how to perform colostomy care before discharge.
Meckel's diverticulum	a) Position the child on her side or with her head elevated when vomiting to prevent aspiration. b) Document the amount and characteristics of vomitus, and describe vomiting behavior to aid in diagnosis of etiology. c) Monitor fluid and electrolyte balance to assess for deficits. d) Provide oral care after the child vomits to prevent damage to teeth from hydrochloric acid contact.	a) Proton pump inhibitors (Prilosec) b) H$_2$ receptor antagonist (Zantac) c) Antibiotics as ordered	Surgical removal of diverticulum	a) Teach the parents signs and symptoms of dehydration. b) Teach the parents to assess the incision and monitor for signs of infection. c) Demonstrate proper hand hygiene techniques. d) Encourage the parents to be active in the care of the child. e) Teach the parents of a child who has a temporary colostomy for Hirschsprung's disease how to perform colostomy care before discharge.

Types of Disorders	NURSING INTERVENTIONS	Medications	Therapeutic Measures	Client Education and Referrals
Intussusception	a) Position the child on her side or with her head elevated when vomiting to prevent aspiration. b) Document the amount and characteristics of vomitus, and describe vomiting behavior to aid in diagnosis of etiology. c) Monitor fluid and electrolyte balance to assess for deficits. d) Provide oral care after the child vomits to prevent damage to teeth from hydrochloric acid contact.	a) Proton pump inhibitors (Prilosec) b) H$_2$ receptor antagonist (Zantac) c) Antibiotics as ordered	Surgical reduction if inflating the bowel with air or administering a barium enema is not successful	a) Teach the parents signs and symptoms of dehydration. b) Teach the parents to assess the incision and monitor for signs of infection. c) Demonstrate proper hand hygiene techniques. d) Encourage the parents to be active in the care of the child. e) Teach the parents of a child who has a temporary colostomy for Hirschsprung's disease how to perform colostomy care before discharge.
Cleft lip (CL) and Cleft palate (CP)	a) **Preoperative nursing care** (1) Assess respiratory status and ease of respiratory effort. (2) Keep suction equipment and bulb syringe at bedside. (3) Encourage the parents to express feelings. (4) Assess ability to suck and swallow. (5) Follow precautions during feedings. (6) Modify feeding techniques utilizing obturators, special nipples, and feeders. (7) Feed in upright position in frequent, small amounts; burp frequently. (8) Monitor I&O. (9) Weigh daily. b) **Postoperative nursing care** (1) Monitor for respiratory distress. (2) Maintain suture integrity. (3) Provide age-appropriate activities. (4) Preserve suture line. (5) Restrain elbows. (6) Avoid sucking. (7) Cleanse suture after each feeding. (8) Maintain airway and prevent aspiration. (9) Provide support to the parents.	Antibiotics and pain medications as ordered	a) Repair usually completed by 12 to 18 months of age to prevent speech problems. b) Surgery may be performed in stages.	a) Teach the parents appropriate feeding and prevention interventions prior to discharge. b) Encourage the parents to verbalize feelings, and offer emotional support.

4. Collaborative Care

 a. **NURSING INTERVENTIONS**

1) Maintain fluid and electrolyte balance.
2) Assess for signs of dehydration.
3) Provide IV fluids.
4) Monitor renal function.
5) Maintain afebrile status.
6) Frequently assess temperature.
7) Encourage clear liquids.
8) Expose skin and avoid excessive clothing.
9) Provide safe care during febrile seizure.
   a) Maintain airway.
   b) Prevent aspiration and injury.
   c) Observe the seizure.

b. Medications

1) Fever management is questionable because fever is considered a part of the body's defense mechanism.
2) Antipyretics, such as acetaminophen (Tylenol) or ibuprofen (Motrin), should be given in weight-appropriate dose.
3) No aspirin is allowed due to the risk of Reye syndrome.
4) Use diazepam (Valium) and/or antipyretics if a febrile seizure occurs.

c. Client Education

    1) Educate parents regarding seizure precautions.

    2) Methods to control fever.

    3) Teach how to prevent dehydration.

    4) Address parental fears about fevers.

    5) Teach how to take an age-appropriate and accurate temperature.

B. Vomiting

1. Contributing Factors: Vomiting causes a loss of hydrochloric acid, which leads to metabolic alkalosis.

    a. Short-term illness such as a virus

    b. Children with GERD

    c. Related to medications or treatments such as chemotherapy

    d. Postoperative nausea

2. Manifestations

    a. Emaciation

    b. Dry skin and mucous membranes

    c. Sunken fontanels or lack of tears in infants

    d. Lethargic

    e. Potential metabolic alkalosis

    f. Poorly perfused

    g. Hyperventilating

3. Diagnostic Procedures: The following may be done for prolonged or unusual emesis:

    a. Upper GI series

    b. CT of abdomen

    c. pH probe

    d. Esophagoscopy

4. Collaborative Care

    a. **NURSING INTERVENTIONS**

      1) Assess and document the following:

        a) Amount, color, and consistency of emesis

        b) Time and frequency of emesis

        c) Relationship to meals or medication

      2) Assess for signs of dehydration.

      3) Maintain fluid and electrolytes.

      4) Adhere to strict I&O and daily weights.

      5) Maintain NPO status until asymptomatic.

      6) Introduce clear liquids slowly and frequently.

      7) Monitor for metabolic alkalosis.

    b. Medications

      1) Antiemetics (Phenergan, Thorazine)

      2) Reglan

      3) Tigan

      4) IV fluids if indicated

C. Gastroenteritis (Diarrhea): Expelled forcefully; Na^+, K^+, and bicarbonate are lost via the stool. Diarrhea is serious in young children because dehydration can occur very rapidly.

1. Contributing Factors

    a. Bacteria (salmonella or shigella)

    b. Viral (rotavirus), allergies

    c. Emotional disturbances

    d. Dietary and malabsorption problems

    e. Chronic nonspecific diarrhea

2. Manifestations

    a. An increase in fluid, frequency and volume of stool

    b. Usually results from increased rate of peristalsis

    c. Stools that are watery, acidic, green in color

    d. Weight is a critical indicator of fluid loss in young children:

      1) 1 g of weight equals 1 mL of body fluid; a weight loss or gain of 1 kg in a 24-hr period represents a fluid shift of 1,000 mL.

    e. The loss of fluid and electrolytes in the diarrhea stool results in dehydration and electrolyte depletion.

3. Diagnostic Procedures

    a. Serum electrolytes

    b. CBC

    c. Blood cultures

    d. Antibiotic therapy is a common cause of diarrhea; obtain a thorough history including dietary habits, family history, recent travel, or exposures to contagious illness.

4. Collaborative Care

    a. **NURSING INTERVENTIONS**

      1) Assess for signs of dehydration or poor skin turgor.

      2) Maintain fluid and electrolyte balance.

      3) Monitor daily weights and strict I&O.

      4) Apply skin barrier (zinc products).

      5) Monitor for metabolic acidosis.

      6) Maintain NPO status until asymptomatic.

      7) Introduce clear liquids slowly and frequently (avoid apple juice).

      8) Administer antidiarrheal as prescribed.

    b. Therapeutic Measures

      1) Mild dehydration (2–9%) without hypernatremia; generally treated with oral rehydrating solutions; critical behaviors that demand immediate attention are persistent diarrhea, weight loss, bloody stools, or physiological changes such as deep breathing, listlessness, or reduced urinary output.

      2) Secondary lactose intolerance may occur following gastroenteritis; child may be maintained temporarily on a lactose-free diet.

D. Respiratory Infections

1. **Acute otitis media** (most prevalent childhood disease)

   a. Manifestations

      1) Middle ear infections are common in children under age 5; breast-fed infants have decreased incidence.

      2) Eustachian tube is shorter, wider, and straighter.

      3) Organisms from nasopharynx have easier access to middle ear.

      4) Tonsils and adenoids are usually enlarged.

      5) Young children have poorly developed immune mechanisms.

      6) Infants and toddlers are supine a large portion of the day.

      7) Usually follows an upper respiratory infection during which the swollen mucosa close off the eustachian tube; the growth of the organism along with the fluid retention in the ear combine to cause the infection.

      8) Most frequently seen bacterial infection in young children; most serious long-term problem associated with otitis is conductive hearing loss, tinnitus, or vertigo.

      9) Manifestations: fever; irritability; pulling, tugging or rubbing the affected ear; anorexia; signs of a upper respiratory infection; older children may report earache or pain when chewing or sucking; purulent discharge may be present.

   b. Diagnostic Procedure

      1) Otitis media: otoscopy reveals an intact tympanic membrane that appears inflamed, bulging, and without a light reflex.

      2) Chronic otitis media: otoscopy reveals dull, gray membrane with visible fluid behind eardrum.

   c. Collaborative Care

      1) **NURSING INTERVENTIONS**

         a) Administer analgesics such as acetaminophen (Tylenol) as needed; apply warm compresses to affected ear; avoid foods that require chewing.

         b) Assess for nonverbal signs of discomfort; changes in behavior can be an early indicator of pain; humidity, clear PO fluids may also be helpful.

      2) Medications

         a) Oral antibiotics; therapy should last 10–14 days.

         b) Oral decongestants such as sympathomimetics (vasoconstriction) or antihistamines (reduce congestion) may be used; analgesics may be prescribed to reduce pain, discomfort.

         c) Following completion of the antibiotic regimen, treatment effectiveness should be evaluated.

      3) Therapeutic Measures

         a) Children with recurrent otitis media should be tested for hearing loss.

         b) Myringotomy (surgical incision of the ear drum) and insertion of pressure-equalizing (PE) tubes may be ordered in cases of recurrent chronic otitis media

      4) Client Education and Referral

         a) Instruct the parents regarding the importance of antibiotic compliance; medication should be taken for 10–14 days (even after manifestations have gone away).

         b) Instruct the parents in feeding techniques to reduce the incidence of ear infection (upright when feeding; breast-feeding offers protection against pathogens).

         c) Eliminate tobacco smoke and known or potential allergens from environment.

         d) Following myringotomy and PE tubes insertion, some drainage from the ears is expected; report obvious bleeding and an abrupt rise in temperature; the ear should be kept dry; avoid activities that require submerging the head in water (use earplugs for bathing).

2. **Epiglottitis**: Acute bacterial infection of the supraglottic structures resulting in obstructive airway problems. Most common causative organism—*H. influenza*, type B. Seen primarily in children 2 to 8 years of age; considered a medical emergency; immediate treatment must be initiated.

   a. Manifestations

      1) Manifestations: abrupt onset with rapid progression to severe respiratory distress, sore throat, stridor, high fever (38.9–40° C [102–104° F]), drooling, dysphagia, muffled voice; tripod position (sit upright, lean forward with mouth open and tongue protruding). ***Must be NPO immediately.***

   b. Diagnosic Procedure

      1) Throat is red, inflamed with a cherry-red epiglottis;

   > **Note:** Under no circumstance should an inspection of the throat be initiated unless emergency equipment is available (trach setup, ET tube); do not take a throat culture.

      2) Lateral neck film (soft-tissue x-ray) reveals swollen epiglottis.

   c. Collaborative Care

      1) **NURSING INTERVENTIONS**

         a) Frequently assess for respiratory distress.

         b) Available oxygen, suction, emergency.

         c) Maintain NPO status.

         d) Do not leave child unattended.

         e) Humidified oxygen

2) Medications

    a) Parenteral therapy with IV antibiotics is begun; PO antibiotics for 10 to 14 days following IV therapy

    b) Steroid therapy—frequently used for anti-inflammatory effects

    c) Bronchodilators

    d) Antibiotics

    e) Antipyretics

3) Therapeutic Measures

    a) Intubation or tracheostomy usually necessary to prevent obstruction; extubation may occur within 3–4 days

4) Parent Education and Referral

    a) Vaccine prevention—*H. influenza* type B conjugate vaccine effective against *H. influenza* epiglottitis

3. **Laryngotracheobronchitis (croup)**: Most common form of croup; peak age is below 5 years; because of smaller airway diameter, child is more prone to significant airway narrowing.

  a. May begin as an upper respiratory infection that proceeds to lower respiratory structures.

  b. Most common causative organisms are parainfluenza viruses.

  c. Manifestations

    1) Narrowing of airway—hoarseness, barking or "seal-like" cough, inspiratory stridor, increasing respiratory distress.

  d. Diagnosic Procedure

    1) Lateral or soft-tissue x-rays of neck

  e. Collaborative Care

    1) **NURSING INTERVENTIONS**

      a) Monitor the child's respiratory status frequently.

      b) Provide humidified oxygen.

      c) Encourage fluids.

      d) Keep environment quiet and calm.

      e) Have suction and emergency intubation equipment available at the bedside.

      f) Assess parental anxiety.

    2) Medications

      a) Humidity with cool mist provides relief by reducing inflamed mucosa.

      b) Aerosol epinephrine (Racepinephrine) may also be used if child is hospitalized.

      c) Corticosteroids may be used for their anti-inflammatory effects with humidified oxygen.

      d) Administer analgesics such as acetaminophen (Tylenol) as needed.

      e) Bronchodilators

4. **Bronchiolitis**

  a. Acute viral infection that primarily affects bronchioles; most commonly seen in infants between 1 and 18 months; occurs in winter and spring months.

  b. Respiratory syncytial virus (RSV) is responsible for half of the documented cases of bronchiolitis; mode of transmission is hand to nose, droplet infections; reinfection common in all ages. The younger the child, the greater the chance of severe lower respiratory disease requiring hospitalization; infants at high risk for severe RSV infection include premature infants, infants with underlying cardiac or respiratory conditions, infants with immune deficit.

  c. Bronchiolar obstruction leads to hyperinflation and air trapping.

  d. Manifestations: Initial manifestations of upper respiratory infection that progress to tachypnea.

    1) Paroxysmal coughing,

    2) Increased restlessness

    3) Nasal flaring

    4) Fever

    5) Cyanosis

    6) Intercostal and substernal retractions

    7) Wheezing and decreased breath sounds indicate severe lower-respiratory tract disease.

  e. Diagnosic Procedures

    1) Manifestations are clinically diagnostic.

    2) RSV is diagnosed using enzyme-linked immunosorbent assay (ELIZA) from nasal secretions.

    3) Chest film will reveal areas of consolidation that are difficult to differentiate from bacterial pneumonia; areas of hyperinflation.

  f. Collaborative Care

    1) **NURSING INTERVENTIONS**

      a) Monitor respiratory status frequently.

      b) Assess oxygen saturation levels and ABGs.

      c) Maintain fluid and electrolyte balance.

      d) Maintain isolation precautions.

      e) Provide teaching for parents.

      f) Prevent recurring infection in children who are under age 2 with the use of palivizumab (Synagis) or IV immunoglobulin.

      g) Use a bulb syringe or humidifier.

      h) Wash hands frequently.

      i) Observe for signs of dehydration

    2) Medications

      a) In serious cases, steroids and inhaled bronchodilators will be administered.

      b) With severe RSV infection, ribavirin (Virazole), an antiviral aerosol, may be administered via oxygen tent or hood; teratogenic effects have been reported, so pregnant caregivers are at risk; strict guidelines exist for use.

c) Bronchodilators

d) Steroids

e) Ribavirin (Virazole)

3) Therapeutic Measures

a) Treated symptomatically; humidity, rest, adequate hydration are main therapeutic interventions; can be successfully treated at home in most cases.

b) Rationale for hospitalization: tachypnea (> 70 breaths/min), severe retractions, change in behavior, hydration problems; at-risk children with chronic or debilitating diseases should be hospitalized.

c) Palivizumab (Synagis) immunization is given to at-risk infants during their first winter. (This includes infants born at less than 32 weeks gestation, a large number of those born between 32 and 35 weeks gestation, and children with chronic lung or heart disease.)

SECTION 9

Nursing Care of the Surgical Child

A. Preoperative Preparation

1. Assess parents' and child's level of understanding.

2. Teach based on developmental level of child.

3. Involve parents and allow discussion.

4. Gather baseline data.

B. Common Surgical Problems

1. **Tonsillectomy and adenoidectomy (T&A)**

   a. Tonsils help protect body from infections; typically enlarged in children

   b. Contributing Factors

   1) Chronic tonsillitis (controversial)

   2) Massive hypertrophy that interferes with breathing (obstructive apnea)

   c. Collaborative Care

    1) **NURSING INTERVENTIONS**

   a) **Preoperative**

   (1) Assess bleeding and coagulation time.

   (2) Confirm child is free from current infection.

   (3) Prepare the child.

   b) **Postoperative**

   (1) Hemorrhage: greatest risk first 48 hr, then 7 days later; manifestations—frequent swallowing or clearing of throat, bright red emesis, oozing from capillary bed, shock (late sign, indicates significant blood loss); prevention—avoid coughing, sneezing, sucking on straw

   (2) Offer cool fluids; ice pops to decrease edema and to relieve pain.

2) Medications

   a) Administer analgesics regularly first 24 hr—acetaminophen (Tylenol); may require rectal or parenteral route due to throat pain

3) Client Education and Referrals

   a) Instruct parents that child may return to school in 1–2 weeks.

   b) Instruct parents on foods to avoid: Avoid red-colored foods. Avoid pretzels, crackers, chips, and dairy products.

2. **Pyloric stenosis**: Congenital hypertrophy of pyloric sphincter

   a. Manifestations

   1) Insidious vomiting occurring 2–3 weeks after birth, increasing in intensity until forceful and projectile (no bile) by about 6 weeks of age

   a) Small, olive-size mass in right-upper quadrant

   b) Weight loss, dehydration

   c) Chronic hunger

   b. Diagnostic Procedure

   1) History and physical signs

   2) Upper gastrointestinal series

   3) Barium swallows under fluoroscopy

   c. Collaborative Care

    1) **NURSING INTERVENTIONS**

   a) **Preoperative**: NPO; daily weights; NG tube for gastric decompression; monitor I&O and specific gravity; monitor emesis

   b) **Postoperative**: position on right side to prevent aspiration; begin oral feedings 4 to 6 hr postoperatively after bowel sounds return; maintain in upright position after feeding in infant seat; start with small, frequent feedings of oral rehydration solution (Pedialyte); monitor for emesis; advance feeding as tolerated

   2) Therapeutic Measures

   a) Correct dehydration, metabolic alkalosis

   b) Pylorus resected

3. **Appendicitis**: Inflammation of vermiform appendix; problem in school-age children

   a. Manifestations

   1) Periumbilical pain radiating to right-lower quadrant; rebound tenderness

   2) Low-grade temperature

   3) Nausea and vomiting

   4) Elevated WBC count: 15,000–20,000/mm^3

   5) May perforate and lead to peritonitis; sudden relief of pain followed by increased pain and rigid abdomen; high fever

b. Collaborative Care

 1) **NURSING INTERVENTIONS**

    a) **Preoperative nursing care**

      (1) Provide pain relief.

      (2) Place in right side-lying position.

      (3) Perform abdominal assessment frequently.

      (4) Maintain NPO status.

      (5) Provide fluid and electrolyte balance.

    b) **Postoperative nursing care**

      (1) Assess vital signs and perform abdominal assessment frequently.

      (2) Monitor for signs of infection.

      (3) Promote mobility.

      (4) Promote respiratory toileting.

  2) Medications

    a) Provide analgesics as ordered.

4. **Intussusception**: Telescoping of the bowel

  a. Manifestations

    1) Colicky pain with knees drawn up

    2) Currant jelly stools

  b. Collaborative Care

 1) **NURSING INTERVENTIONS**

    a) Prepare for procedure.

    b) Provide routine postoperative abdominal surgical care.

  2) Therapeutic Measures

    a) Barium enema: diagnostic; may reduce intussusception by hydrostatic pressure

    b) Bowel resection if barium enema does not reduce

5. **Hirschsprung's disease** (megacolon): Congenital absence of parasympathetic ganglion in distal colon; bowel proximal to a ganglionic section becomes enlarged

  a. Manifestations

    1) In newborn: failure to pass meconium within 24 hr after birth

    2) In older child: recurrent abdominal distension; chronic constipation with ribbon-like stools; diarrhea; bile-stained emesis

  b. Collaborative Care

 1) **NURSING INTERVENTIONS**

    a) Provide colostomy care (same as adult).

    b) Check stoma for color.

    c) Change dressings frequently (abdominal, perineal).

    d) Monitor accurate I&O.

    e) Avoid incision irritation (keep diapers low).

  2) Therapeutic Measures

    a) Cleansing enemas with antibiotics preoperatively

    b) Temporary colostomy

    c) Bowel resection to remove aganglionic portion

  3) Parent Education and Referral

    a) Encourage independence based on age of child.

    b) Discuss diet and hydration.

6. **Hernias**: Most common inguinal and umbilical

  a. Always consider developmental level (mutilation fears) when preparing child.

  b. Usually repaired in ambulatory surgery setting.

 1) **NURSING INTERVENTIONS**

  2) Care for surgical site.

  3) Note manifestations of an infection.

SECTION 10

Nursing Care for Childhood Accidents

A. Ingestions

1. General information

  a. Provide emergency care—ABCs.

  b. Identify substance; save evidence of poison.

  c. Call poison control center for treatment advice.

  d. Remove substance.

    1) Activated charcoal

    2) Gastric lavage

    3) Specific antidote

  e. Provide supportive therapy.

  f. Educate parents about childproof environment.

  g. Provide anticipatory guidance.

    1) Infants and toddlers: at risk because everything goes into the mouth

    2) Adolescents: at risk for intentional ingestion

  h. Types of ingestions: See Overview of Common Accidental Ingestion table.

B. Burns

1. Manifestations

  a. Due to the difference in proportions of head, trunk, and limbs, burn percentages are rated differently for children.

  b. Manifestations vary based on the TBSA, type and depth of burn.

  c. Due to the high percentage of extracellular fluids in the child, fluid loss can quickly lead to hypovolemic shock.

2. Collaborative Care

 a. **NURSING INTERVENTIONS**

  1) Similar to adult

  2) Monitor for signs of infection

  3) Monitor I&O

  4) Dressing changes using sterile technique

Overview of Common Accidental Ingestion

Ingestion	Manifestations	Treatment	NURSING INTER–VENTIONS
Salicylate (Aspirin)	• Tinnitus • Hyperpyrexia • Seizures • Bleeding • Hyperventilation	• Emesis • Hydration • Vitamin K • Activated charcoal	• Anticipatory guidance • Bleeding precautions • Counseling if suicide attempt
Acetaminophen (Tylenol)	• Liver necrosis in 2–5 days • Nausea • Vomiting • Pain in right upper quadrant • Jaundice • Coagulation abnormalities • Hepatotoxic	• Emesis • Mucomyst (antidote)	• Counseling if suicide attempt • Liver assessment
Lead (paint, soil near heavily traveled roads, household dust)	• Developmental regression • Impaired growth (encephalopathy) • Irritability • Increased clumsiness	• Chelation therapy—to remove heavy metals • Promote hydration	• Neurological assessment • Diet high in calcium, iron • Educate the parents to wash the child's hands and toys, and to frequently remove lead dust • Lead abatement
Hydrocarbons (kerosene, turpentine, gasoline)	• Burning in the mouth • Choking and gagging • CNS depression	• Do not induce emesis • Activated charcoal • Gastric lavage	• If vomiting, reduce aspiration
Corrosives (drain or oven cleaner, chlorine bleach, battery acid)	• Burning in the mouth • White, swollen mucous membranes • Violent vomiting	• Do not induce emesis • Dilute toxin with water • Activated charcoal	• Keep warm and inactive

b. Medications
   1) Administer antibiotics
   2) Administer IV Fluids
   3) Administer Analgesics
   4) Administer nutritional supplements as ordered. Children are likely to resist eating enough calories to sustain healing and growth needs Parenteral or enteral feedings are usually necessary.

c. Client Education and Referrals
   1) Teach parents how to recognize signs and symptoms of infection
   2) Incorporate play into the physical or occupational therapy regimens for improved success.
   3) Consider psychosocial needs of the child.
   4) Adjustment and transition back to school may be very difficult for the child who has sustained a disfiguring burn.
   5) Ensure parents understand all instructions and have necessary follow up appointments.

C. Fractures

1. Manifestations

   a. Due to immaturity of bones and incomplete ossification, greenstick (incomplete) fractures are commonly seen.

   b. Fractures to the epiphysis (growth plate) are of greater concern, as growth in limb can be stunted depending on the amount of injury.

2. Collaborative Care

   a. Therapeutic Measures
      1) Similar to adult, although pediatric fractures often have shorter healing times
      2) May use cast (plaster or, more commonly, fiberglass), soft splint, traction, or bracing

D. Child Abuse

1. Types

   a. Physical neglect: failure to provide necessities of life

   b. Physical abuse: deliberate infliction of injury

   c. Emotional neglect: failure to provide emotional nurturing

   d. Emotional abuse: deliberate assault on child's self-esteem

   e. Sexual abuse: use of child to meet adult's sexual needs

   f. Munchausen syndrome by proxy (MSBP): a disorder in which a caregiver (usually parent) falsely reports or intentionally causes symptoms in her own child to seek attention

2. Contributing Factors

   a. Parental
      1) Poor self-esteem
      2) Abused as a child
      3) Lack of knowledge
      4) Lack of support system, poor coping skills

b. Child
   1) Unwanted pregnancy or sex
   2) Difficult temperament, hyperactive

c. Environment
   1) Chronic stress
   2) Socioeconomic factors

3. Manifestations of Abuse and Neglect

a. Physical neglect
   1) Failure to thrive: disruption in maternal–infant bonding; poor feeding behaviors; mother does not respond to infant's cues; weight less than 5th percentile; developmental delay
   2) Poor health care, lack of immunizations
   3) Failure to meet basic needs: malnutrition, poor hygiene

b. Physical abuse
   1) Bruises: not on bony prominences, in varying degrees of healing; with patterns
   2) Burns: with immersion lines, in patterns
   3) Fractures: spiral, twisting
   4) Shaken baby: unconscious infant with retinal hemorrhage and no external signs of trauma
   5) Conflicting stories given by parents, child, or others
   6) History incompatible with physical findings or developmentally improbable
   7) Delay in seeking medical attention

c. Emotional neglect and abuse
   1) Extremes of behavior
   2) Poor self-esteem

d. Sexual abuse
   1) Bruising of the genitalia
   2) STD
   3) Sudden change in behavior, regressive behavior

e. Munchausen syndrome by proxy
   1) Victims usually under age 6
   2) May have lasting emotional impact
   3) Increased risk for child to develop Munchausen syndrome as adult
   4) Parent well versed in medical knowledge

4. Collaborative Care

a. **NURSING INTERVENTIONS**
   1) Document suspected findings.
   2) Do not leave child unattended.
   3) Establish trust with child.

b. Referrals
   1) Refer psychiatric consult.
   2) Notify Social Services or policy specific to you institution

A. Immune Disorders

1. **Eczema**: Inflammation of the skin not due to a specific etiology. Known as atopic dermatitis.

a. Contributing Factors
   1) Etiology: Unknown but appears to be related to abnormal function of the skin, including alterations in perspiration, peripheral vascular function, and heat intolerance
   2) Family history of eczema, allergy, asthma, or allergic rhinitis

b. Manifestations
   1) Unknown but appears to be related to abnormal function of the skin, including alterations in perspiration, peripheral vascular function, and heat intolerance
   2) Family history of eczema, allergy, asthma, or allergic rhinitis
   3) Papules are red and oozing; predominantly on face and extensor surfaces in infants, flexural areas in children (knees, wrists, antecubital fossa)
   4) Lesions eventually become scaly
   5) Pruritus may lead to secondary infection

c. Collaborative Care
   1) **NURSING INTERVENTIONS**
     a) Maintain skin integrity.
     b) Educate parents to control dry skin to minimize itching.
     c) Use nonsoap cleanser.
     d) Apply lubricating creams.
     e) Advise parents that the child may be more comfortable in cotton, long-sleeved clothing.
     f) Instruct parents to launder with a nonsoap or hypoallergenic cleanser.
     g) Fingernails and toenails should be kept short to prevent scratching.
     h) Assess developmental needs.
     i) Provide a hypoallergenic diet.
     j) Provide parental support and education.
     k) Encourage elimination diet (milk, eggs, chocolate, wheat).
   2) Medications
     a) Topical steroids: triamcinolone (Kenalog); avoid chronic use
     b) Diphenhydramine HCl (Benadryl) or hydroxyzine HCl (Atarax): reduces itching
     c) Antibiotics if secondary infection occurs

2. **Bronchial asthma**: Chronic inflammatory disorder of the airways involving mast cells, eosinophils, and T lymphocytes. Inflammation causes recurrent episodes of wheezing, breathlessness, chest tightness, and cough. Also known as reactive airway disease. A chronic condition with acute exacerbations.

   a. Contributing Factors
      1) In response to allergen or trigger, acute hyperactive changes occur in reactive (lower) airways.
         a) Spasm of smooth muscle
         b) Edema of mucous membranes
         c) Thick, tenacious mucus
         d) Severe, sudden dyspnea
   b. Potential Triggers
      1) Foods
      2) Inhalants (secondhand smoke)
      3) Infection
      4) Vigorous activity
      5) Stress, anxiety
      6) Allergens (pet dander, dust)
      7) Cold air
   c. Manifestations
      1) Paroxysmal, hacking nonproductive cough
      2) Prolonged expiratory phase with expiratory wheeze
      3) Respiratory distress, anxiety
      4) Complications
         a) Pneumonia
         b) Atelectasis
   d. Collaborative Care
      1) **NURSING INTERVENTIONS**
         a) Avoid allergens and triggers.
         b) Teach correct use of metered-dose inhaler (with spacer device).
         c) Plan activities that require stop-and-start energy.
         d) Teach use of a peak-flow meter to monitor airway compliance.
      2) Medications
         a) Bronchodilators: albuterol (Proventil) useful for acute attack; salmeterol (Serevent) for chronic daily use, not for acute attack via nebulizer or metered-dose inhaler
         b) Inhaled corticosteroids: effective in reducing airway hyper-reactivity; for chronic daily use, not acute attack; avoid chronic oral steroids that can stunt growth
         c) Cromolyn sodium (Intal): mast-cell inhibitor; reduces allergic response; for chronic daily use, not acute attack
      3) Client Education and Referral
         a) Chronic (home) management of child

3. **Status asthmaticus**: Severe respiratory distress requiring hospitalization
   a. Medications
      1) Bronchodilators
      2) Epinephrine (Adrenalin): subcutaneous
      3) Assist with monitoring of aminophylline (Phyllocontin): IV drip
      4) Steroids: IV
      5) Inhalants: bronchodilators; albuterol (Proventil), metaproterenol (Alupent)
      6) Antibiotics: prophylactic
      7) Hydration
      8) Oxygen therapy

4. **Rheumatic fever**: An inflammatory disease that involves the joints, skin, brain, serous surfaces, and heart; usually occurs 2–6 weeks after an upper respiratory infection with group A beta-hemolytic strep. Cardiac valve damage is the most significant complication. Sequelae include scarring and damage to mitral valve.
   a. Manifestations
      1) Arthralgia; low-grade fever that spikes in the afternoon; hot, red, swollen joints (polyarthritis); tachycardia with precordial friction rub; subcutaneous nodules; truncal rash (erythema marginatum)
      2) Chorea
         a) Sudden, involuntary movements with involuntary facial grimaces
         b) Muscle weakness and speech disturbances
         c) Is transitory; reassure parents that chorea will self-resolve
   b. Diagnosis Procedure
      1) Elevated or rising antistreptolysin O (ASO) titer with elevated erythrocyte sedimentation rate (ESR)
      2) Jones criteria (presence of two major, or one major and two minor manifestations)
   c. Collaborative Care
      1) **NURSING INTERVENTIONS**
         a) Assess vital signs.
         b) Control joint pain and inflammation with massage and alternating hot and cold applications.
         c) Provide bed rest in acute febrile phase.
         d) Initiate seizure precautions if child is experiencing chorea.
         e) Ensure bed rest in the acute phase.
      2) Medications
         a) Provide prophylactic antibiotics with all dental work
         b) Administer antibiotics and anti-inflammatory medications as prescribed.

3) Client Education
  a) Instruct parents about the importance of follow-up.
  b) Instruct parents that the child will require prophylactic antibiotics when at risk for infection.
  c) Instruct parents that the child will require prophylactic antibiotics when at risk for infection.

B. Musculoskeletal Disorders

1. **Scoliosis**: Lateral curvature of the spine; most common form is idiopathic, seen (predominately) in adolescent females; unknown etiology. Acquired scoliosis; associated with deformity resulting from other neuromuscular disorders

  a. Contributing Factors
    1) No apparent cause identified
  b. Diagnosic Procedure
    1) Screening exam in school: child flexes at waist; one scapula more prominent
    2) Spinal x-ray
  c. Collaborative Care
    1) **NURSING INTERVENTIONS**
      a) Provide postoperative nursing care.
      b) Log roll for first 24 hr.
      c) Perform neurovascular assessments frequently.
      d) Promote pulmonary toileting.
      e) Provide pain management.
      f) Encourage age-appropriate activities.
    2) Therapeutic Measures
      a) Mild scoliosis (< 20° curvature): observation, encourage physical exercise
      b) Moderate scoliosis (20–40° curvature): fitted Milwaukee brace
      c) Goal is to prevent worsening of curve
      d) Severe scoliosis (> 40° curvature): requires surgery
      e) Spinal fusion with instrumentation
      f) Requires prolonged immobilization in cast, brace, or body jacket
    3) Client Education and Referral
      a) Address developmental needs of client.
      b) Provide client teaching—skin care, commitment of therapy, and fashion concerns.
      c) Reinforce the importance of compliance with all follow up appointments.
      d) Reinforce the importance of prophylactic antibiotics prior to any dental work or other invasive procedures.

2. **Juvenile rheumatoid arthritis (JRA)**: Autoimmune, inflammatory disease affecting the joints occurring most often in girls. Early diagnosis essential due to long-term complications (blindness, contracture); early onset often associated with spontaneous permanent remission

  a. Classification
    1) Systemic (fever, rash, and organomegaly in addition to joint involvement)
    2) Polyarticular (many joints)
    3) Pauciarticular (few joints)
  b. Manifestations
    1) Swelling, thickening of joint
    2) Pain, stiffness, impaired range of motion
    3) Lethargy, weight loss
    4) Supportive treatment to maintain joint mobility
  c. Collaborative Care
    1) **NURSING INTERVENTIONS**
      a) Promote mobility and range of motion.
      b) Encourage nutritional intake.
      c) Provide pain relief (medication, heat, and cold).
      d) Monitor for exacerbation of symptoms.
    2) Medications
      a) NSAIDs
      b) Methotrexate
      c) Corticosteroids

C. Endocrine Disorders

1. **Type 1 diabetes mellitus**: Diabetes mellitus is characterized by chronic hyperglycemia due to problems with insulin secretion and/or the effectiveness of endogenous insulin (insulin resistance). Diabetes mellitus is a contributing factor for the development of cardiovascular disease, hypertension, renal failure, blindness, and stroke as individuals age.

  a. Contributing Factors
    1) May be autoimmune response to environmental factors
    2) Genetics can predispose a person to the occurrence of type 1 and type 2 diabetes mellitus.
    3) Toxins and viruses can predispose an individual to diabetes by destroying the beta cells, leading to type 1 diabetes mellitus.
    4) Obesity
    5) Physical inactivity
    6) High triglycerides (greater than 250 mg/dL)
    7) Hypertension may lead to the development of insulin resistance and type 2 diabetes mellitus.
  b. Manifestations
    1) Blood glucose alterations
      a) Hypoglycemia: Blood glucose level less than 70 mg/dL

Effects of Hypoglycemia

Autonomic Nervous System Responses Rapid Onset	Impaired Cerebral Function Gradual Onset
• Hunger, lightheadedness, and shakiness • Nausea • Anxiety and irritability • Pale, cool skin • Diaphoresis • Irritability • Normal or shallow respirations • Tachycardia and palpitations	• Strange or unusual feelings • Decreasing level of consciousness • Difficulty in thinking and inability to concentrate • Change in emotional behavior • Slurred speech • Headache and blurred vision • Seizures leading to coma

  b) Hyperglycemia: Blood glucose levels usually greater than 250 mg/dL
   (1) Thirst
   (2) Frequent urination
   (3) Hunger
   (4) Skin that is warm, dry, and flushed with poor turgor
   (5) Dry mucous membranes
   (6) Soft eyeballs
   (7) Weakness
   (8) Malaise
   (9) Rapid, weak pulse; hypotension
   (10) Rapid, deep respirations with acetone/fruity odor due to ketones (Kussmaul respirations)

 c. Diagnostic Procedures
  1) Laboratory tests: Diagnostic criteria for diabetes include two findings (on separate days) of one of the following:
   a) Symptoms of diabetes plus a casual plasma glucose concentration of greater than 200 mg/dL (without regard to time since last meal)
    (1) A fasting blood glucose greater than 126 mg/dL
    (2) A 2-hour glucose of greater than 200 mg/dL with an oral glucose tolerance test
   b) Fasting blood glucose
    (1) Ensure that the child has fasted (no food or drink other than water) for 8 hr prior to the blood draw. Antidiabetic medications should be postponed until after the level is drawn.
   c) Oral glucose tolerance test
    (1) Instruct the client to consume a balanced diet for the 3 days prior to the test. Then instruct the client to fast for the 10–12 hr prior to the test. A fasting blood glucose level is drawn at the start of the test. The client is then instructed to consume a specified amount of

glucose. Blood glucose levels are drawn every 30 min for 2 hr. The child must be assessed for hypoglycemia throughout the procedure.
   d) Glycosylated hemoglobin (HbA1c)
    (1) The expected reference range is 4–6%, but an acceptable target for children who have diabetes may be 6.5–8% with a total target goal of less than 7%.
   e) Self-monitored blood glucose (SMBG)
    (1) Follow or ensure that the child follows the proper procedure for blood sample collection and use of a glucose meter.
    (2) Supplemental short-acting insulin may be prescribed for elevated pre-meal glucose levels.
    (3) Instruct the child to check the accuracy of the strips with the control solution provided.
    (4) Advise the child to keep a record of the SMBG that includes time, date, serum glucose level, insulin dose, food intake, and other events that may alter glucose metabolism, such as activity level or illness.

 d. Collaborative Care
  1) **NURSING INTERVENTIONS**
   a) Monitor the following:
    (1) Blood glucose levels and factors affecting levels (other medications)
    (2) I&O and weight
    (3) Skin integrity and healing status of any wounds, paying close attention to the feet and folds of the skin
    (4) Sensory alterations (tingling, numbness)
    (5) Visual alterations
    (6) Presence of recurrent infections
    (7) Dietary practices
    (8) Exercise patterns
    (9) The child's proficiency at self-monitoring blood glucose
    (10) The child's proficiency at self-administering medication
   b) Foot Care: Follow agency policy for nail care. Some protocols allow for trimming toenails straight across with clippers and filing edges with a nail file. If clippers or scissors are contraindicated, the child should file the nails straight across.
  2) Medication Administration
   a) Most children are on an insulin regimen that frequently consists of more than one type of insulin (rapid, short, intermediate, and/or long acting). Insulin given in this manner is administered one or more times per day and based on a child's blood glucose level.

b) Some children are given an insulin pump, which is a small pump that is worn externally, contains insulin, and delivers insulin as programmed via a needle inserted into the subcutaneous tissue. The catheter should be changed at least every 3 days.

c) The rate of onset, peak, and duration of action vary for each different type of insulin.

d) Observe the child perform self-administration of insulin and offer additional instruction as indicated. (See the Pharmacology section.)

3) Client Education and Referrals

a) Teach proper foot care.

(1) Inspect feet daily. Wash feet daily with mild soap and warm water.

(2) Pat feet dry gently, especially between the toes.

(3) Use mild foot powder (powder with cornstarch) on sweaty feet.

(4) Do not use commercial remedies for the removal of calluses or corns.

(5) Perform nail care after a bath/shower if possible.

(6) Separate overlapping toes with cotton or lamb's wool.

(7) Avoid open-toe, open-heel shoes. Leather shoes are preferred to plastic ones.

(8) Wear slippers with soles.

(9) Do not go barefoot.

(10) Shake out shoes before putting them on.

(11) Wear clean, absorbent socks or stockings that are made of cotton or wool and have not been mended.

(12) Do not use hot water bottles or heating pads to warm feet.

(13) Wear socks for warmth.

(14) Avoid prolonged sitting, standing, and crossing of legs.

(15) Teach the child to cleanse cuts with warm water and mild soap, gently dry, and apply a dry dressing.

(16) Instruct the child and parents to monitor healing and to seek intervention promptly.

b) Provide nutritional guidelines.

(1) Plan meals to achieve appropriate timing of food intake, activity, onset, and peak of insulin. Calories and food composition should be similar each day.

(2) Eat at regular intervals and do not skip meals.

(3) Count grams of carbohydrates consumed.

(4) Recognize that 15 g of carbohydrates is equal to 1 carbohydrate exchange.

(5) Restrict calories and increase physical activity as appropriate to facilitate weight loss (for children who are obese or to prevent obesity).

(6) Include fiber in the diet to increase carbohydrate metabolism and to help control cholesterol levels.

(7) Avoid concentrated sweets.

(8) Use artificial sweeteners.

(9) Keep fat content below 30% of the total caloric intake.

(10) Teach the child appropriate techniques for SMBG, including obtaining blood samples, recording and responding to results, and correctly handling supplies and equipment.

c) Teach the child guidelines to follow when sick.

(1) Monitor blood glucose levels every 3–4 hr.

(2) Continue to take insulin or oral antidiabetic agents.

(3) Consume 4 oz of sugar-free, non-caffeinated liquid every 0.5 hr to prevent dehydration.

(4) Meet carbohydrate needs by eating soft foods if possible. If not, consume liquids that are equal to the usual carbohydrate content.

(5) Test urine for ketones and report if abnormal (should be negative to small).

(6) Rest.

d) Call the health care provider if:

(1) Blood glucose is higher than 240 mg/dL

(2) Fever higher than 38.9° C (102° F), fever does not respond to acetaminophen (Tylenol), or fever lasts more than 12 hr

(3) Disorientation or confusion occurs

(4) Rapid breathing is experienced

(5) Vomiting occurs more than once

(6) Diarrhea occurs more than five times or for longer than 24 hr

(7) Liquids cannot be tolerated

(8) Illness lasts longer than 2 days

e) Teach the child measures to take in response to signs and symptoms of hypoglycemia, which include

(1) Shakiness

(2) Diaphoresis

(3) Anxiety

(4) Nervousness

(5) Chills

(6) Nausea

(7) Headache

(8) Weakness

(9) Confusion

f) Teach the child and parents signs and symptoms of hypoglycemia and measures to take in response to hypoglycemia. Follow guidelines outlined by the health care provider/diabetes educator. Guidelines may include:

    (1) For hypoglycemia, treat with 15–20 g carbohydrates.

    (2) Recheck blood glucose in 15 min.

    (3) If still low (less than 70 mg/dL), give 15–20 g more of carbohydrates. Examples: 4 oz orange juice, 2 oz grape juice, 8 oz milk, glucose tablets per manufacturer's suggestion to equal 15 g of carbohydrates.

    (4) Recheck blood glucose in 15 min.

    (5) If blood glucose is within normal limits, take 7 g protein (if the next meal is more than an hour away). Examples: 1 oz of cheese (1 string cheese), 2 tablespoons of peanut butter, or 8 oz of milk

    (6) If the child is unconscious or unable to swallow, administer glucagon SC or IM and notify the health care provider. Administer liquid with glucose as soon as tolerated. Watch for vomiting and take precaution against aspiration.

g) Teach the child and parents signs and symptoms of hyperglycemia (hot, dry skin and fruity breath) and measures to take in response to hyperglycemia. Follow guidelines outlined by the health care provider/diabetes educator. Guidelines may include:

    (1) Encourage oral fluid intake.

    (2) Administer insulin as prescribed.

    (3) Restrict exercise when blood glucose levels are greater than 250 mg/dL.

    (4) Test urine for ketones and report if findings are abnormal.

    (5) Consult the health care provider if symptoms progress.

h) Encourage the child to wear a medical identification wristband.

i) Provide information regarding self-administration of insulin.

    (1) Rotate injection sites (prevent lipohypertrophy) within one anatomic site (prevent day-to-day changes in absorption rates).

    (2) Inject at a 90° angle (45° angle if thin). Aspiration for blood is not necessary.

    (3) When mixing a rapid- or short-acting insulin with a longer-acting insulin, draw up the shorter-acting insulin into the syringe first and then the longer-acting insulin (this reduces the risk of introducing the longer-acting insulin into the vial of the shorter-acting insulin).

e. Referrals

    1) Refer the child to a diabetes educator for comprehensive education in diabetes management.

2. **Diabetic ketoacidosis (DKA)**: An acute, life-threatening condition characterized by hyperglycemia (greater than 300 mg/dL), resulting in the breakdown of body fat for energy and an accumulation of ketones in the blood and urine. The onset is rapid, and the mortality rate is high.

  a. Contributing Factors

    1) Insufficient insulin (usually failure to take the appropriate dose)

    2) Acute stress (as from trauma or surgery)

    3) Poor management of acute illness

  b. Manifestations

    1) Blood glucose level greater than 300

    2) Reports of nausea, vomiting, and/or abdominal pain (DKA/metabolic acidosis)

    3) Reports of frequent urination, thirst, and hunger (3 P's—Polyuria, Polydipsia, and Polyphagia)

    4) Reports of confusion

    5) Change in mental status

    6) Signs of dehydration (e.g., dry mucous membranes, weight loss, sunken eyeballs resulting from fluid loss such as polyuria)

    7) Kussmaul respiration pattern, rapid and deep respirations, fruity scent to the breath (DKA/metabolic acidosis)

  c. Collaborative Care

    1) **NURSING INTERVENTIONS**

      a) Provide rapid isotonic fluid (0.9% sodium chloride) replacement to maintain perfusion to vital organs. Often large quantities are required to replace losses.

      b) Monitor the child for evidence of fluid volume excess.

      c) Follow with a hypotonic fluid (0.45% sodium chloride) to continue replacing losses to total body fluid.

      d) When serum glucose levels approach 250 mg/dL, add glucose to IV fluids to minimize the risk of cerebral edema associated with drastic changes in serum osmolality.

    2) Medications

      a) Administer regular insulin 0.1 unit/kg as an IV bolus dose and then follow with a continuous intravenous infusion of regular insulin at 0.1 unit/kg/hr.

D. Hematological Disorders

1. **Hemophilia**: Group of bleeding disorders that includes a deficiency in one of the factors necessary for coagulation of the blood.

   a. Contributing Factors
   1) Deficiency of clotting factors
   2) Sex-linked recessive trait more common in males
   3) Factor VIII and IX are most common deficiencies
   4) Hemarthrosis (bleeding into joint cavities), bruises easily

   b. Manifestations
   1) Bleeding into subcutaneous and intramuscular tissue
   2) Hemarthrosis characterized by swelling, warmth, redness, pain, and loss of movement in joints
   3) Bruising

   c. Collaborative Care
    1) **NURSING INTERVENTIONS**
   a) Control bleeding.
   b) Provide supportive therapy.
   c) Immobilize joint.
   d) Provide ice packs.
   2) Medications
   a) Administer Cryoprecipitate (transfusion that replaces missing clotting factor)
   b) Risk for AIDS and/or hepatitis is decreased because of screening, but does still exist.
   3) Client Education
   a) Safety is directed toward developmental level to prevent injury, bleeding.
   b) Avoid contact sports (difficult for children).
   c) Childproof environment.
   d) Avoid aspirin.
   e) Provide parental education and support

2. **Sickle cell anemia**: Disease in which hemoglobin A is partly replaced by abnormal sickle hemoglobin S. Accounts for elongated shape of RBCs. Sickling increases blood viscosity, which causes further sickling and RBC destruction.

   a. Contributing Factors
   1) Sickling occurs in response to
   a) Infection, stress
   b) Dehydration
   c) Decreased oxygen
   d) High altitude

   b. Types of crisis
   1) Vaso-occlusive: "hand-foot syndrome" caused by stasis of blood in capillaries; schema and infarction
   2) Sequestration: pooling of large amounts of blood in liver, spleen; hypovolemia and shock

   c. Manifestations
   1) Shortness of breath, fatigue
   2) Tachycardia, pallor, jaundice
   3) Lethargy, irritability, weakness
   4) Pain, nausea, vomiting, anorexia
   5) Swelling, fever

   d. Collaborative Care
   1) **NURSING INTERVENTIONS**
   a) Provide hydration.
   b) Administer analgesics, antibiotics as prescribed.
   c) Reduce stress of hospitalization.
   d) Provide parental support.
   2) Medications
   a) Analgesics
   3) Therapeutic Measures
   a) Eliminate cause of crisis.
   b) Blood transfusions
   (1) Monitor complications:
   (a) Anemia
   (b) Splenic sequestration
   (c) Cerebrovascular accidents

E. Renal Disorders

1. Glomerulonephritis
2. Nephrotic syndrome
   See the Renal Disorders table below.

F. Metabolic Disorders

1. **Cystic fibrosis (CF)**: A genetic disease that affects salt and water movement in and out of body cells. Thick mucus causes blockages of small tubes and ducts in the body. Primarily affects the lungs and digestive system.

   a. Contributing Factors
   1) Inherited disease
   2) Requires inheritance of two mutated CF genes, one from each parent

   b. Manifestations
   1) Chronic respiratory infection
   2) Accumulation of sticky, thick mucus in the lungs, adventitious or decreased breath sounds, wheezing and chronic cough with blood streaking, changes in color and amount of sputum
   3) Stools pale or clay colored, foul smelling, float on surface of water
   4) Weight loss, failure to thrive in infants, abdominal swelling
   5) Excessive salt in sweat, dehydration
   6) Abdominal pain, flatulence
   7) Fatigue
   8) Clubbing of fingertips

   c. Collaborative Care
   1) **NURSING INTERVENTIONS**
   a) Assess respiratory status; oxygenation, color, and amount of sputum.

Renal Disorders

	Nephrotic Syndrome	Acute Glomerulonephritis
Other Names	Childhood nephrosis	Poststreptococcal glomerulonephritis
Contributing Factors	Cause unknown; likely autoimmune	Antigen–antibody reaction secondary to infection elsewhere in the body; usually a streptococcus ß-hemolytic, group A of the upper respiratory tract
Incidence	Average age of onset about 2.5 years; more common in boys	Two-thirds of cases are in children who are under 4–7 years; more common in boys
Pathology	Increased permeability of the glomerular membrane to protein	Inflammation of the kidneys; damage to the glomeruli allows excretion of RBCs
Manifestations	Edema—appears insidiously; usually first noticed in the eyes and can advance to the legs, arms, back, peritoneal cavity, and scrotum; massive proteinuria; anorexia; pallor	Periorbital edema—appears insidiously; tea-colored urine from hematuria; hypertension; oliguria
Blood Pressure	Usually normal; transient elevation may occur early	Varying degrees of hypertension may be present; when blood pressure is elevated, cerebral manifestations may occur as a result of vasospasm; these may include headache, drowsiness, diplopia, vomiting, convulsions
Diagnostic Procedures	Urine shows heavy hematuria	Urine contains RBCs; has a high specific gravity
Diagnostic Lab	Involves reduction in protein (mainly albumin); gamma globulin is reduced; during the active stages of the disease, the sedimentation rate is greatly increased	BUN value is elevated; anemia (reduction in circulating RBCs, in Hgb, or both) tends to develop rapidly
Medications and Treatments	Prednisone (Deltasone) Furosemide (Lasix) Salt-poor albumin	Antibiotics for strep infection Diuretics and antihypertensives used to remove accumulated fluid and manage hypertension. **NURSING INTERVENTIONS** • Monitor blood pressure. • Monitor I&O. • Monitor for electrolyte imbalances, such as hypokalemia. Observe for side effects of medications. Corticosteroids
NURSING INTERVENTIONS	Control edema; provide skin care; prevent infection; monitor nutrition (low sodium, high protein, high potassium); monitor urine for proteinuria; monitor for side effects from steroid therapy. Provide rest. Monitor I&O. Monitor urine for specific gravity and protein. Monitor daily weights; weigh the child on the same scale with the same amount of clothing. Monitor edema and measure abdominal girth daily. Measure at the widest area, usually at or above the umbilicus. Assess degree of pitting, color, and texture of skin. Monitor and prevent infection. Assist the child to turn, cough, and deep breathe to prevent pulmonary involvement. Monitor vital signs, especially temperature, for changes secondary to infection. Maintain good hand hygiene. Administer antibiotic therapy as prescribed.	Monitor I&O. Monitor daily weights Weigh the child on the same scale with the same amount of clothing daily. Monitor vital signs. Monitor neurological status and observe for behavior changes, especially in children who have edema, hypertension, and gross hematuria. Implement seizure precautions if condition indicates. Encourage adequate nutritional intake within restriction guidelines. A regular diet with elimination of high-sodium foods will be appropriate for most. Restrict foods high in potassium during periods of oliguria. Provide small, frequent meals of favorite foods due to a decrease in appetite. Manage fluid restrictions as prescribed. Fluids may be restricted during periods of edema and hypertension.

(continued)

Renal Disorders (continued)

	Nephrotic Syndrome	Acute Glomerulonephritis
NURSING INTERVENTIONS *(continued)*	Encourage nutritional intake within restriction guidelines. Salt and fluids may be restricted during the edematous phase. Increase protein in diet to replace protein losses. Cluster care to provide for rest periods. Assess skin for breakdown areas. Prevent pressure sores. Avoid use of urinary collection bags in very young children. Pad bony prominences or use a specialty mattress to reduce breakdown of skin. Encourage frequent turning and repositioning of the child. Keep the child's skin dry. Elevate edematous body parts.	Monitor skin for breakdown areas and prevent pressure sores. Encourage frequent turning and repositioning. Keep skin dry. Pad bony prominences and use a specialty mattress. Elevate edematous body parts. Assess tolerance for activity. Provide for frequent rest periods. Monitor and prevent infection. Advise the child to turn, cough, and deep breathe to prevent pulmonary involvement. Monitor vital signs, especially temperature, for changes secondary to infection. Maintain good hand hygiene.
Collaborative Care	Refer the child for dietary consultation if indicated. Provide for age-appropriate diversional activities. Consult child life specialist. Cluster care to facilitate rest and tolerance of activity. Provide emotional support.	Refer the child for dietary consultation if indicated. Provide for age-appropriate diversional activities. Consult Child Life Specialist. Cluster care to facilitate rest and tolerance of activity. Provide emotional support.
Client Education	Encourage the child to eat food high in potassium if potassium-sparing diuretics are not used. Inform the child and family that dizziness can occur with the use of antihypertensives. Encourage the child to verbalize feelings related to body image. Educate the child regarding appropriate dietary management. Educate the family about the need for follow-up care. The child should be seen by the provider weekly for several weeks and then monthly until the disease is fully resolved.	Encourage the child to eat food high in potassium if potassium-sparing diuretics are not used. Inform the child and family that dizziness can occur with the use of antihypertensives. Encourage the child to verbalize feelings related to body image. Educate the child regarding appropriate dietary management. Educate the family about the need for follow-up care. The child should be seen by the provider weekly for several weeks and then monthly until the disease is fully resolved.

b) Assess daily weight and I&O.

c) Provided consistent, scheduled chest physiotherapy and postural drainage with cough and deep breathing.

d) Provide small frequent feedings with pancreatic enzymes with each meal.

e) Provide parental education and emotional support.

f) Teach parents how to avoid exposing the child to infection, and to avoid environments containing smoke.

2) Medications

a) Hypoglycemic agents: Monitor blood glucose levels and administer hypoglycemic agents as prescribed.

b) Bronchodilators (inhalers)

(1) Short-acting ß$_2$-agonists, such as albuterol (Proventil), provide rapid relief.

(2) Cholinergic antagonists (anticholinergics), such as ipratropium (Atrovent), block the parasympathetic nervous system, providing relief of acute bronchospasms.

(3) Instruct the child and family in the proper use of an MDI, DPI, or nebulizer.

(4) Monitor the child for tremors and tachycardia when he is taking albuterol.

(5) Observe the child for dry mouth when taking ipratropium.

c) Antibiotics

(1) Antibiotics are used to treat bacterial infections.

(2) Advise parents that the child should finish the full course of antibiotics.

d) Dornase alfa (Pulmozyme)

(1) Decreases the viscosity of mucus and improves lung function

(2) Monitor the child for improvement in PFTs.

(3) Instruct the child in the use of a nebulizer.

(4) Instruct the child to use once daily.

e) Pancreatic enzymes: pancrelipase (Pancrease)

(1) Used to treat pancreatic insufficiency associated with cystic fibrosis

(2) Capsules should be given with all meals.

(3) Capsules can be swallowed whole or sprinkled on food.

3) Therapeutic Measures

a) Pulmonary postural drainage, aerosol therapy, and treatment with antibiotics for infection

b) Pancreatic enzymes with meals and supplementation of fat-soluble vitamins—A, D, E, K (twice the normal daily age requirement). Give pancreatic enzymes in food.

c) Free use of salt

d) Possible lung transplantation

4) Client Education

a) Ensure that the family has information regarding access to medical equipment.

b) Provide teaching about equipment prior to discharge.

c) Instruct the family in ways to provide CPT and breathing exercises. For example, a child can stand on her head by using a large, cushioned chair placed against a wall.

d) Promote regular primary care provider visits.

e) Emphasize the need for up-to-date immunizations with the addition of an initial seasonal influenza vaccine at 6 months of age and then yearly.

f) Promote regular physical activity.

g) Encourage the family to participate in a support group and use community resources.

5) Referrals

a) Respiratory therapy, social services, and dieticians may be involved in the care of the child who has cystic fibrosis.

2. **Celiac disease**: Disease of digestive system that damages the small intestine and interferes with the absorption of nutrients and food, particularly gluten products due to an inborn error of metabolism (fat and glucen intolerance)

a. Manifestations

1) Diarrhea

2) Large bulky stools

3) Anemia

4) Delayed growth and development

5) Frequent infection

6) Malabsorption of vitamin D

b. Diagnostic Procedure

1) Bowel biopsy

2) Sweat test

c. Collaborative Care

1) **NURSING INTERVENTIONS**

a) Monitor weight and dietary intake.

b) Monitor I&O during acute episodes of diarrhea.

c) Provide gluten-free diet.

2) Medications

a) Administer fat-soluble vitamins A, D, E, and K.

3) Therapeutic Measures

a) Provide emotional support.

b) Provide dietary referral.

4) Client Education

a) Instruct the parents to avoid giving the child foods made with gluten; also, avoid barley, rye, oats, wheat (BROW diet).

SECTION 12
Nursing Care of the Child with an Oncology Disorder

A. **Leukemia:** A term for a group of malignancies that affect the bone marrow and lymphatic system; causes bone marrow dysfunction that leads to anemia and neutropenia. Acute lymphocytic leukemia (ALL) is the most common childhood cancer. Peak incidence is 2 to 6 years of age and is more common in boys older than 1 year. Incidence may be related to environmental exposures. Characterized by proliferation of immature WBCs.

1. Classification

a. Acute lymphocytic (ALL)

b. Acute nonlymphoid (ANLL)

c. Acute myelogenous leukemia (AML)

d. Complications (secondary to bone marrow depression)

1) Infection

2) Intracranial hemorrhage

3) Secondary cancer or relapse

2. Manifestatinos

a. Leukemic infiltrate

b. Limb and joint pain

c. Lymphadenopathy

d. CNS involvement

e. Hepatosplenomegaly/bleeding tendencies

f. History of frequent infection and fever

g. Decreased platelet and RBC count

h. Increased immature WBCs

i. Anemia, pallor, and fatigue from decreased RBCs, headache

j. Low-grade fever

k. Petechiae and epistaxis from decreased platelets

3. Diagnosic Procedure: Bone marrow aspiration reveals hypercellular marrow, abnormal cells.

4. Collaborative Care

 a. **NURSING INTERVENTIONS**

    1) Take complete history and perform physical assessment.

    2) Monitor for anorexia, headache, and fatigue.

    3) Assess vital signs and oxygenation.

    4) Monitor CBC, temperature fluctuations.

    5) Assess for infection.

    6) Weigh daily.

    7) Assess I&O.

    8) Provide support care related to chemotherapy.

    9) Provide anticipatory guidance to child and family.

    10) Provide emotional support and appropriate referrals.

    11) Provide instruction for complex home care management.

b. Medications

    1) Chemotherapy

        a) Purine antagonists: 6-mercaptopurine (Purinethol) (may affect kidneys)

        b) Alkylating agents: cyclophosphamide (Cytoxan) (causes chemical cystitis)

        c) Folic acid antagonists: methotrexate (Folex)

        d) Plant alkaloid: vincristine sulfate (Oncovin) (neurotoxic)

        e) Steroids: prednisone (Prelone)

        f) Enzymes: L-asparaginase (Elspar)

c. Therapeutic Measures

    1) Lumbar puncture for analysis of CSF

    2) Ultrasound for liver and spleen infiltration

    3) Baseline liver and kidney function studies

    4) Radiation therapy for CNS involvement

B. Nephroblastoma (Wilms' tumor): Type of renal cancer with a peak age of 3 years

1. Contributing Factors

    a. Certain genetic conditions or birth defects can increase risk. Arises from embryonal tissue.

    b. Children at risk should be screened for Wilms' tumor every 3 months until age of 8.

2. Manifestations

    a. Most common clinical sign is swelling; mass within the abdomen

    b. Anemia, hypertension, hematuria

3. Diagnostic Procedure

    a. IV pyelogram

    b. Computerized tomography

    c. Bone marrow to rule out metastasis

4. Collaborative Care

 a. **NURSING INTERVENTIONS**

    1) Preoperative care

        a) Support parents, and keep explanations simple.

        b) Monitor blood pressure due to excess renin production.

        c) Prevent rupture of encapsulated tumor.

        d) Post sign on bed: DO NOT PALPATE ABDOMEN.

        e) Bathe and handle child gently.

    2) Postoperative care

        a) Assess vital signs, respiratory status, and oxygenation status.

        b) Monitor blood pressure.

        c) Assess dressing for bleeding.

        d) Provide pain management.

        e) Monitor urinary output and kidney function; dipstick urine for protein or blood.

        f) Provide age-appropriate developmental support and emotional support to parents.

b. Therapeutic Measures

    1) Nephrectomy and adrenalectomy

    2) Radiation and chemotherapy determined by staging

C. Neuroblastoma: Malignancy that occurs in the adrenal gland, sympathetic chain of the retroperitoneal area, head, neck, or pelvis area. Most frequently seen in children less than 2 years.

1. Contributing Factors

    a. An embryonal malignancy of the sympathetic nervous system arising from neuroblasts (pluripotent sympathetic cells)

    b. Frequently called "silent" tumor because by the time of diagnosis, metastasis has occurred

2. Manifestations

    a. Abdominal mass, urinary retention and frequency, lymphadenopathy, generalized weakness, and malaise

    b. Primary site is abdomen, most often in flank area

3. Diagnostic Procedures

    a. Computerized tomography

    b. Bone marrow to determine metastasis

    c. Excessive catecholamine production

4. Collaborative Care

 a. **NURSING INTERVENTIONS**

    1) Assess vital signs, and height and weight.

    2) Monitor I&O and nutritional status.

    3) Assess for developmental delays related to illness.

    4) Provide education and support to child and family.

    5) Make appropriate referrals.

    6) Provide age-appropriate diversional activities.

b. Medications

    1) Administer chemotherapeutic agents as prescribed and according to established protocols.

c. Therapeutic Measures

    1) Surgery to remove as much of the tumor as possible and determine staging

    2) Chemotherapy and radiation determined by staging of tumor

D. Hodgkin's Lymphoma: Cancer of the lymphatic system primarily affecting adolescents and young adults; originates in the lymphoid system. Metastasis may include spleen, liver, bone marrow, and lungs.

1. Diagnosic Procedure

    a. Computerized axial tomography

    b. Lymph node biopsy, exploratory laparotomy (to stage)

2. Collaborative Care

 a. **NURSING INTERVENTIONS**

    1) Assess vital signs, and height and weight.

    2) Monitor I&O and nutritional status.

    3) Assess for developmental delays related to illness.

b. Medications

    1) Administer chemotherapeutic agents as prescribed and according to established protocols.

c. Therapeutic Measures

    1) Radiation and chemotherapy determined by clinical staging

    2) Surgical laparotomy

    3) Splenectomy

d. Client education

    1) Provide education and support to child and family with a splenectomy regarding increased susceptibility to infection and chronic illness.

    2) Make appropriate referrals.

SECTION 13

Nursing Care of the Child with an Infectious Disease

A. Prevention

1. Immunizations

    a. Schedule recommendations established by CDC and reviewed by American Academy of Pediatrics

    b. Contraindication with active illness and fever greater than 438.3° C (101° F)

    c. Precautions

      1) Hepatitis B: allergy to baker's yeast, liver disease

      2) DTaP: delay 30 days after immunosuppression

      3) Hib: delay if child is ill

      4) MMR: do not administer if child is allergic to eggs, neomycin, gelatin. Also, do not give to pregnant women or those who expect to get pregnant in 3 months

      5) Varicella: do not administer if allergic to neomycin or gelatin

      6) Pneumococcal: sensitivity to diphtheria may cause anaphylaxis

      7) Influenza: do not administer if child is allergic to eggs; encourage those undergoing immunosuppressive therapy to receive a flu shot

      8) Meningococcal: unknown impact on pregnancy

B. Communicability

1. Communicable diseases are most contagious prior to the onset of manifestations or rash and in the early prodromal period.

2. Most require respiratory isolation if the child requires hospitalization.

3. Most are preventable through immunization or other measures.

C. Common childhood infections

1. See Communicable Diseases Guide

SECTION 14

CPR Guidelines for Children and Infants

A. Key BLS Components

Note: Always refer to the American Heart Association for the Most current updates and guidelines.

1. Child: Use AED as soon as available; use child pads or a child system for children ages 1 to 8, if available; if child pads are not available, use adult AED and pads.

2. Infant: AED is not recommended for infants less than 1 year of age.

B. Obstructed Airway

1. With a responsive victim:

    a. Infant: Use a combination of back blows and chest thrusts.

    b. Child and Adolescent: Use abdominal thrusts and Heimlich maneuver.

2. Remove large debris in oral cavity.

3. Do not reach into mouth of an infant unless the object is visible.

4. Place recovered child into recovery position.

5. Use calm approach with victim.

6. Administer oxygen as prescribed.

Communicable Diseases Guide

Transmission	Incubation	Manifestations	Treatment and 🩺 NURSING INTERVENTIONS	Prevention
Meningitis Viral or bacterial (*H. influenza*—3 months to 3 years; meningococcal meningitis)				
Direct invasion via otitis media, upper respiratory infection, head injury	2–10 days	Onset abrupt with fever, headache, irritability, altered level of consciousness, nuchal rigidity, increased intracranial pressure; must do lumbar puncture to isolate organism	Isolate; reduce environmental stimuli; monitor hydration; seizure precautions; IV antibiotcis	Rifampin given to contacts of client with meningococcal meningitis as prophylaxis
Mumps Viral (paramyxovirus)				
Saliva, direct contact or droplet	14–21 days	Prodromal stage—headache, malaise, anorexia, followed by earache; parotitis 3 days later with pain/tenderness	Symptomatic and supportive; analgesics; antipyretics; hydration	MMR
***Pediculosis capitis* (head lice)** Pediculus humanus capitis				
Sharing of personal items (hair ornaments, caps, hats)	Eggs hatch in 7–10 days	Intense itching; can visually see nits attached to base of hair shafts; differentiate from dandruff	Do not share personal items. Shampoo with anti-lice products; wash linens and clothing in hot water	Caution children about sharing hair items
Pertussis (whooping cough) *Bordetella pertussis*				
Respiratory droplets and direct contact	7–21 days	Initially "cold" manifesations; progresses to spasms or paroxysmal coughing (whooping cough)	Antibiotics; corticosteroids; supportive care; isolation; stay with child during coughing spells	DtaP
Rabies Viral				
Contact with saliva of infected animal	1–3 months or as short as 10 days	Prodromal—malaise, sore throat followed by hypersensitivity, excitation, convulsions, paralysis; high mortality	Irrigate wound; psychological follow-up	Avoid contact with wild animals; rabies shot (given after exposure)
Reye syndrome Viral				
Unknown—preceded by viral infection and associated with the use of aspirin	Unknown	Prodromal—malaise, cough, upper respiratory infection. 1–3 days after fever—decreased level of consciousness, hepatic and cerebral dysfunction; high mortality	Monitor live function; peak age 4–11 years; neuro assessments; intracranial pressure monitoring	Avoid the use of aspirin in adolescents and children
Rheumatic fever Group A beta-hemolytic strep				
Nasopharyngeal secretions; direct contact with infected person or droplet spread	1–3 weeks after acute infection, develops inflammatory disease	Carditis, arthritis, chorea (involuntary ataxic movements), subcutaneous nodules, erythema marginatum (rash)	Bed rest in acute phase to decrease cardiac workload; full course of antibiotics (penicillin/erythromycin); high dose of aspirin therapy (monitor for toxicity tinnitus)	Adequate, prompt treatment of strep infection (must finish entire course of therapy)
Roseola (exanthem subitum) Viral (human herpes virus type 6)				
Unknown (limited to children 6 months to 2 years of age)	Unknown	Persistent high fever for 3–4 days; precipitous drop in fever with appearance of rash (rose-pink maculopapule on trunk, then spreading to neck, face, and extremities); lasts 1–2 days	Antipyretics to control temperature and prevent febrile seizures; hydrate	None

Transmission	Incubation	Manifestations	Treatment and NURSING INTERVENTIONS	Prevention
Rubella (German measles) Viral (rubella virus)				
Nasopharyngeal secretions—direct contact, indirect via freshly contaminated nasopharyngeal secretions or urine	14–21 days	Prodromal phase; absent in children, present in adults; rash; first face and rapidly spreads downward to neck, arms, trunk, and legs; teratogenic to fetus	No treatment necessary; isolate child from pregnant women; women of childbearing years should have rubella titer done	MMR
Rubeola (measles) Viral				
Respiratory—droplets	10–21 days	Prodromal stage—fever and malaise, coryza, conjunctivitis, Koplik spots (spots with blue/white center on buccal mucosa opposite molars); rash that starts on the face, spreads downward, may desquamate (peel)	Antipyretics to control temperature and prevent seizures; dim lights if photophobia; respiratory precautions	MMR
Scarlet fever Group A beta-hemolytic strep				
Nasopharyngeal secretions, direct contact with infected person or droplet spread	2–4 days	Prodromal stage—abrupt high fever, pulse increased, vomiting, chills, malaise, abdominal pain; enanthema —tonsils enlarged, edematous reddened, covered with patches of exudate; strawberry tongue; exanthema—rash appears 12 hr after prodromal signs	Full course of antibiotics (penicillin/erythromycin); isolate; monitor for rheumatic fever; glomerulonephritis hydrate	Adequte, prompt treatment of strep infection (must finish entire course of therapy)
Tetanus *Clostridium tetani*				
Deep puncture, not contagious, "anaerobic"	7–14 days	Gradual stiffening of voluntary muscles until rigid (lockjaw, rigid abdomen); sensitive to stimuli; clear sensorium	Eliminate stimuli; monitor respirations, blood gases; muscle relaxants; monitor hydration	DtaP, Td

UNIT 7

Pharmacology

SECTION 1

Review of Calculations and Conversions

Basic medication dose conversion and calculation skills are essential to providing safe nursing care. Standard conversions are used to solve dosage calculation problems. Nurses are responsible for the administration of the correct amount of medication based on the type of medication being administered.

A. Standard Conversion Factors

1. 1 mg = 1,000 mcg
2. 1 g = 1,000 mg
3. 1 kg = 1,000 g
4. 1 kg = 2.2 lb
5. 60 mg = 1 g
6. 30 mL = 1 oz
7. 1 L = 1,000 mL
8. 5 mL = 1 tsp
9. 15 mL = 1 tbsp
10. 1 tbsp = 3 tsp

B. Temperature Conversions

1. $37.0°\,C = 98.6°\,F$
2. $°C = (F - 32) \times 5/9$
3. $°F = (C \times 9/5) + 32$

C. Calculations for IV Administration

1. Number of hours = total volume/mL/hr
2. gtts per min = total volume × gtts/mL in administration set/total number of minutes

D. Calculations for Dosage

1. Dosage on hand (H)/mL = Dosage desired (D)/mL

E. Fill-in-the-Blank Question Format

1. An NCLEX® alternate-test item where the answer is placed in the box below a question.

F. Practice Test Questions (answers on the following page)

1. A client has the following food for lunch: 8 oz. of ice chips, 1 cup of tea, 1 cup of coffee, and 240 mL of milk. The client drinks all of the tea and coffee and half of the milk. The total intake for lunch is

   _____.

2. A client has a prescription for 0.25 mg of lanoxin (Digoxin). The dose on hand is 0.5-mg tablets of lanoxin. How many tablets will the client receive?

3. A client's IV infusion rate is 75 mL/hr. How many hours will it take for a 500-mL bag of IV fluid to infuse?

4. The IV rate is 100 mL/hr and the administration set is 15 drops/mL. How many drops per minute will deliver the required fluids?

5. A preschool child is prescribed 5 mL of ampicillin (Polycillin Pediatric) for otitis media every 6 hr. When preparing the child for discharge, the nurse should tell the child's mother to give how much ampicillin every 6 hr?

6. A client has a prescription for heparin sodium (Heparin) 7,000 units IV. The vial contains 10,000 units/mL. How many milliliters of heparin will the nurse administer?

7. A nurse is preparing 300,000 units of procaine penicillin (Wycillin). The vial contains 1,500,000 units/2 mL. How many milliliters will the nurse administer?

8. A client weighs 180 lb and has a prescription for 0.5 mL of medication per kilogram of body weight. How many milliliters of medication will the client receive?

9. A client is receiving dextrose 5% in water at 50 mL/hr in one IV and D5W 75 mL/hr in another IV. The client also receives IV piggyback medication every 8 hr prepared in 100 mL of fluid. What is the total amount of IV fluid the client will receive in 8 hours?

10. The IV administration set delivers 10 drops/mL. The rate of flow in drops/min for 1,000 mL dextrose 5% in water to infuse in 8 hr is _____.

11. When measuring a client's output, the nurse records 300 mL of urine at 0800, 450 mL of liquid stool at 1130, 225 mL of urine at 1300, and 35 mL of emesis at 1430. What is the client's total output for this shift?

12. A client receiving an IV infusion has a prescription for 1,000 mL in 12 hr. Using a microdrip system that delivers 60 microdrops/mL, the nurse should regulate the infusion for how many drops per minute?

    A. 45
    B. 68
    C. 83
    D. 96

13. A client's temperature is 100° F. What is this temperature in degrees centigrade?

14. A nurse has available meperidine (Demerol) 50 mg/mL. The order is to administer meperidine 35 mg. How many milliliters will the nurse safely administer?

15. A nurse is preparing an IV antibiotic in 100 mL of dextrose 5% in water to infuse over 20 min. The infusion set is calibrated for 10 gtts/mL. What drip rate should the nurse use?

G. Test Answers

1. 720
2. 0.5
3. 6.6 hrs
4. 25 tsp.
5. 1
6. 0.7
7. 0.4
8. 41
9. 1,100
10. 21
11. 1,010
12. C (83)
13. 37.7
14. 0.7
15. 50

SECTION 2

Pharmacology

Medication Actions, Interactions, and Reactions

A. Medication Properties (pharmacokinetics): The absorption, distribution, metabolism, and excretion of a medication; describes the onset of action, peak level, duration of action, and bioavailability

B. Medication Interaction: When a medication is given with another medication and alters the effect of either or both medications

C. Adverse Reactions: Negative effects experienced by a client as the result of a specific medication, which may be hazardous, may be tolerated, or may subside with continued use

Pharmacotherapy Across the Life Span

A. Medications and Pregnancy: A majority of medications cross the placental barrier, thereby increasing the risk of teratogenicity; all medications should be given with extreme caution to ensure safety to the developing fetus

B. Medications and Breast-feeding: Most medications taken by a mother who is breast-feeding appear in breast milk. Medication levels tend to be the highest in the newborn immediately after the medication is administered to the mother. Mothers who are breast-feeding are advised to breast-feed before taking the medication.

C. Medication in Children: Pharmacokinetics are influenced by a child's age, size, and maturity of the targeted organ. To reduce the risk of toxicity, these factors must be considered: safe calculation of the child's dosage mg/kg/day, medication that is age-appropriate, monitoring of IV medications to prevent fluid overload (no more than 2 hr of IV therapy with a fluid-control device), and the administration of inhalants using a metered-space device.

D. Intramuscular Injections for Children

1. EMLA or LMX cream may be applied topically if time permits and is congruent with facility practice guidelines.
2. Vastus lateralis (anterolateral thigh) is the site for IM injections in children who are < 2 years of age.
3. Needle length must be sufficient to penetrate the subcutaneous tissue and deposit the medication in the body of the muscle.
4. Maximum dose is not to exceed 0.5 mL for small infants and no more than 1mL for small children.

E. Medication in Older Adults: Age-related changes impact therapeutic effects of medications in older adult clients. Older adult clients experience twice as many adverse effects as younger adults due to aging body systems. Confusion, lethargy, falls, and weakness may be mistaken for senility, rather than adverse reactions. If the adverse reaction is not identified, unnecessary medication may be prescribed to treat complications caused by the medication. As the client continues to receive medications, the risk for toxicity increases, especially in cases of polypharmacy.

1. Toxicity in older adults: a greater risk when taking diuretics, antihypertensives, digoxin, steroids, anticoagulants, hypnotics, and over-the-counter medications

Safe Medication Administration

The RN is prepared to administer medications using the enteral, parenteral and transcutaneous routes.

The RN must assess the client's:

1. past history with drug administration, including side effects, allergies, and adverse effects,
2. current drug regimen for potential interactions, and
3. physiologic status as compared to baseline assessment data.

The RN follows the six rights of medication administration (right client, right drug, right dose, right route, right time, and right documentation) to protect the safety of the client and follow the scope of practice to maintain professional licensure.

Laboratory Profiles in Pharmacology

Laboratory testing may be indicated for specific medications. The nurse is accountable for collaborating with the healthcare provider in ensuring client safety when laboratory testing is ordered.

A. Therapeutic Drug Monitoring

1. Definition: Measures blood drug levels to determine effective drug dosages and prevent drug toxicity. The test may also be used to identify noncompliance with medication regimens.

   a. Blood testing is preferred because it provides information about current therapeutic levels, whereas urine levels reflect the presence of a drug over several days.

B. **Peak levels** reflect the highest concentration.

   1. Average times used for drawing peak levels

Average Times for Drawing Peak Levels

Route of Administration	Time Specimen Is Drawn After Administration
Oral intake	1–2 hr
Intramuscular	1 hr
Intravenous	30 min

C. **Trough levels** reflect the lowest concentration or residual level and are usually obtained within 15 min prior to administration of the next scheduled dose. The scheduled dose of medication should not be administered until the trough level is confirmed.

NOTE: The timing for drawing a peak and trough level varies based on the half-life (time required for the body to decrease the drug blood level by 50%) for the drug.

D. **Culture and Sensitivity:** Cultures are obtained to detect the presence of pathogens within the specimen collected. If a culture produces organisms, testing is performed in the laboratory to identify the appropriate antibiotic therapy (sensitivity).

NOTE: When ordered, cultures should be obtained PRIOR to initiating antibiotic therapy (definitive therapy). When cultures cannot be drawn prior to initiating antibiotic therapy, the provider will order a broad-spectrum antibiotic (empirical therapy). Monitoring culture results is imperative to ensure the proper antimicrobial treatment.

Intravenous Therapy

A. **Definition:** Administration of fluids via an intravenous catheter (peripheral or central vein access) for the purpose of providing medication, fluid, electrolyte, or nutrient replacement

B. **Guidelines for Safe IV Administration**

   1. Review medication guidelines for precautions related to IV administration for compatibility, rate of administration, necessity of infusion pump, and serious adverse reactions.

   2. Never administer medications through tubing being used for blood administration.

   3. Implement standard precautions and follow policies related to IV site changes.

   4. Fluids should be infused within 24 hr (discard unused portion) to prevent infection.

   5. Maintain patency of IV access.

C. **Prevent complications associated with IV infusion.**

Complications Associated with IV Infusion

Complication	NURSING INTERVENTIONS
Infiltration	**Prevention:** use smallest catheter for prescribed therapy, stabilize port-access, assess blood return
	Treatment: stop infusion, remove peripheral catheters, apply cold compress, elevate extremity, insert new catheter in opposite extremity
Extravasation	**Prevention:** know vesicant potential before giving medication
	Treatment: stop infusion, d/c administration set, aspirate drug if possible, apply cold compress, document condition of site (may photograph)
Phlebitis/ thrombophlebitis	**Prevention:** rotate sites every 72–96 hr, secure catheter, use aseptic technique; for PICCs avoid excessive activity with the extremity
	Treatment: stop infusion, remove peripheral IV catheters, apply heat compress, insert new catheter in opposite extremity
Hematoma	**Prevention:** avoid veins not easily seen or palpated, obtain hemostasis after insertion
	Treatment: remove IV device and apply light pressure if bleeding, monitor for signs of phlebitis and treat
Venous spasm	**Prevention:** allow time for vein diameter to return after tourniquet removed, infuse fluids at room temperature
	Treatment: temporarily slow infusion rate, apply warm compress

Total Parenteral Nutrition (TPN)

Definition: Hypertonic solution containing dextrose, proteins, electrolytes, minerals, trace elements, and insulin prescribed according to the client's needs and administered via central venous device (PICC line, subclavian, or internal jugular vein)

A. **Care and Maintenance of TPN**

   1. Before administering, verify prescription and solution with another nurse.

   2. Administer via infusion pump.

   3. Monitor client's weight daily.

   4. Monitor and record client's I&O, noting fluid balance.

   5. Monitor serum glucose levels every 4 hr.

   6. Monitor for signs of infection.

   7. Change the dressing every 48–72 hr per facility protocol.

   8. Change IV tubing and fluid every 24 hr.

   9. If TPN solution is temporarily unavailable, administer 10% dextrose water to prevent complications.

B. Complications of Central Venous Catheters

Complications of Central Venous Catheters

Complication	NURSING INTERVENTIONS
Pneumothorax (during insertion)	**Prevention:** use ultrasound to locate veins, avoid subclavian insertion when possible **Treatment:** administer oxygen, assist provider with chest tube insertion
Air embolism	**Prevention:** have client lie flat when changing administration set or needleless connectors, ask client to perform Valsalva maneuver if possible **Treatment:** place client in left lateral Trendelenburg, administer oxygen
Lumen occlusion	**Prevention:** flush promptly with NS between, before, and after each medication **Treatment:** use thrombolytic enzymes
Bloodstream infection	**Prevention:** maintain sterile technique **Treatment:** change entire infusion system, notify provider, obtain cultures, and administer antibiotics

Medications for the Cardiovascular System

Antihypertensives

Treatment for clients with hypertension includes lifestyle modification and medications.

 NURSING INTERVENTIONS for all clients taking antihypertensive medications include:

1. Assess weight, VS, hydration status.
2. Assess blood pressure in supine, sitting, and standing positions.
3. Assess laboratory profiles: renal function, coagulation.
4. Teach client to take medication at same time each day.
5. Clients should avoid hot tubs, saunas.
6. Do not discontinue medication abruptly.
7. Prevent orthostatic hypotension.

Angiotensin-Converting Enzyme (ACE) Inhibitors and Angiotensin II Receptor Blockers (ARBS)

Action:
- ACE inhibitors: block the conversion of angiotensin I to angiotensin II in the lungs
- ARBs: selectively block the binding of angiotensin II to AT_1 receptors found in tissues

ACE Inhibitors and ARBs

ACE Inhibitors	ARBs
captopril (Capoten)	losartan (Cozaar)
enalapril (Vasotec)	valsartan (Diovan)
enalaprilat (Vasotec IV)—intravenous route	irbesartan (Avapro)
fosinopril (Monopril)	
lisinopril (Prinivil)	

A. Therapeutic use: hypertension, heart failure, MI, diabetic nephropathy

B. Precautions/Interactions
1. If client is on diuretic therapy, must stop 24–48 hr prior to ACE medication.
2. Monitor potassium levels.

C. Side Effects/Adverse Effects
1. Persistent non-productive cough with ACE inhibitors
2. Angioedema; hypotension
3. Should not be used in 2nd and 3rd trimester of pregnancy

 D. NURSING INTERVENTIONS and Client Education
1. Captopril should be taken 1 hr before meals.
2. Monitor blood pressure.
3. Monitor for angioedema and promptly administer epinephrine 0.5 mL of 1:1,000 solution subcutaneously.

Calcium Channel Blockers

Action: Slows movement of calcium into smooth-muscle cells, resulting in arterial dilation and decreased blood pressure

Medications:
- **nifedipine (Adalat, Procardia)**
- **verapamil (Calan)**
- **diltiazem (Cardizem)**
- **amlodipine (Norvasc)**

A. Therapeutic Use
1. Angina, hypertension
2. Verapamil and diltiazem may be used for atrial fibrillation, atrial flutter, or SVT.

B. Precautions/Interactions
1. Use cautiously in clients taking digoxin and beta-blockers.
2. Contraindicated for clients with heart failure, heart block, or bradycardia.
3. Do not consume grapefruit juice (toxic effects).

C. Side Effects/Adverse Effects
1. Constipation
2. Reflex tachycardia
3. Peripheral edema
4. Toxicity

 D. NURSING INTERVENTIONS and Client Education
1. Do not crush (or chew) sustained-release tablets.
2. IV administration inject over 2–3 min.
3. Slowly taper dose if discontinuing.
4. Monitor heart rate and blood pressure.

Alpha Adrenergic Blockers (Sympatholytics)

Action: Selectively inhibit alpha-1 adrenergic receptors, resulting in peripheral arterial and venous dilation that lowers blood pressure

Medications:
- prazosin (Minipress)
- doxazosin mesylate (Cardura)

A. Therapeutic Use

1. Primary hypertension
2. Cardura may be used in treatment of BPH.

B. Precautions/Interactions

1. Increased risk of hypotension and syncope if given with other antihypertensives, beta blockers, or diuretics.
2. NSAIDs may decrease the effect of prazosin.

C. Side Effects/Adverse Effects

1. Dizziness
2. Fainting

D. NURSING INTERVENTIONS and Client Education

1. Monitor heart rate and blood pressure.
2. Take drug at bedtime to minimize effects of hypotension.
3. Advise to notify prescriber immediately about adverse reactions.
4. Consult prescriber before taking **any OTC medications**.

Centrally Acting Alpha-2 Agonists

Action: Stimulate alpha-adrenergic receptors (alpha 1) in the brain to reduce peripheral vascular resistance, heart rate, systolic and diastolic blood pressure

Medications:
- clonidine (Catapres)
- guanfacine HCl (Tenex)
- methyldopa (Aldomet)

A. Therapeutic Use

1. Primary hypertension—may be used in combination with diuretics or other antihypertensives
2. Hypertensive crisis
3. Severe cancer pain (parenteral administration via epidural)

B. Precautions/Interactions

1. Contraindicated with anticoagulant therapy, hepatic failure.
2. Do not give to clients taking MAOIs.
3. Do not administer methyldopa through IV line with barbiturates or sulfonamides.
4. Use cautiously in CVA, MI, diabetes, major depression, or chronic renal failure.
5. Do not use during lactation.

C. Side Effects/Adverse Effects

1. Dry mouth
2. Drowsiness and sedation (resolves over time)
3. Rebound hypertension
4. Black or sore tongue
5. Leukopenia

D. NURSING INTERVENTIONS and Client Education

1. Monitor for adverse CNS effects.
2. Monitor CBC, heart rate, and blood pressure.
3. Assess for weight gain or edema.
4. Monitor closely for rebound hypertension when medication is discontinued (48 hr).
5. Instruct to never skip a dose.
6. Take at bedtime to minimize effects of hypotension.
7. Notify prescriber of any involuntary jerky movements, prolonged dizziness, rash, yellowing of skin.

Beta Adrenergic Blockers (Sympatholytics)

Action: Inhibit stimulation of receptor sites resulting in decreased cardiac excitability, cardiac output, myocardial oxygen demand; lower blood pressure by decreasing release of renin in the kidney

> **NOTE:**
> - **Beta-1** receptors are primarily in the cardiac and renal tissues
> - **Beta-2** receptors are found primarily in the lungs, gastrointestinal tract, liver, uterus, vascular smooth muscle, and skeletal muscle

Medications: May be "selective" or "non-selective"
- Cardioselective Beta-1 Medications
  - metoprolol (Lopressor)
  - atenolol (Tenormin)
  - metoprolol succinate (Toprol XL)
- NONselective (Beta-1 and Beta-2) Medications
  - propranolol (Inderal)
  - nadolol (Corgard)
  - labetalol (Normodyne)

A. Therapeutic Use

1. Primary hypertension
2. Angina
3. Tachydysrhythmias, heart failure, and MI

B. Precautions/Interactions

1. Contraindicated in clients with AV block and sinus bradycardia.
2. Do not administer NONselective beta blockers to clients with asthma, bronchospasm, or heart failure.
3. Propanolol may mask signs of hypoglycemia in diabetic clients.
4. Do not administer labetolol in same IV line with furosemide.

C. Side Effects/Adverse Effects

1. Bradycardia
2. Nasal stuffiness
3. AV block
4. Rebound myocardium excitation if stopped abruptly
5. Bronchospasm

 D. NURSING INTERVENTIONS and Client Education

1. Administer 1–2 times daily as prescribed.
2. Do not discontinue without consulting provider.
3. Do not crush (or chew) extended-release tablets.
4. Hold medication and notify provider if SBP < 100 or pulse < 50.
5. Monitor diabetic clients for signs of hypoglycemia.

Vasodilators

Action: Direct vasodilation of arteries and veins resulting in rapid reduction of blood pressure (decreased preload and afterload)

Medications:

- nitroglycerin (Nitrostat IV)
- nicardipine (Cardene)
- clevidipine (Cleviprex)
- enalaprilat (Vasotec IV)
- esmolol HCl (Brevibloc)

A. Therapeutic Use

1. Hypertensive emergencies

B. Precautions/Interactions

1. Clients with hepatic or renal disease
2. Older adults
3. Electrolyte imbalances

C. Side Effects/Adverse Effects

1. Dizziness
2. Headache
3. Profound hypotension
4. Cyanide toxicity
5. Thiocyanate poisoning

D. NURSING INTERVENTIONS and Client Education

1. Nitroprusside may not be mixed with any medication.
2. Apply protective cover to container.
3. Discard unused fluid after 24 hr.
4. Provide continuous ECG and blood pressure monitoring.

Cardiac Glycosides

Used in the treatment of clients with cardiac failure or ineffective pumping mechanism of the heart muscle.

Action: (1) Increase the force and velocity of myocardial contractions to improve stroke volume and cardiac output, and (2) slow the conduction rate, allowing for increased ventricular filling.

Medications:

- digoxin (Lanoxin, Lanoxicaps, Digitek)

A. Therapeutic Uses

1. Heart failure
2. Atrial fibrillation

B. Precautions/Interactions

1. Thiazide or loop diuretics increase risk of hypokalemia and precipitate digoxin toxicity.
2. ACE, ARBs increase risk of hyperkalemia.
3. Verapamil (Calan) increases risk of toxicity.

C. Side Effects/Adverse Effects

1. Digoxin toxicity: GI effects (anorexia, N/V, abdominal pain); CNS effects (fatigue, weakness, diplopia, blurred vision, yellow-green or white halos around objects)

D. NURSING INTERVENTIONS and Client Education

1. Assess apical pulse for 1 min prior to administration.
2. Notify provider if HR < 60 (adult), < 70 (child), < 90 (infant).
3. Monitor for signs of digoxin toxicity, hypokalemia, and hypomagnesemia.
4. Notify provider of any sudden increase in pulse rate that previously had been normal or low.
5. Maintain therapeutic digoxin level 0.8–2.0 ng/mL.

E. Management of Digoxin Toxicity

1. Discontinue digoxin and potassium-sparing medications.
2. Treat dysrhythmias with phenytoin (Dilantin) or lidocaine.
3. Treat bradycardia with atropine.
4. For excess overdose, administer Digibind to prevent absorption.

Medication to Treat Angina

The use of organic nitrates, beta adrenergic-blocking agents, and calcium channel blockers to treat pain related to imbalances between myocardial oxygen supply and demand

Organic Nitrates

Action: (1) Relax peripheral vascular smooth muscles, resulting in dilation of arteries and veins, thus reducing venous blood return (reduced preload) to the heart, which in turn leads to decreased oxygen demands on the heart; (2) increase myocardial oxygen supply by dilating large coronary arteries and redistributing blood flow.

Medications:

- Nitrostat (Sublingual)
- Nitrolingual (Translingual spray)
- Nitro-Bid (Topical ointment)
- Nitro-Dur (Transderm patch)

A. Therapeutic Use

1. Acute angina attack
2. Prophylaxis of chronic stable or variant angina

B. Precautions/Interactions

1. Contraindicated in clients with head injury
2. Hypotensive risk with antihypertensive medications
3. Erectile dysfunction meds = life-threatening hypotension

C. Side Effects/Adverse Effects

1. Headache
2. Orthostatic hypotension
3. Reflex tachycardia
4. Tolerance

D. NURSING INTERVENTIONS and Client Education

1. Nitrostat/Nitrolingual
   a. Administer sublingual.
   b. Repeat in 5 min if no relief and call 9-1-1; may take up to 3 doses.
   c. Keep Nitrostat in original dark container.
   d. Nitrolingual may be used prophylactically 5–10 min before exercise.
   e. Do not shake Nitrolingual canister (forms bubbles).
   f. Replace NTG tablets every 6 months.
   g. Wear medical alert identification.
2. Nitro-Bid (topical ointment)
   a. Wear gloves for administration.
   b. Do not massage or rub area.
   c. Apply to area without hair (chest, flank, or upper arm preferable).
   d. Cover the area where the patch is placed with a clear plastic wrap, and tape in place.
   e. Gradually reduce the dose and frequency of application over 4–6 weeks.

3. Nitro-Dur (transderm patch)
   a. Skin irritation may alter drug absorption.
   b. Optimal locations for patch are upper chest or side; pelvis; and inner, upper arm.
   c. Rotate skin sites daily.

Antidysrhythmic Agents

Action: Antidysrhythmic agents are complex agents with multiple mechanisms of action. They are classified according to their effects on the electrical conduction system of the heart (Class I, II, III, IV).

Medications:

- adenosine (Adenocard): slows conduction time through the AV node, interrupts AV node pathways to restore NSR
- amiodarone (Cordorone): prolongs repolarization, relaxes smooth muscles, decreases vascular resistance
- atropine: increases firing of the sinoatrial node (SA) and conduction through the atrioventricular node (AV) of the heart, opposes the actions of the vagus nerve by blocking acetylcholine receptor sites

A. Precautions/Interactions

1. Toxicity is major concern due to additive effects.
2. Caution is needed when used with an AV block.
3. Caution is needed when using anticholinergic medications.

Antidysrhythmic Agents

Medication	Therapeutic Use	Side Effects/ Adverse Effects	NURSING INTERVENTIONS
Adenosine	Convert SVT to sinus rhythm	• Flushing, nausea • Bronchospasm, prolonged asystole	• Rapid IV (1–2 sec) push • Flush immediately with NS
Amniodarone	V-Fib, unstable ventricular tachycardia	• Bradycardia • Cardiogenic shock • Pulmonary disorders	• Incompatible with heparin • May be given in PO maintenance dose • Monitor for respiratory complications
Atropine	Asystole, bradycardia, known exposure to chemical nerve agent (AtroPEN)	• When used for life-threatening emergency, has no contraindications	• Asystole: a single dose of 3 mg not be repeated unless the rhythm changes to bradycardia or pulseless electrical activity

Antilipemic Medications

Action: Aid in lowering low-density lipoprotein (LDL) levels and increase high-density lipoprotein (HDL) levels. Therapy includes diet, exercise, and weight control.

A. Therapeutic Uses

1. Primary hypercholesterolemia
2. Prevention of coronary events
3. Protection against MI and stroke in clients with diabetes

B. Precautions/Interactions

1. Contraindicated in liver disease
2. Used with caution in renal dysfunction

C. Side Effects/Adverse Effects

1. Muscle aches
2. Hepatotoxicity
3. Myopathy
4. Rhabdomyolysis
5. Peripheral neuropathy

D. NURSING INTERVENTIONS and Client Education

1. Take medication in the evening (cholesterol synthesis increases).
2. Monitor liver and renal function laboratory profiles.
3. Low-fat/high-fiber diet.
4. Note dietary precautions with specific classes.

Statin Medications

Action: Interfere with hepatic enzyme HMG COA to reduce formation of cholesterol precursors

Medications:

- simvastatin (Zocor)
- lovastatin (Mevacor)
- dravastatin sodium (Pravachol)
- rosuvastatin (Crestor)
- fluvastatin (Lescol, Lescol XL)

A. Precautions/Interactions

1. Prolonged bleeding in clients taking warfarin (Coumadin)
2. Multiple drug interactions: digoxin, warfarin, thyroid hormones, thiazide diuretics, phenobarbital, NSAIDs, tetracycline, beta-blocking agents, gemfibrozil, glipizide, glyburide, oral contraceptives, and phenytoin

B. NURSING INTERVENTIONS and Client Education

1. Do not administer with grapefruit juice.

Cholesterol Absorption Inhibitor

Action: Inhibits the absorption of cholesterol secreted in the bile and from food. Often used in combination with other antilipemic medications.

Medication:

- ezetimibe (Zetia)

A. NURSING INTERVENTIONS and Client Education

1. Take 1 hr before or 4 hr after other antilipedmics.

Medications for the Respiratory System

Medications used to treat chronic inflammatory conditions caused by asthma, bronchitis, and emphysema.

Treatment for chronic respiratory disorders often includes multiple drug therapies. When administered as inhalation therapies, the following guidelines should be implemented:

1. If taking inhaled glucocorticoid, advise to take the beta-2 agonist before the glucocorticoid to increase steroid absorption.
2. Instruct on procedures for inhalation:
   a. Remove the mouthpiece cap.
   b. If appropriate for medication, shake container.
   c. Stand up or sit upright; breathe out deeply.
   d. Place the mouthpiece between teeth, and close lips tightly around the inhaler.
   e. Start to breathe in slowly and activate the inhaler once, and continue breathing in slowly for several more seconds (slow long, steady inhalation is better than a quick short breaths).
   f. Hold breath for 5–10 seconds.
   g. Breathe in/out normally.
3. Examine mouth for irritation.
4. Perform frequent oral care.

Beta-2 Adrenergic Agonists

Action: Promote bronchodilation by activating beta-2 receptors in bronchial smooth muscle

Beta-2 Adrenergic Agonists

Medication	Route/Onset	Use
albuterol (Proventil, Ventolin)	Inhaled (short-acting) Few minutes	Acute bronchospasm
formoterol (Foradil) salmeterol (Serevent)	Inhaled (long-acting) 15–20 min, lasts 12 hr	Long-term control of asthma
terbutaline (Brethine)	Oral, long-acting	Long-term control of asthma

A. Precautions/Interactions

1. Contraindicated for clients with tachydysrhythmias.
2. Caution: diabetes, hyperthyroidism, heart disease, hypertension, angina.
3. Beta blockers will reduce effects.
4. MAOIs will increase effects.

B. Side Effects/Adverse Effects

1. Tachycardia, palpitations
2. Tremors

 ## C. NURSING INTERVENTIONS and Client Education

1. Caution against using salmeterol more frequently than every 12 hr.

Methylxanthines

Action: Relaxation of bronchial smooth muscle resulting in bronchodilation

Medications:
- aminophylline (Truphylline)
- theophylline (Theodur, Theolair, Theo-42)

A. Therapeutic Uses

1. Relief of bronchospasm
2. Long-term control of asthma

B. Precautions/Interactions

1. Contraindicated with active peptic ulcer disease.
2. Caution: diabetes, hyperthyroidism, heart disease, hypertension, angina.
3. Do not mix parenteral form with other medications.
4. Phenobarbital and phenytoin decrease theophylline levels.
5. Caffeine, furosemide, cimetidine, fluroquinolones, acetaminophen and phenylbutazone falsely elevate therapeutic levels.

C. Side Effects/Adverse Effects

1. Irritability and restlessness
2. Toxic effects: tachycardia, tachypnea, seizures

 ## D. NURSING INTERVENTIONS and Client Education

1. Monitor therapeutic level *Aminophylline*: 10–20 mcg/mL
2. Monitor therapeutic level *Theophylline*: 10–20 mcg/mL
3. Avoid caffeine intake.
4. Monitor for signs of toxicity.
5. Smoking will decrease effects.
6. Alcohol abuse will increase effects.

E. Treatment of Toxicity

1. Stop parenteral infusion
2. Activated charcoal to decrease absorption in oral overdose

3. Lidocaine for dysrhythmias
4. Diazepam to control seizures

Inhaled Anticholinergics

Action: muscarinic receptor blocker resulting in bronchodilation

Medications:
- ipratropium (Atrovent)
- tiotropium (Spiriva)

A. Therapeutic Uses

1. Prevent bronchospasm
2. Manage allergen- or exercise-induced asthma
3. COPD

B. Precautions/Interactions

1. Contraindicated for clients with peanut allergy (contains soy lecithin)
2. Extreme caution with narrow-angle glaucoma and BPH
3. Not used for treatment of acute bronchospasms

C. Side Effects/Adverse Effects

1. Dry mouth and eyes
2. Urinary retention

 ## D. NURSING INTERVENTIONS and Client Education

1. Instruct client that maximum effects may take up to 2 weeks.
2. Shake inhaler well before administration.
3. When using 2 different inhaled medications, wait 5 min between.
4. If administered via nebulizer, use within 1 hr of reconstitution.

Glucocorticoids

Action: Prevent inflammatory response by suppression of airway mucus production, suppression of immune responses and adrenal function

Medications:

Glucocorticoids

Oral	Inhalation	Intravenous
prednisone (Deltasone)	beclometha-sone dipropionate (QVAR)	hydrocortisone sodium succinate (Solu-Cortef)
prednisolone (Prelone)	budesonide (Pulmicort Flexhaler)	methylpredniso-lone sodium succi-nate (Solu-Medrol)
betamethasone (Celestone)	fluticasone pro-pionate (Advair, Flovent)	betamethasone sodium phosphate (Betnesol, Cele-stone Phosphate)
	triamcinolone ace-tonide (Azmacort)	

A. Respiratory Therapeutic Uses

1. Short term
   a. IV agents: status asthmaticus
   b. Oral: treatment of symptoms following an acute asthma attack
2. Long term
   a. Inhaled: prophylaxis of asthma
   b. Oral: treatment of chronic asthma

B. Precautions/Interactions

1. Diabetic clients may require higher doses.
2. Never stop medication abruptly.

C. Side Effects/Adverse Effects

1. Euphoria, insomnia, psychotic behavior
2. Hyperglycemia
3. Peptic ulcer
4. Fluid retention
5. Withdrawal symptoms

D. NURSING INTERVENTIONS and Client Education

1. Assess client activity and behavior.
2. Administer medication with meals.
3. Teach client symptoms to report.
4. Do not take with NSAIDs.
5. Teach client about gradual reduction of dose to prevent Addisonian crisis.

Leukotriene Modifiers

Action: Prevent effects of leukotriene resulting in decreased inflammation, bronchoconstriction, airway edema, and mucus production

Medications:
- montelukast (Singulair)
- zileuton (Zyflo)
- zafirlukast (Accolate)

A. Therapeutic Uses

1. Long-term management of asthma in adults and children > 15 years old
2. Prevention of exercise-induced bronchospasm

B. Precautions/Interactions

1. Do not use for acute asthma attack.
2. Zileuton or zafirlukast: high risk of liver disease, increased warfarin effects, and theophylline toxicity.
3. Phenobarbital will decrease circulating levels of montelukast.
4. Chewable tablets contain phenylalanine.

C. Side Effects/Adverse Effects

1. Elevated liver enzymes (zileuton or zafirlukast)
2. Warfarin and theophylline toxicity (zileuton or zafirlukast)

D. NURSING INTERVENTIONS and Client Education

1. Never abruptly substitute for corticosteroid therapy.
2. Teach client to take daily.
3. Do not decrease or stop taking other prescribed asthma drugs until instructed.
4. If using oral granules, pour directly into mouth or mix with cold soft foods (never liquids).
5. Use open packets within 15 min.

Antitussives, Expectorants, Mucolytics

Antitussives, Expectorants, Mucolytics

Class/Drug	Action	Therapeutic Use
Antitussives: hydrocodone, codeine	Suppress cough through action in the CNS	Chronic nonproductive cough
Expectorants: guaifenesin (Mucinex)	Promote increased mucous secretion to increase cough production	Often combined with other agents to manage respiratory disorders
Mucolytics: acetylcysteine (Mucomyst, Acetadote), hypertonic saline	Enhance the flow of secretions in the respiratory tract	• Acute and chronic pulmonary disorders with copious secretions • Cystic fibrosis • Antidote for acetaminophen poisoning

A. Precautions/Interactions

1. Only saline solutions should be used in children < 2 years old.
2. Opioid antitussives have potential for abuse.
3. Caution with OTC medications—potentiate effects.

B. Side Effects/Adverse Effects

1. Drowsiness
2. Dizziness
3. Aspiration and bronchospasm risk with mucolytics
4. Constipation

C. NURSING INTERVENTIONS and Client Education

1. Monitor cough frequency, effort, and ability to expectorate.
2. Monitor character, tenacity of secretions.
3. Auscultate for adventitious lung sounds.
4. Teach client why multiple therapies are needed.
5. Promote fluid intake.

Decongestants, Antihistamines

Class/Drug	Action	Therapeutic Use
Decongestants • Phenylephrine (Sudafed) • Ephedrine (Pretz-D) • Naphazoline (Privine) • Phenylpropanolamine	Stimulate alpha-1 adrenergic receptors, causing reduced inflammation of nasal membranes	Allergic rhinitis Sinusitis Common cold
Antihistamines • diphenhydramine (Benadryl) • loratadine (Claritin) • cetirizine (Zyrtec) • fexofenadine (Allegra) • desloratadine (Clarinex)	Decrease allergic response by competing for histamine receptor sites	Relieve/prevent hypersensitivity reactions

A. Precautions/Interactions

1. Use cautiously in clients with glaucoma, PUD, and urinary retention.
2. Children may have symptoms of excitation, hallucinations, incoordination, and seizures.
3. Avoid alcohol intake.
4. Products containing pseudoephedrine should not be used longer than 7 days.

B. Side Effects/Adverse Effects

1. Anticholinergic effects
2. Drowsiness

C. NURSING INTERVENTIONS and Client Education

1. Assess for hypokalemia.
2. Monitor BP.
3. Teach client to manage anticholinergic effects.
4. Advise to take at night.

Medications for the Endocrine System

Oral Hypoglycemics

Used in conjunction with diet and exercise to control glucose levels in clients with type 2 diabetes mellitus

A. Precautions/Interactions

1. Caution in clients with renal, hepatic, or cardiac disorders.
2. Generally avoided during pregnancy and lactation. Instruct client to discuss with prescriber.

Oral Hypoglycemics

Medications	Action	Precautions/Interactions
Alpha-glucosidase inhibitors Acarbose (Precose) Miglitol (Glyset)	Slows carbohydrate absorption and digestion	Contraindicated in clients with intestinal disease due to increased gas formation
Biguanides • metformin (Glucophage)	Reduces gluconeogenesis Increases uptake of glucose by muscles	Withhold 48 hr prior to and 48 hr after a test with contrast media Contraindicated in clients with severe infection, shock, hypoxic conditions
Gliptins • sitagliptin (Januvia)	Promotes release of insulin, lowers glucagon secretion and slows gastric emptying	Caution with impaired renal function—dose will be reduced
Meglitinides • repaglinide (Prandin) • nateglinide (Starlix)	Reduces production of glucose within the liver through suppression of gluconeogenesis Increases muscle uptake and use of glucose	Should not be used with NPH insulin due to risk of angina
Sulfonylureas • glipizide (Glucotrol) • glyburide (Dia-Beta, Micronase)	Promotes release of insulin from the pancreas	Extreme high risk of hypoglycemia in clients with renal, hepatic, or adrenal disorders
Thiazolidinediones • rosiglitazone (Avandia) • pioglitazone (Actos)	Decreases insulin resistance	High risk of CHF due to fluid retention

B. NURSING INTERVENTIONS and Client Education

1. Teach signs and management for hypoglycemia, especially with sulfonylureas.
2. Encourage diet and exercise to follow ADA recommendations.
3. Monitor glycosylated hemoglobin (HgA1C).
4. Refer to diabetic nurse educator.

Insulin

Various forms of insulin are available to manage diabetes. The medications vary in onset, peak, and duration.

Insulin

Classification	Drug Name	Onset	Peak	Duration
Rapid-acting	lispro (Humalog)	< 15 min	0.5–1 hr	3–4 hr
Short-acting	regular (Humulin R)	0.5–1 hr	2–3 hr	5–7 hr
Intermediate	NPH (Humulin N)	1–2 hr	4–12 hr	18–24 hr
Long-acting	i glargine (Lantus)	1 hr	none	10.5–24 hr

A. Therapeutic Uses

1. Glycemic control of diabetes mellitus (type 1, type 2, gestational) to prevent complications
2. Clients taking oral hypoglycemic agents may require insulin therapy when:
   a. Undergoing diagnostic tests
   b. Pregnant
   c. Severe renal or liver disease is present
   d. Oral agents are inefficient
   e. Treatment of hyperkalemia

B. Precautions/Interactions

1. When mixing regular with NPH insulin, draw up regular first.
2. Do not mix other insulins with lispro, glargine, or combination 70/30.
3. Only regular insulin is given IV (only in normal saline).
4. Administer glargine at bedtime.

C. Side Effects/Adverse Effects

1. Hypo/hyperglycemia
2. Lipodystrophy

D. NURSING INTERVENTIONS and Client Education

1. Monitor serum glucose levels before meals and at bedtime or patterned schedule-specific to client.
2. Roll vial of insulin (except regular) to mix; do NOT shake.
3. Instruct client to rotate injection sites to prevent lipodystrophy.
4. Teach signs and management for hypo/hyperglycemia.
5. Encourage diet and exercise to follow ADA recommendations.
6. Monitor glycosylated hemoglobin (HgA1c).
7. Refer to diabetic nurse educator.

Glycemic Agent

Action: Initiates regulatory processes to promote breakdown of glycogen to glucose in the liver, resulting in increased serum glucose levels

Medication:
- Glucagon (GlucaGen)

A. Therapeutic Uses

1. Emergency treatment of severe hypoglycemia

B. Precautions/Interactions

1. Do not mix with sodium chloride or dextrose solutions.

C. Side Effects/Adverse Effects

1. Nausea and vomiting
2. Rebound hypoglycemia

D. NURSING INTERVENTIONS and Client Education

1. Administer medication for unresponsive client.
2. Monitor blood glucose levels.
3. Instruct client to self-monitor for early signs of hypoglycemia.
4. Instruct client to wear medical alert ID.
5. Advise client to teach family members how to administer medication.
6. Provide carbohydrates when client awakens from hypoglycemic reaction.

Thyroid Hormone

Action: Stimulates metabolism of all body systems by accelerating the rate of cellular oxygenation

Medication:
- levothyroxine/T_4 (Synthroid)

A. Therapeutic Uses

1. Hypothyroidism
2. Emergency treatment of myxedema coma

B. Precautions/Interactions

1. Overmedication can result in signs of hyperthyroidism.

C. Side Effects/Adverse Effects

1. Tachycardia
2. Restlessness
3. Diarrhea
4. Weight loss
5. Decreased bone density
6. Heat intolerance
7. Insomnia

D. NURSING INTERVENTIONS and Client Education

1. Monitor the client's cardiac system.
2. Therapy initiated with low doses; advance to higher dosages, while monitoring laboratory values.
3. Monitor T_4 and TSH levels.
4. Take in early morning.

Thyroid Hormone Antagonist

Action: Inhibits synthesis of thyroid hormone

Medication:
- methimazole (Tapazole)

A. Therapeutic Uses

1. Hyperthyroidism
2. Preoperative thyroidectomy
3. Thyrotoxic crisis
4. Thyroid storm

B. Precautions/Interactions

1. Administer with caution to clients with bone marrow depression, hepatic disease, or bleeding disorders.
2. Discontinue prior to radioactive iodine uptake testing.
3. Contraindicated with breast-feeding.

C. Side Effects/Adverse Effects

1. Skin rash, pruritus
2. Abnormal hair loss
3. GI upset
4. Paresthesias
5. Periorbital edema
6. Joint and muscle pain
7. Jaundice
8. Agranulocytosis
9. Thrombocytopenia

D. NURSING INTERVENTIONS and Client Education

1. Administer with food at the same time each day.
2. Increase fluids to 3 L/day.
3. Instruct client to avoid OTC products containing iodine.
4. Instruct client to take medication as prescribed.
5. If discontinuing dose must be tapered off.
6. Monitor client for therapeutic response: weight gain, decreased pulse, blood pressure, and T_4 levels.
7. Monitor client for signs of overdose: periorbital edema, cold intolerance, mental depression.

Anterior Pituitary/Growth Hormones

Action: Increase production of insulin-like growth factor throughout the body

Medications:
- somatropin (Genotropin, Nutropin)
- somatrem (Protropin)

A. Therapeutic Use

1. Treat growth hormone deficiencies
2. Turner's syndrome

B. Precautions/Interactions

1. Contraindicated in clients who are severely obese.
2. Therapy must be discontinued prior to epiphyseal closure.
3. Avoid concurrent use of glucocorticoids.

C. Side Effects/Adverse Effects

1. Hyperglycemia
2. Hypothyroidism

D. NURSING INTERVENTIONS and Client Education

1. Monitor growth patterns.
2. Reconstitute medication (do not shake).
3. Administer subcutaneous per protocol.
4. Dose is individualized.

Posterior Pituitary Hormones/Antidiuretic Hormones

Action: Promote reabsorption of water with the kidneys; vasoconstriction of vascular smooth muscle

Medications:
- desmopressin (DDAV): oral, intranasal, subcutaneous, IV
- pitressin (Vasopressin): intranasal, subcutaneous, IV

A. Therapeutic Uses

1. Treat diabetes insipidus
2. Cardiac arrest
3. Nocturnal enuresis

B. Precautions/Interactions

1. Contraindicated in clients with chronic nephritis or high risk for myocardial infarction

C. Side Effects/Adverse Effects

1. Hyponatremia
2. Seizures
3. Coma

D. NURSING INTERVENTIONS and Client Education

1. Monitor urine specific gravity.
2. Monitor blood pressure.
3. Monitor urinary output.
4. Prevent hyponatremia due to water intoxication.
5. Instruct for use of nasal spray.

Adrenal Hormone Replacement

Action: Anti-inflammatory suppresses immune response

Medications:

- dexamethasone (Decadron)
- hydrocortisone (Solu-Cortef)
- fludrocortisone acetate (Florinef)
- prednisone (Meticorten)

A. Therapeutic Uses

1. Acute and chronic replacement for adrenocortical insufficiency (Addison's disease)
2. Inflammation, allergic reactions, cancer

B. Precautions/Interactions

1. Adrenal suppression when administered for inflammation, allergic reactions
2. Contraindicated in clients with systemic fungal infection
3. Caution in client's with hypertension, gastric ulcers, diabetes, osteoporosis
4. Requires higher doses in acute illness or extreme stress

C. Side Effects/Adverse Effects

1. Adrenal suppression when administered for inflammation, allergic reactions
2. Infection
3. Hyperglycemia
4. Osteoporosis
5. GI bleeding
6. Fluid retention

D. NURSING INTERVENTIONS and Client Education

1. Do not skip doses.
2. Monitor blood pressure.
3. Monitor fluid and electrolytes (F&E) balance, weight, and output.
4. Monitor for signs of bleeding and GI discomforts.
5. Teach client to take calcium supplements and maintain vitamin D levels.
6. Give with food.
7. Taper off dose regimen when discontinuing medication.
8. Provide immunoprotection.

Medications for the Hematologic System

Blood and Blood Products

- Whole blood
- Packed red blood cells (PRBCs)
- Platelet concentrations

Administration of Blood Products

Time Completed	Action/ Therapeutic Use	Monitor for Reaction
Whole blood 2–4 hr	Replace volume: • Hemorrhage • Surgery • Trauma • Burns • Shock	• Acute hemolytic • Febrile • Anaphylactic • Mild allergic • Hypervolemia • Sepsis
PRBCs 2–4 hr	Increase available RBC Severe anemia Hemoglobinopathies Hemolytic anemia Erythroblastosis fetalis	• Acute hemolytic • Febrile • Anaphylactic • Mild allergic • Sepsis
Platelets 15–30 min	Increase platelet count Active bleeding (platelets < 80,000 mm3) thrombocytopenia (platelets < 20,000 mm3) Aplastic anemia Bone marrow suppression	• Febrile • Sepsis
FFP 30–60 min	Replace clotting factors: • Hemorrhage • Burns • Shock • TTP • Reverse effects of warfarin	• Acute hemolytic • Febrile • Anaphylactic • Mild allergic • Hypervolemia • Sepsis
Pheresed granulocytes 45–60 min	Severe neutropenia (< 500) Neonatal sepsis Neutrophil dysfunction	• Acute hemolytic • Febrile • Anaphylactic • Mild allergic • Hypervolemia • Sepsis
Albumin • 5% (1–10 mL/min) • 25% (4 mL/min)	Expand volume via oncotic changes Hypovolemia Hypoalbuminemia Burns Severe nephrosis Hemolytic disease of NB	• Risk for hypervolemia and pulmonary edema

A. NURSING INTERVENTIONS and Client Education

1. Client ID, name, and blood type must be verified by two nurses.
2. Prior to administration, assess baseline vital signs, including temperature.
3. Establish IV access, 20-gauge or larger catheter.
4. Must have 0.9% sodium chloride primed tubing.
5. For the first 15 min, stay with the client and infuse slowly; monitor/intervene for any reaction.
   a. Stop blood immediately and take the client's vital signs.
   b. Infuse 0.9% sodium chloride.
   c. Notify the health care provider.
   d. Follow facility policy (send urine sample, CBC, and bag and tubing to laboratory for analysis).
6. Complete infusion of product within 4 hr.

Hematopoietic Growth Factors

Action: Stimulate the bone marrow to synthesize the specific blood cells

Hematopoietic Growth Factors

Medication	Therapeutic Uses	Side Effects/ Adverse Effects	NURSING INTERVENTIONS
epoetin alfa (Procrit)	Stimulate RBC production Anemia related to: • CRF • retrovir therapy • chemotherapy	Hypertension	Subcutaneous or IV • Do not agitate vial • Monitor Hct
filgrastim (Neupogen) injection pegfilgrastim (Neulasta) IV over 2–4 hr	Stimulate WBC production Neutropenia related to cancer	• Bone pain • Leukocytosis	• Subcutaneous or IV • Do not agitate vial • Monitor CBC
oprelvekin (Neumega)	Stimulate platelet production Thrombocytopenia related to cancer	• Fluid retention • Papilledema • Cardiac dysrhythmia	• Administer within 6–24 hr after chemotherapy • Subcutaneous

Iron Preparations

A. Oral

1. Dilute liquid preparations with juice or water and administer with a plastic straw or medication dosing syringe (avoid contact with client's teeth).
2. Encourage orange juice fortified with vitamin D (facilitates absorption) after orange juice (Vitamin C facilitates absorption)
3. Avoid antacids, coffee, tea, dairy products, or whole grain breads concurrently and for 1 hr after administration due to decreased absorption.
4. Monitor the client for constipation and gastrointestinal upset.

B. Intramuscular

1. Use a large-bore needle (19 to 20 gauge, 3-inch needle).
2. Change needle after drawing up from vial.
3. Z-track (ventro-gluteal preferable) **NEVER** in deltoid muscle
4. Do not massage injection site.

Anticoagulants

Heparin Sodium and Enoxaparin (Lovenox) (Parenteral Medications)

Action:

- Modify or inhibit clotting factors or cellular properties to prevent clot formation
- Enoxaparin (Lovenox) prevents conversion of prothrombin to thrombin by inactivating coagulation enzymes.

A. Therapeutic Uses

1. Evolving stroke
2. Pulmonary embolism
3. Massive DVT
4. Cardiac catheterization
5. MI
6. DIC

B. Precautions/Interactions

1. Must be given subcutaneous or IV
2. Incompatible with many drugs (any bicarbonate base)
3. Avoid NSAIDs, aspirin, or medications containing salicylates

C. Side Effects/Adverse Effects

1. Hemorrhage
2. Heparin-induced thrombocytopenia
3. Toxicity/overdose

D. NURSING INTERVENTIONS and Client Education

1. Clients receiving heparin: Monitor APTT every 4–6 hr for IV administration (normal range is 16–40); therapeutic range is 1.5–2.5 times the control alert value > 100.

2. Monitor for signs of bleeding.

3. Safety precautions to prevent bleeding.

4. Administer subcutaneous heparin to abdomen, 2 inches from umbilicus (do not aspirate or massage).

5. Rotate injection sites and observe for bleeding or hematoma.

6. Administer protamine sulfate for heparin toxicity (1 mg neutralizes 100 units of heparin).

Warfarin (Coumadin) (Oral Medication)

Action: Prevents the synthesis of coagulation factors VII, IX, X and prothrombin

A. Therapeutic Uses

1. Venous thrombosis

2. Thrombus prevention for clients with atrial fibrillation or prosthetic heart valves

3. Prevention of recurrent MI

4. Transient ischemic attacks (TIAs)

B. Precautions/Interactions

1. Not safe for use during pregnancy

2. Contraindications: thrombocytopenia, vitamin K deficiency, liver disease, alcoholism

3. Decreased effects with phenobarbital, carbamazepine (Tegretol), phenytoin (Dilantin), oral contraceptives

4. Food sources high in vitamin K may decrease effects

C. Side Effects/Adverse Effects

1. Hemorrhage

2. Toxicity/overdose

D. NURSING INTERVENTIONS and Client Education

1. Administer once daily.

2. Monitor INR (therapeutic levels 2–3) or PT (normal range is 11–14 and therapeutic level is 18-24 sec.); may be altered based on therapeutic indication.

3. Teach client that bleeding risk remains up to 5 days after discontinued therapy.

4. Teach client to avoid NSAIDs and medications with aspirin.

5. Teach client to wear medical alert bracelet.

6. Client may be on home self-monitor for PT/INR.

7. Teach measures to prevent injury and bleeding.

8. Administer vitamin K for warfarin toxicity.

Dabigatran (Pradaxa) (Oral Medication)

Action: Prevents thrombus formation by directly inhibiting thrombin formation

A. Therapeutic Use

1. Reduces the risk of stroke and embolism for clients with non-valvular atrial fibrillation

B. Precautions/Interactions

1. Caution when client is making a change in medication if currently receiving warfarin. (Must discontinue warfarin and start Pradaxa when INR is below 2.0)

2. When possible, discontinue 1–2 days prior to surgical procedures.

C. Side Effects/ Adverse Effects

1. Bleeding

2. GI discomfort

D. NURSING INTERVENTIONS and Client Education

1. Teach client to take medication daily and avoid skipping doses.

2. If a dose is missed, it should not be taken within 6 hr of the next scheduled dose.

3. Tablets should not be crushed, broken, or chewed.

4. Teach client to avoid NSAIDs and medications with aspirin.

5. Teach client to monitor for signs of GI bleeding.

Antiplatelet Medications

Action: Prevent platelets from aggregating (clumping together) by inhibiting enzymes and factors that normally promote clotting

Medications:

- aspirin (Ecotrin)
- abciximab (ReoPro)
- clopidogrel (Plavix)
- ticlopidine (Ticlid)
- pentoxifylline (Trental)
- dipyridamole (Persantine)

A. Therapeutic Uses

1. Prevention of acute myocardial infarction or acute coronary syndromes

2. Prevention of stroke

3. Intermittent claudication

B. Precautions/Interactions

1. Contraindicated in thrombocytopenia

2. Caution with PUD

C. Side Effects/Adverse Effects

1. Prolonged bleeding

2. Gastric bleeding

3. Thrombocytopenia

D. NURSING INTERVENTIONS and Client Education

1. Monitor for signs of prolonged bleeding.

2. Teach client to report tarry stool, ecchymosis.

Thrombolytic Medications

Action: Dissolve clots that have already formed by converting plasminogen to plasmin, which destroys fibrinogen and other clotting factors

Medications:

- alteplase (Activase, tPA)
- tenecteplase (TNKase)
- reteplase (Retavase)

A. Therapeutic Uses

1. Acute myocardial infarction
2. Deep vein thrombosis (DVT)
3. Massive pulmonary emboli (PE)
4. Ischemic stroke (alteplase)

B. Precautions/Interactions

1. Contraindicated for intracranial hemorrhage, active internal bleeding, aortic dissection, brain tumors
2. Caution when using in clients with severe hypertension
3. Concurrent use of anticoagulants or antiplatelet medications increases risk for bleeding

C. Side Effects/Adverse Effects

1. Serious bleeding risks from recent wounds, puncture sites, weakened vessels
2. Hypotension
3. Possible anaphylactic reaction

D. NURSING INTERVENTIONS and Client Education

1. Administration must take place within 4–6 hr of symptom onset.
2. Continuous monitoring is required.
3. Clients will begin anticoagulant therapy to prevent repeated thrombotic event.

Medications for the Gastrointestinal System

Antacids

Action: Neutralize gastric acid and inactivate pepsin

Medications for the Gastrointestinal System

Medication	Side Effects/Adverse Effects
aluminum hydroxide (Amphojel)	Constipation Hypophosphatemia
magnesium hydroxide (Milk of Magnesia)	Diarrhea Hypermagnesemia Renal impairment
sodium bicarbonate	Constipation

A. Therapeutic Uses

1. Peptic ulcer disease
2. GERD

B. NURSING INTERVENTIONS and Client Education

1. Do not administer to clients with GI perforation or obstruction.
2. Clients with renal impairment should only use aluminum-based preparations.
3. Other medications should be taken 1 hr before or after antacids.
4. Require repeated doses up to 7 times per day—1 hr and 3 hr after meals and at bedtime.

Antisecretory/Blocking Agents

Action: Prevent or block selected receptors within the stomach

Therapeutic Uses:

1. Gastric and peptic ulcers
2. GERD
3. Zollinger-Ellison syndrome

Proton Pump Inhibitors

Medications:

- omeprazole (Prilosec)
- lansoprazole (Prevacid)
- rabeprazole sodium (AcipHex)
- esomeprazole (Nexium)

A. Precautions/Interactions

1. Omeprazole promotes increased risk for infection; use with caution in COPD.
2. Digoxin levels may be increased with omeprazole.
3. Long-term therapy has increased risk of gastric cancer and osteoporosis.

B. Side Effects/ Adverse Effects

1. Low incidence of diarrhea, nausea, and vomiting

C. NURSING INTERVENTIONS and Client Education

1. Do not crush, chew, or break tablets.
2. Notify prescriber of any sign of GI bleeding.
3. Teach client to take medication as scheduled.

Histamine-2 Receptor Antagonists

Medications:

- ranitidine hydrochloride (Zantac)
- cimetidine (Tagamet)
- nizatindine (Axid)
- famotidine (Pepcid)

A. Precautions/Interactions

1. May cause toxicity for clients taking phenytoin, warfarin, theophylline, and lidocaine.
2. Cimetidine promotes increased risk for infection; use with caution in COPD.

B. Side Effects/Adverse Effects

1. Decreased libido/impotence
2. Lethargy, depression, confusion

C. NURSING INTERVENTIONS and Client Education

1. Instruct clients to seek appropriate health care (many take OTC preparations).
2. Instruct client to follow medication regimen.
3. Ranitidine can be taken with or without food.
4. Instruct client to modify diet as prescribed.

Mucosal Protectants

Sucralfate (Carafate)

Action: Adheres to injured gastric ulcers upon contact with gastric acids; protective action for up to 6 hr; has no systemic effects

A. Therapeutic Use

1. Gastric and duodenal ulcers
2. GERD

B. NURSING INTERVENTIONS and Client Education

1. Administer on an empty stomach at least 1 hr before meals.
2. Do not administer within 30 min of other antacids.

Antiemetics

Action: Multiple classifications of medications that affect the GI tract or the "vomiting center" of the brain to reduce nausea/vomiting

A. Therapeutic Uses

1. Postoperative
2. Chemotherapy
3. Reduce N/V associated with disease process

Antiemetics

Medication	Side Effects/ Adverse Effects	NURSING INTERVENTIONS
promethazine (Phenergan)	• Drowsiness • Anticholinergic effects • EPS • Potentiates effects when given with narcotics	• Monitor VS • Safety precautions • IM—large muscle
metoclo-pramide (Reglan)	• Drowsiness • Anticholinergic effects • Restlessness • EPS • Tardive dyskinesia	• Instruct client about rapid GI emptying • Discontinue with signs of EPS
ondansetron (Zofran)	• Headache • EPS	• Administer tablets 30 min prior to chemo-therapy and 1–2 hr before radiation
Scopolamine	• Blurred vision • Sedation • Anticholinergic effects	• Do not use with angle-closure glaucoma • Apply transdermal patches behind ear • Use lubricating eye drops

Antidiarrheals

Action: Activate opioid receptors in the GI tract to decrease intestinal motility and to increase the absorption of fluid and sodium in the intestine

Medications:
• diphenoxylate plus atropine (Lomotil)
• loperamide (Imodium)

A. Precautions/Interactions

1. Increased risk of megacolon for IBS clients

B. NURSING INTERVENTIONS and Client Education

1. Monitor F&E.
2. Avoid caffeine intake (increases GI motility).

Stool Softeners/Laxatives

Stool Softeners/Laxatives

Medication	Therapeutic Uses
psyllium (Metamucil)	Decrease diarrhea (bulk forming)
docusate sodium (Colace)	Relieve constipation (surfactant)
bisacodyl (Dulcolax)	Pre-procedure colon evacuation (stimulant)
magnesium hydroxide (Milk of Magnesia)	Prevent painful elimination (low-dose osmotic) Promote rapid evacuation (high-dose osmotic)

A. NURSING INTERVENTIONS and Client Education

1. Contraindicated with fecal impaction, bowel obstruction, and acute surgical abdomen.
2. Encourage regular exercise and promote regular bowel elimination.
3. Monitor for chronic laxative use/abuse.
4. Provide adequate fluid intake.

Medications Affecting the Urinary System

Diuretics

Action: Increase the amount of fluid excretion via the renal system

Diuretics

Loop	Thiazide	Potassium Sparing
furosemide (Lasix) bumetanide (Bumex)	hydrochlorothia-zide (Hydrodiuril) chlorothiazide (Diuril)	spironolactone (Aldactone) triamterene (Dyrenium)

A. Therapeutic Use

1. Pulmonary edema caused by heart failure
2. Edema unresponsive to other diuretics (liver disease, renal dysfunction, hypertension, heart failure)

B. Precautions/Interactions

1. Use cautiously in diabetic clients.
2. Contraindicated in pregnancy.
3. NSAIDs reduce diuretic effect.

C. Side Effects/Adverse Effects

1. Loop and Thiazide Diuretics
   a. Hypovolemia
   b. Ototoxicity
   c. Hypokalemia
   d. Hyponatremia
   e. Hyperglycemia
   f. Digoxin toxicity
   g. Lithium toxicity
2. Potassium-Sparing Diuretics
   a. Hyperkalemia
   b. Endocrine effects (impotence, menstrual irregularities)

D. NURSING INTERVENTIONS and Client Education

1. Monitor I&O.
2. Monitor VS.
3. Monitor for F&E imbalances.
4. Administer early morning to prevent nocturia.
5. Instruct clients taking loop/thiazide diuretics to increase intake of foods high in potassium.
6. Instruct clients taking potassium-sparing diuretics to avoid salt substitutes.

Osmotic Diuretics

Action: Pull fluid back into the vascular and extravascular space by increasing serum osmolality to promote osmotic changes

Medication:
- Mannitol (Osmitrol)

A. Therapeutic Uses

1. Prevent renal failure related to hypovolemia
2. Decrease intracranial pressure related to cerebral edema
3. Decrease intraocular pressure

B. Precautions/Interactions

1. Caution heart failure
2. May increase digoxin levels due to hypokalemia

C. Side Effects/Adverse Effects

1. Pulmonary edema
2. F&E imbalances
3. Thirst, dry mouth

D. NURSING INTERVENTIONS and Client Education

1. Monitor daily weight, I&O, and electrolytes.
2. Monitor for signs of hypovolemia.
3. Monitor neurological status.

Alpha-Adrenergic Blockers for Urinary Hesitancy
Tamsulosin (Flomax)

Action: Inhibits smooth muscle contraction in the prostate, which improves the rate of urine flow for clients with BPH

A. Precautions/Interactions

1. Must "rule out" bladder cancer prior to administering tamsulosin

Bethanechol (Urecholine)

Action: Increases detrusor muscle tone to allow strong start to voiding for clients with postoperative urinary hesitancy

A. Precautions/Interactions

1. Do not administer IV or IM.

Alpha-Adrenergic Blockers

Medication	Side Effects/Adverse Effects	NURSING INTERVENTIONS and Client Education
tamsulosin (Flomax)	May cause decreased libido, reduced ejaculate	Take 30 min after meal at same time each day Teach client to contact prescriber if > 4 doses are missed
bethanechol (Urecholine)	Excessive salivation, tearing	Administer on empty stomach

Anticholinergic Medications for Overactive Bladder

Action: Antispasmodic actions to decrease detrusor muscle spasms and contractions

Medications:
- oxybutynin (Ditropan, Gelnique)
- tolterodine (Detrol)
- darifenacin (Enablex)
- solifenacin (Vesicare)
- trospium (Sanctura)
- fesoterodine (Toviaz)

A. Therapeutic Use

1. Urinary incontinence
2. Urinary urgency and frequency

B. Precautions/Interactions

1. Do not use for clients with intestinal obstruction.

C. Side Effects/Adverse Effects

1. Anticholinergic symptoms
2. Drowsiness
3. Dyspepsia

D. NURSING INTERVENTIONS and Client Education

1. Administer medication with a full glass of water.
2. Instruct client that full effects may take 1–2 months.
3. Instruct client to manage anticholinergic side effects.
4. Instruct client to report constipation lasting > 3 days.

Sexual Dysfunction

Action: enhances the effect of nitric oxide to promote relaxation of penile muscles allowing increased blood flow to produce an erection

Medications

- Sildenafil (Viagra)
- Tadalafil (Cialis)
- Vardenafil (Levitra)

A. Therapeutic Uses

1. Erectile Dysfunction
2. Sexual Dysfunction in women (unlabeled use)

B. Precautions/Interactions

1. Contraindicated for clients taking nitrate drugs, anticoagulants, alpha blockers for BPH or antihypertensives
2. Contraindicated for clients with medical history including stroke, uncontrolled diabetes, hypo/hypertension and heart failure

C. Side Effects/Adverse Effects

- headache
- heartburn
- diarrhea
- flushing
- nosebleeds
- difficulty falling asleep or staying asleep
- paresthesias
- muscle aches
- changes in color vision
- sensitivity to light

D. Nursing Interventions and Client Education

1. Drug is administered 1 hr before sexual activity; do not use more than once daily
2. Instruct client to notify provider of all medications currently taken including herbal preparations
3. Instruct client to avoid intake of any organic nitrates
4. Instruct client to stop taking medication and notify prescriber immediately for any of the following: erection lasting > 4 hours, any loss of vision and unusal bleeding problems

Medications for the Immune System

Immunizations

Action: Stimulate production of antibodies to prevent illness

Childhood Immunizations*

Type	Side Effects/Adverse Effects Risk in Addition to Localized Inflammation	Contraindication
DTaP Tdap	Fever and irritability Seizures	Occurrence of seizures within 3 days of vaccine
Hib	Low-grade fever	Children < 6 yrs
Rotavirus		Infant with diarrhea and vomiting Immunocompromised
IPV	Allergic reaction	Allergy to "mycin" drugs
MMR	Joint pain Anaphylaxis Thrombocytopenia	Allergy to gelatin and neomycin Immunocompromised
Varicella	Vesicles on skin Pruritus	Pregnancy Allergy to gelatin and neomycin Immunocompromised
Seasonal influenza	Fever	Nasal spray contraindicated for child < 2 and adults > 50 years History of Guillain-Barré
Hepatitis A, B	Anaphylaxis	Hep A: pregnancy Hep B: allergy to yeast
Meningococcal (MCV4) Students entering college		History of Guillain-Barré
HPV (up to age 26)		Pregnancy Allergy to yeast

*Schedule is determined by the Centers for Disease Control and Prevention.

Adult Immunizations (Ages 18 Years and Older)*

Type	Schedule
Tetanus booster	Every 10 years
MMR	1 or 2 doses at ages 19 to 49
Varicella	2 doses if no history of disease
Pneumococcal (PPSV)	Once after age 65 Also recommended for immuno-compromised, COPD, living in long-term care facility
Hepatitis A	2 doses for high-risk clients
Hepatitis B	3 doses for high-risk clients
Seasonal influenza	Annually
Meningococcal (MCV4)	Adults > 56 years Repeat every 5 years for high-risk clients
Herpes zoster	Over age 60

*Schedule is determined by the Centers for Disease Control and Prevention.

A. NURSING INTERVENTIONS and Client Education

1. Consult CDC guidelines for schedule of administration.
2. Educate clients about the purpose of immunizations and keeping records.
3. Instruct parents to avoid administration of aspirin for management of side effects in children.
4. Instruct clients regarding side/adverse effects and management.

Antimicrobials

Action: Inhibit growth, destroy or otherwise control replication of microbes

Multigeneration Antibiotics

Class	Therapeutic Use	Precautions
Aminoglycosides • amikacin (Amikin) • vancomycin (Vancocin) • gentamicin sulfate (Garamycin) • streptomycin	Septicemia, meningitis, pneumonia	High risk for ototoxity, nephrotoxicity Monitor creatinine and BUN Peak and trough levels Therapeutic range: gentamicin 4–12 mcg/dL, vancomycin 20–40 mcg/dL
Cephalosporins • cephalexin (Keflex) • cefaclor (Celor) • cefotaxime (Claforan)	Upper respiratory, skin, urinary infections Used as prophylaxis for clients at risk	Cross-sensitivity with penicillins Monitor for signs of *Clostridium difficile*
Fluroquinolones • ciprofloxacin (Cipro) • levofloxacin (Levaquin)	Bronchitis, chlamydia, gonorrhea, PID, UTI, pneumonia, prostatitis, sinusitis	Caution with hepatic, renal, or seizure disorders
Macrolides • azithromycin (Zithromax) • clarithromycin (Biaxin) • erythromycin (E-mycin)	Upper respiratory infections, sinusitis, Legionnaires' disease, whooping cough, acute diphtheria, chlamydia	Used for clients with PCN allergy Administer with meals
Nitrofurantoin (Macrodantin)	UTI	Broad spectrum Contraindicated in renal dysfunction Urine will have brown discoloration
Penicillins • amoxicillin (Amoxil) • ampicillin (Omnipen)	Pneumonia, upper respiratory infections, septicemia, endocarditis, rheumatic fever, GYN infections	Hypersensitivity with possible anaphylaxis
Sulfonamides • trimethoprim-sulfamethoxazole (Bactrim, Septra)	UT, bronchitis, otitis media	Consume at least 3 L fluid per day Use backup contraceptives Avoid sun exposure
Tetracyclines • doxycycline calcium (Vibramycin) • tetracycline HCl (Sumycin)	Fungal, bacterial, protozoal, rickettsial infections	Consume at least 3 L fluid per day Use backup contraceptives Avoid sun exposure Permanent tooth discoloration if given to children < 8 yr

Special Classes of Antifungals, Antimicrobials, and Antiprotozoals

Class	Therapeutic Use	Precautions
Antifungal • fluconazole (Diflucan)	Candidiasis infections	Monitor hepatic and renal function Refrigerate suspensions Increased risk of bleeding for clients taking anticoagulants
Antimalarials • hydroxychloro-quine (Plaquenil) • quinine sulfate (Quinine)	Prevent malarial attacks, rheumatoid arthritis Systemic lupus	Increased risk of psoriasis Monitor for drug-induced retinopathy
Antiprotozoal • metronidazole (Flagyl)	Trichomoniasis and giardiasis, *Clostridium difficile*, amebic dysentery, PID, vaginosis	Take with food Do not consume alcohol during therapy or 48 hr after completion of regimen
Antituberculars • isoniazid (INH) • rifampin (Rifadin)	Prevention and treatment of TB Latent TB INH: 6–9 months Active TB: multiple therapy up to 24 months	Risk of neuropathies and hepatotoxicity Consume foods high in vitamin B_6 Avoid foods with tyramine (INH) Increased risk of phenytoin (Dilantin) toxicity (INH) Avoid alcohol Discoloration of urine, saliva, sweat, and tears (rifampin)
Antiretrovirals • acyclovir (Zovirax) • valacyclovir HCl (Valtrex) • Zidovudine (AZT, Retrovir)	Genital herpes, shingles, HIV	Acyclovir and valacyclovir: administer with food Zidovudine: empty stomach Increase fluid intake Begin therapy with first onset of symptoms

 A. NURSING INTERVENTIONS and Client Education

1. Assess history of medication allergies including treatment.
2. Monitor client for signs of medication reaction.
3. Monitor client for signs of secondary infections.
4. Administer medications at appropriate time intervals to maintain therapeutic effects.
5. If C&S is ordered, perform test before initiating therapy.
6. Instruct client to complete entire medication regimen.

Medications for the Musculoskeletal System

Bisphosphonates

Action: Decrease the number and action of osteoclasts, resulting in bone resorption

Medications:
- ibandronate sodium (Boniva): daily
- risedronate (Actonel): weekly
- zoledronate (Reclast, Zometa): IV monthly

A. Therapeutic Use

1. Prevention and treatment of osteoporosis
2. Paget's disease
3. Hypercalcemia related to malignancy

B. Precautions/Interactions

1. Contraindicated during lactation
2. Clients with esophageal stricture or difficulty swallowing may only use zoledronate
3. Absorption is decreased when taken with calcium supplements, antacids, orange juice, and caffeine

C. Side Effects/Adverse Effects

1. Musculoskeletal pain
2. Esophagitis and GI discomfort
3. Pain in the jaw with zoledronate

D. NURSING INTERVENTIONS and Client Education

1. Administer medication in the morning on an empty stomach.
2. Instruct client to consume at least 8 oz. of water (not carbonated).
3. Client must remain sitting or standing for 30 min after taking medication.
4. Consume adequate amounts of vitamin D.

Antirheumatics

Action: Provide symptomatic relief and delay in disease progression by inhibiting or modulating inflammatory processes

Antirheumatics

Category	Medications	Action
Disease-modifying antirheumatic drugs (DMARDs)	• methotrexate (Theumatrex) • hydroxychloroquine (Plaquenil) • etanercept (Enbrel) • infliximab (Remicade) • adalimumab (Humira)	Interrupt complex immune responses, preventing disease progression
Glucocorticoids	• prednisone (Deltasone) • prednisolone (Prelone)	Decrease inflammation by suppressing leukocytes and fibroblasts, and reversing capillary permeability
NSAIDs	• ibuprofen (Advil, Motrin) • diclofenac (Voltaren) • indomethacin (Indocin) • naproxen (Naprosyn) • celecoxib (Celebrex)	Inhibit prostaglandin synthesis resulting in decreased inflammatory responses

DMARDs

A. Therapeutic Use

1. Slow joint degeneration and progression of rheumatoid arthritis

B. Precautions/Interactions

1. Methotrexate: Contraindicated in pregnancy, renal or liver failure, psoriasis, alcoholism, or hematologic dyscrasias

C. Side Effects/Adverse Effects

1. Methotrexate: Increased risk of infection, bone marrow suppression, GI ulceration
2. Hydroxychloroquine: retinal damage (blindness)

D. NURSING INTERVENTIONS and Client Education

1. Instruct client about measures to prevent infection.
2. Monitor liver function tests.
3. Instruct client to use reliable contraception.
4. Instruct client that initial effects may take 3–6 weeks and full therapeutic effects make take several months.
5. Administer with food.
6. Instruct clients taking hydroxychloroquine about the critical importance of retinal examination every 6 months.

Glucocorticoids

A. Therapeutic Use

1. Provide symptomatic relief of inflammation and pain

B. Precautions/Interactions

1. Contraindicated in systemic fungal infection.
2. Do not administer live virus vaccines during therapy.
3. Should only be used for a short duration.

C. Side Effects/Adverse Effects

1. Risk of infection
2. Osteoporosis
3. Adrenal suppression
4. Fluid retention
5. GI discomfort
6. Hyperglycemia
7. Hypokalemia

D. NURSING INTERVENTIONS and Client Education

1. Do not skip doses.
2. Monitor blood pressure.
3. Monitor F&E balance and weight.
4. Monitor for signs of bleeding, GI discomforts.
5. Teach client to take calcium supplements and maintain vitamin D levels.
6. Give with food.
7. Never stop abruptly.
8. Provide immunoprotection.

NSAIDs

A. Therapeutic Use

1. Provide rapid, symptomatic relief of inflammation and pain

B. Precautions/Interactions

1. Hypersensitivity to aspirin or other NSAIDs
2. May increase the risk of MI and stroke

C. Side Effects/Adverse Effects

1. GI discomforts
2. GI ulceration
3. Liver impairment
4. Photosensivity

D. NURSING INTERVENTIONS and Client Education

1. Administer with food and full glass of water.
2. Avoid lying down for 30 min after administration.
3. Instruct client to use only as needed for symptoms to reduce risk of GI ulceration.
4. Instruct client to use sunscreen.

Antigout

Antigout Medications

Medication	Action	Therapeutic Use
allopurinol (Zyloprim)	Inhibits uric acid production	Chronic gouty arthritis
colchicine (Colcrys)	Inhibits processes to prevent leukocytes from invading joints	Acute gouty arthritis

A. Precautions/Interactions

1. Caution in clients with renal, cardiac, or gastrointestinal dysfunction

B. Side Effects/Adverse Effects

1. GI distress
2. Hepatitis

C. NURSING INTERVENTIONS and Client Education

1. Instruct client to avoid foods high in purines to reduce uric acid.
2. Monitor CBC and uric acid levels.
3. Instruct clients to avoid aspirin.
4. Administer with meals.

Medications for the Nervous System

Mental Health

Antianxiety Medications

Action: Increase the efficacy of GABA to reduce anxiety

Medications:

- alprazolam (Xanax)
- buspirone (BuSpar)
- chlordiazepoxide (Librium)
- clonazepam (Klonopin)
- diazepam (Valium)
- lorazepam (Ativan)

A. Therapeutic Use

1. Generalized anxiety disorder and panic disorder
2. Insomnia
3. Alcohol withdrawal
4. Induction of anesthesia

B. Precautions/Interactions

1. Diazepam and buspirone are used with caution in clients with substance abuse and liver disease.
2. Buspirone is contraindicated for clients taking MAOIs.

C. Side Effects/Adverse Effects

1. CNS depression
2. Paradoxical response (insomnia, excitation, euphoria)
3. Withdrawal symptoms (not with buspirone)
4. Risk of abuse and potential for overdose

D. NURSING INTERVENTIONS and Client Education

1. Monitor vital signs.
2. Instruct clients to never abruptly discontinue medication.
3. Monitor clients for side/adverse effects.
4. Instruct clients to avoid alcohol.
5. Treat overdose with flumazenil (Romazicon).

Antidepressants

Action:

- **SSRI** inhibits serotonin reuptake.
- **Tricyclic** blocks reuptake of norepinephrine and serotonin.
- **MAOI** increases norepinephrine, dopamine, and serotonin by blocking MAO-A.

Antidepressants

Class	Precautions/ Interactions	Side Effects/ Adverse Effects
SSRI • duloxetine (Cymbalta) • fluoxetine (Prozac) • escitalopram (Lexapro) • fluvoxamine (Luvox) • paroxetine (Paxil, Pexeva) • sertraline (Zoloft)	1. Must avoid alcohol 2. Do not discontinue abruptly 3. Monitor for serotonin syndrome (agitation, confusion, hallucinations) within first 72 hr	1. Weight gain 2. Sexual dysfunction 3. Fatigue 4. Drowsiness
Tricyclic • amitriptyline (Elavil) • clomipramine (Anafranil) • doxepin (Sinequan) • imipramine (Tofranil)	1. Do not administer with MAOIs or St. John's wort 2. Must avoid alcohol 3. Contraindicated for clients with seizure disorder	1. Anticholingeric effects 2. Sedation 3. Toxicity 4. Decreased seizure threshold
MAOI • isocarboxazid (Marplan) • tranylcypromine (Parnate)	1. Must avoid foods containing tyramine 2. Antihypertensives have additive hypotensive effect 3. Contraindicated for clients taking SSRIs, tricyclics, heart failure, CVA, renal insufficiency	1. CNS stimulation 2. Orthostatic hypotension 3. Hypertensive crisis with intake of tyramine, SSRIs, and tricyclics 4. Orthostatic hypotension

A. NURSING INTERVENTIONS and Client Education

1. Assess client for suicidal risk.
2. Instruct client to take on daily basis and never miss a dose.
3. Instruct client about therapeutic effects and time of onset.
4. Instruct client to avoid discontinuing drug abruptly.
5. Instruct client to take SSRIs in the morning to minimize sleep disturbances.
6. Provide clients taking MAOIs a list of foods containing tyramine.
7. Advise clients to avoid taking other medications without consulting provider.

Bipolar Disorder Medications

Action: produces neurochemical changes in the brain to control acute mania, depression and incidence of suicide

Medication:

- lithium carbonate (Eskalith, Lithobid)

A. Therapeutic Uses

1. Bipolar disorder
2. Alcoholism
3. Bulimia
4. Schizophrenia

B. Precautions/Interactions

1. Use cautiously in clients with renal dysfunction, heart disease, hyponatremia, and dehydration.
   a. NSAIDs or aspirin will increase lithium levels.
   b. Monitor serum sodium levels.

C. Side Effects/Adverse Effects

1. GI distress
2. Fine hand tremors
3. Polyuria
4. Weight gain
5. Renal toxicity

D. NURSING INTERVENTIONS and Client Education

1. Monitor therapeutic levels (0.4–1.0 mEq/L).
2. Monitor serum sodium levels.
3. Instruct clients that therapeutic effects begin in 7–14 days.
4. Doses must be administered 2–3 times daily per prescriber.
5. Provide nutritional counseling to include food sources for sodium.
6. Administer with food to decrease GI distress.

Antipsychotic Medications

Action: Block dopamine, acetylcholine, histamine, and norepinephrine receptors in the brain and periphery

Medications:

- Conventional
  - chlorpromazine (Thorazine)
  - fluphenazine (Prolixin)
  - haloperidol (Haldol)
  - thiothixene (Navane)
- Atypical (less severe side/adverse effects)
  - aripiprazole (Abilify)
  - clozapine (clozaril)
  - olanzapine (Zyprexa)
  - paliperidone (Invega)
  - quetiapine (Seroquel)
  - ziprasidone (Geodon)

A. Therapeutic Use

1. Acute and chronic psychosis
2. Schizophrenia
3. Manic phase of bipolar disorders
4. Tourette's syndrome
5. Delusional and schizoaffective disorders
6. Dementia

B. Interactions/Precautions

1. Contraindicated for clients with severe depression, Parkinson's disease, prolactin-dependent cancer, and severe hypotension.
2. Use with caution in clients with glaucoma, paralytic ileus, prostate enlargement, or seizure disorder.

C. Side Effects/Adverse Effects

1. Sedation
2. Extrapyramidal effects (administer Cogentin)
3. Anticholinergic effects
4. Tardive dyskinesia
5. Agranulocytosis
6. Neuroleptic malignant syndrome
7. Seizures (may require increased dose of antiseizure meds)

D. NURSING INTERVENTIONS and Client Education

1. Monitor for side effects within 5 hr to 5 days of administration.
2. Advise client of potential side effects.
3. Monitor CBC.
4. Encourage fluids.
5. Stop medication for signs of neuroleptic malignant syndrome.

Attention Deficit Hyperactive Disorder Medications

Action: Increase attention span and reduce impulsive behavior and hyperactivity

- **Stimulants** increase levels of norepinephrine, serotonin, and dopamine into the CNS.
- **Nonstimulants** increase levels of norepinephrine into the CNS.

Attention Deficit Hyperactive Disorder Medications

Class/Medication	Side Effects	NURSING INTERVENTIONS and Client Education
Stimulants • **Dextroamphetamine and Amphetamine** Adderall/ Adderall XR) • methylphenidate (Daytrana—transdermal) • methylphenidate (Concerta, Ritalin)	Mood changes Insomnia Anxiety	1. Administer in early morning 2. Do not abruptly discontinue 3. Monitor for signs of abuse 4. Monitor for signs of agitation
Nonstimulants • atomoxetine (Strattera) • guanfacine (Intuiv): may also be used in treatment of Asperger's syndrome	GI upset Constipation Fatigue	1. Take medication daily 2. Do not crush or chew 3. Instruct client to immediately report worsening of anxiety, agitation 4. Do not take with MAOIs

Sedative/Hypnotic Medications

Action: Slow neuronal activity in the brain to induce sedation/sleep

Medications:
- eszopiclone (Lunesta)
- temazepam (Restoril)
- zolpidem tarate (Ambien)

A. Therapeutic Use

1. Short-term insomnia
2. Difficulty falling or staying asleep

B. Precautions/Interactions

1. Use cautiously in clients with severe mental depression

C. Side Effects/Adverse Effects

1. Dry mouth
2. Decreased libido
3. Respiratory depression

D. NURSING INTERVENTIONS and Client Education

1. Instruct client to take immediately before bedtime as medication has abrupt onset of sleep.
2. Instruct client to avoid alcohol.
3. Warn client and caregivers of potential for sleep activities without recall; notify prescriber immediately.

Abstinence Maintenance Medications

Disulfiram (Antabuse)

Action: Interferes with hepatic oxidation of alcohol, resulting in elevation of blood acetaldehyde levels

A. Therapeutic Use

1. Adjunct to maintain sobriety in treatment of alcoholism

B. Interactions/Precautions

1. INH will increase risk of adverse CNS effects for clients taking disulfiram.
2. Ingestion of large amounts of alcohol may cause respiratory depression, arrhythmias, and cardiac arrest.
3. Adjust medication doses of warfarin and phenytoin.

C. Side Effects/Adverse Effects

1. Drowsiness
2. Headache
3. Metallic taste

D. NURSING INTERVENTIONS and Client Education

1. Do not give within 14 days of client's ingestion of alcohol-containing substances.
2. Instruct client that consumption of alcohol while taking disulfiram will result in flushing, throbbing in head and neck, throbbing headache, respiratory difficulty, nausea, copious vomiting, sweating, thirst, chest pain, palpitation, dyspnea, hyperventilation, tachycardia, hypotension, syncope, marked uneasiness, weakness, vertigo, blurred vision, and confusion.
3. Instruct client that undesirable effects last 30 min to several hours when alcohol is consumed.
4. Instruct client the effects of disulfiram may stay in the body for weeks after therapy is discontinued.
5. Instruct client therapy may last for months to years.

Methadone (Dolophine)

Action: Binds with opiate receptors in CNS to produce analgesic and euphoric effects

A. Therapeutic Use

1. Prevents withdrawal symptoms in patients who were addicted to opiate drugs

B. Precautions/Interactions

1. Should not be used in clients with severe asthma, chronic respiratory disease, or history of head injury

C. Side Effects/Adverse Effects

1. Sedation
2. Respiratory depression
3. Paradoxical CNS excitation

 D. NURSING INTERVENTIONS and Client Education

1. Monitor clients for signs of drug tolerance and psychological dependence.
2. Monitor pancreatic enzymes, as drug may cause biliary spasms.
3. Instruct client that methadone must be slowly reduced to produce detoxification.
4. Client must be monitored through treatment center.

Chronic Neurological Disorders

Cholinesterase Inhibitors

Action: Prevent cholinesterase from inactivating acetylcholine, resulting in improved transmission of nerve impulses

Medications:
- neostigmine (Prostigmin)
- ambenonium (Mytelase)
- edrophonium (Tensilon)

A. Therapeutic Use

1. Myasthenia gravis

B. Precautions/Interactions

1. Do not administer if SBP < 90 mm Hg.

C. Side Effects/Adverse Effects

1. Slow heart rate
2. Chest pain, weak pulse, increased sweating, and dizziness
3. Client feeling like he or she might pass out
4. Weak or shallow breathing
5. Urinating more than usual
6. Seizures
7. Trouble swallowing

 D. NURSING INTERVENTIONS and Client Education

1. Dose must be individualized.
2. Instruct client to keep individual diary to record side effects.
3. Advise client to wear medic-alert bracelet.
4. Monitor for cholinergic crisis.

Anti-Parkinson's

Action: Increase dopamine to minimize tremors and rigidity

Medications:
- benztropine (Cogentin)
- carbidopa/levodopa (Sinemet)
- levodopa (Dopar)

A. Therapeutic Use

1. Parkinson's disease

B. Precautions/Interactions

1. Do not use levodopa within 2 weeks of MAOI use.
2. Pyridoxine (vitamin B$_6$) decreases effects of levodopa.
3. Benztropine is contraindicated in clients with narrow-angle glaucoma.
4. Must discontinue 6–8 hr before anesthesia.

C. Side Effects/Adverse Effects

1. Muscle twitching (especially eyelid spasms)
2. Headache
3. Dizziness
4. Dark urine
5. Agitation

 D. NURSING INTERVENTIONS and Client Education

1. Instruct family members to assist with medication regimen.
2. Instruct client to notify prescriber if sudden loss of the medication effects should occur.
3. Instruct client it may take 4–6 weeks to reach maximum therapeutic effects.
4. Monitor closely for signs of adverse reactions.
5. Instruct client to avoid high-protein meals and snacks.
6. Keep medication away from heat, light, and moisture. If pills become darkened, they have lost potency and must be discarded.

Antiseizure

Action: Slows rates of neuronal activity in the brain by blocking specific channels responsible for neuron firing, which results in an elevation of the seizure threshold

Medications:
- carbamazepine (Tegretol)
- gabapentin (Neurontin)
- phenobarbital (Luminal)
- phenytoin (Dilantin)
- valproic acid (Depakote)

A. Therapeutic Use

1. Prevent and/or control seizure activity

Antiseizure Medications

Medication	Precautions/ Interactions	Side Effects/ Adverse Effects
carbamazepine (Tegretol)	Contraindicated in clients with bone marrow suppression or bleeding disorders Warfarin therapy will decrease effectiveness	Anemia, leukopenia, Stevens-Johnson syndrome
gabapentin (Neurontin)	Do not abruptly discontinue	Dizziness, ataxia, somnolence, hypertension, bruising
phenobarbital (Luminal)	Contraindicated in history of drug addiction	Drowsiness, hypotension, respiratory depression
phenytoin (Dilantin)	Causes increased excretion of digoxin, warfarin, oral contraceptives	Gingival hypertrophy, diplopia, drowsiness, hirsutism
valproic acid (Depakote)	Contraindicated in liver disease, pregnancy	Hepatotoxicty, teratogenic effects, pancreatitis

B. NURSING INTERVENTIONS and Client Education

1. Monitor clients for therapeutic effects.
2. Monitor clients taking phenytoin for toxic effects, including serum levels for toxicity (therapeutic range 10–20 mcg/mL).
3. Instruct clients regarding the importance of compliance; drug is treatment not a cure.
4. Individualize treatment regimen.
5. Instruct client regarding side effects/adverse effects.
6. Drug therapy for status epilepticus: intravenous phenytoin and valium.

Ophthalmologic Medications (Antiglaucoma)

Action: Reduction of aqueous humor

Medications:
- levobunolol (Betagan)
- pilocarpine HCl (Pilocar)
- timolol maleate (Timoptic)

A. Precautions/Interactions

1. Caution in clients taking oral beta blocker or calcium channel blocker

B. Side Effects/Adverse Effects

1. Blurred vision
2. Photophobia
3. Dry eyes
4. May have systemic effects of beta blockade

C. NURSING INTERVENTIONS and Client Education

1. Instruct to use sterile technique when handling applicator portion of the container.
2. Hold gentle pressure on the nasolacrimal duct for 30–60 seconds immediately after instilling drops.
3. Monitor pulse rate/rhythm for clients taking oral beta or calcium channel blocker.

Medications for Pain and Inflammation

NSAIDs (see Medications for the Musculoskeletal System)

Acetaminophen

Action: Slows production of prostaglandins in the CNS

A. Therapeutic Use

1. Analgesic
2. Antipyretic

B. Precautions/Interactions

1. Caution in clients who consume 3 or more alcoholic beverages per day
2. Concurrent use of rifampin, INH, carbamazepine, and barbiturates may increase hepatotoxic effects
3. Slows the metabolism of warfarin

C. Side Effects/Adverse Effects

1. Nausea and vomiting
2. Long-term therapy: hemolytic anemia, leukopenia, neutropenia, and thrombocytopenia

D. NURSING INTERVENTIONS and Client Education

1. Monitor liver function.
2. Monitor renal function.
3. Instruct client to not exceed recommended dose (adult 4,000 mg/24 hr).
4. Instruct client to recognize signs of hepatotoxicity.
5. Administration to children should be based on age, not to exceed 5 doses per day (READ LABELS CAREFULLY).
6. Treat acetaminophen overdose with acetylcysteine (Mucomyst).

Opioid Analgesics

Action: Bind with opiate receptors in the CNS to alter the perception of and emotional response to pain

Medications:
- fentanyl (Sublimaze, Duragesic)
- hydromorphone (Dilaudid)
- morphine sulfate
- meperidine (Demerol)
- codeine, oxycodone (OxyContin)

A. Therapeutic Use

1. Relief of moderate to severe pain
2. Sedation

B. Precautions/Interactions

1. Morphine is contraindicated after biliary tract surgery.
2. Meperidine is contraindicated in clients with renal failure.
3. Monitor for potentiate effects when given with barbiturates, benzodiazepines, phenothiazines, hypnotics, and sedatives.

C. Side Effects/Adverse Effects

1. Orthostatic hypotension
2. Constipation
3. Urinary retention
4. Blurred vision
5. Respiratory depression
6. Abstinence syndrome

 D. NURSING INTERVENTIONS and Client Education

1. Monitor vital signs.
2. Monitor for respiratory depression.
3. Instruct client regarding administration if PCA pump.
4. Administer naloxone (Narcan) for clients with respiratory depression.

Medications for the Reproductive System

Contraception

The nurse should consider the following when providing client education and support regarding contraception. Factors that influence one's choice of a contraceptive include the following:

- Age and health status, including risk for STD
- Religion and culture
- Plans for future conception
- Frequency of intercourse
- Number of sexual partners
- Personal concerns about availability, spontaneity, ease of use

Contraceptives

Method	Considerations for Use	Client Education
Rhythm method	Develop "fertile awareness" by noting • Cervical mucus changes • Menstrual cycle pattern • Basal temperature	• Do not have sexual intercourse during "fertile periods" • Low reliability for preventing pregnancy

Method	Considerations for Use	Client Education
Oral contraceptives	• Pill is taken daily • Side effects: breast tenderness, bleeding, nausea/vomiting	• Antibiotic therapy reduces effectiveness • Avoid smoking
ethinyl estradiol and norelgestromin (Ortho Evra) contraceptive patch	Replace patch each week for 3 weeks	• Apply patch to buttocks, abdomen, upper torso, upper/outer arm • Period will begin on week 4 (no patch)
medroxyprogesterone (Depo-Provera)	Injection is administered every 3 months during menstrual cycle	• Use backup form of birth control for 7 days after first injection • Fertility "returns" approximately 1 year after stopping
Emergency contraception	• A larger-than-normal dose of oral contraceptive • Can be taken no later than 72 hr after unprotected sex • Second dose is repeated 12 hr later • Antiemetics may be needed	• Should discuss options with provider • Should never be used as the primary method of birth control
etonogestrel, ethinyl estradiol vaginal ring (NuvaRing)	Placed deep into the vagina once every 3 weeks	• One size fits most women • If "falls out," rinse in warm water and replace within 5 hr • Remove ring during week 4; menses should begin
Intrauterine device (IUD)	• Contraindicated for women with diabetes or history of PID • High risk of infection • May have cramping and heavier periods	• Hormonal IUD effective for up to 7 years • Copper IUD effective for up to 12 years • Must monitor for signs of infection • Verify "string" is present
Cervical cap	• Use with spermicide • Fit by prescriber • Pap smear every 3 months • Increased risk of vaginal infections	• Leave in place 6 hr after intercourse but not longer than 48 hr

Method	Considerations for Use	Client Education
Cervical diaphragm	• Use with spermicide • Fitted by prescriber • Refitted after childbirth or weight gain/loss	• Leave in place 6 hr after intercourse
Condom	Use with spermicide	• Protects against STDs • Apply and remove correctly • Use only water-soluble lubricants
Spermicides	Available as: • Cream • Foam • Gel • Suppository • Film	• Should use with barrier method • Can insert up to 1 hr before intercourse

 A. NURSING INTERVENTIONS and Client Education

1. Discuss conception and contraceptive plans with client to include reliability, benefits, and risks.
2. Instruct client to maintain regular health screening visits.
3. Instruct client about measures to prevent PID, STDs.
4. Explain that contraceptive decisions may change over the life span.
5. Teach clients unreliable forms of birth control including coitus interruptus (withdrawal), douching, and breast-feeding.

Oxytocic

Cervical "Ripening"

Action: Prostaglandins cause cervical softening in preparation for cervical dilation and effacement.

Medication:
• dinoprostone cervical gel (Cervidil)

A. Precautions/Interactions

1. Contraindicated in clients with genital herpes, ruptured membranes, or placenta previa

B. Side Effects/Adverse Effects

1. Nausea
2. Stomach pain
3. Back pain
4. Feeling of warmth in the vaginal area

 C. NURSING INTERVENTIONS and Client Education

1. Maintain client on bed rest for 1 to 2 hr after insertion.
2. Monitor and record maternal vital signs and fetal heart rate.
3. Monitor for uterine contractions.
4. Remove by gently pulling the netted string and discard.
5. Oxytocin augmentation may be initiated as needed.
6. Assess Bishop's Score for 6 and greater to begin induction.

Oxytocin (Pitocin)

Action: Stimulates uterine contractions for the purpose of induction or augmentation of labor

A. Therapeutic Use

1. Antepartum for Contraction Stress Test (CST)
2. Intrapartum for induction or augmentation of labor
3. Postpartum to promote uterine involution

B. Precautions/Interactions

1. Contraindicated with placental insufficiency
2. Bishop Score of 6 and greater when planning induction

C. Side Effects/Adverse Effects

1. Intense uterine contractions
2. Uterine hyperstimulation (contraction > 90 sec.)
3. Uterine rupture

 D. NURSING INTERVENTIONS and Client Education

1. Administer as secondary infusion via infusion pump for induction or augmentation.
2. Continuously monitor uterine contractions and fetal heart rate.
3. Discontinue oxytocin with any signs of uterine hyperstimulation.
4. Administer oxygen via facemask 10 L for signs of hyperstimulation.
5. When used in postpartum, monitor client for uterine bleeding.

Methylergonovine (Methergine)

Action: Acts directly on the uterine muscle to stimulate forceful contractions

A. Therapeutic Use

1. Postpartum hemorrhage

B. Precautions/Interactions

1. Use with extreme caution in clients with hypertension, preeclampsia, heart disease, venoatrial shunts, mitral valve stenosis, sepsis, or hepatic or renal impairment

C. Side Effects/Adverse Effects

1. Potent vasoconstriction
2. Hypertension
3. Headache

 D. NURSING INTERVENTIONS

1. Continuously monitor blood pressure.
2. Assess uterine bleeding and uterine tone.

Tocolytics

Action: Act on uterine muscle to cease contractions

A. Therapeutic Use

1. Stop preterm labor

Tocolytics

Medication	Side Effects/ Adverse Effects	NURSING INTERVENTIONS
terbutaline sulfate (Brethine) ritrodrine HCl (Yutopar)	• Nervousness • Tremulousness • Headache • Nausea and vomiting • Hyperglycemia • Severe palpitations • Chest pain • Pulmonary edema	1. Monitor contractions and FHT 2. Monitor VS 3. Do not administer if pulse rate > 140 or client has chest pain 4. Administer beta blocking agent as antidote
nifedipine (Procardia)	• Hypotension • Fatigue • Nausea • Flushing • Uteroplacental perfusion complications	1. Monitor BP 2. Avoid concurrent use with magnesium sulfate 3. Monitor contractions and FHT 4. Prevent complication with hypotension
magnesium sulfate	• Warmth • Flushing • Respiratory Depression • Diminished DTRs • Decreased urine output • Pulmonary edema	1. Monitor VS and DTRs 2. Monitor magnesium levels (therapeutic range is 4–8 mg/dL) 3. Administer via infusion pump in diluted form 4. Use indwelling catheter to monitor urinary elimination 5. Administer calcium gluconate 10% if available for signs of toxicity

Antenatal Steroids

Action: Stimulate production of surfactant in fetus between 24 and 34 weeks gestation

A. Therapeutic Use

1. Promote fetal lung maturity in preterm labor when delivery is likely

B. Side Effects/Adverse Effects

1. Fluid retention
2. Elevated blood pressure

 C. NURSING INTERVENTIONS and Client Education

1. Administer 2 doses (usually IM) 24 hr apart (repeat doses not recommended).
2. Provide emotional support to family.

Medications for the Postpartum Client

Rho(D) Immune Globulin (RhoGAM)

Action: Suppresses the stimulation of active immunity by Rh-positive foreign red blood cells that enter the maternal circulation at the time of delivery

A. Therapeutic Use

1. Rh factor incompatibility to prevent sensitization for subsequent pregnancies

B. Precautions

1. Confirm that the mother is Rh-negative.
2. Never administer the IGIM full-dose or microdose products intravenously.
3. Never administer to a neonate.

C. NURSING INTERVENTIONS and Client Education

1. RhoGAM is administered as an injection after any event where fetal cells can mix with maternal blood, including:
   a. Miscarriage
   b. Ectopic pregnancy
   c. Induced abortion
   d. Amniocentesis
   e. Chorionic villus sampling (CVS)
   f. Abdominal trauma

Varicella Vaccine

A. Women who are not immune to varicella should be immunized in the postpartum period.

B. Instruct client to use reliable form of contraception and avoid pregnancy for 3 months.

Antidote/Reversal Agents

- Acetaminophen: acetylcysteine (Mucomyst)
- Benzodiazepine: flumazenil (Ramazicon)
- Curare: edrophonium (Tensilon)
- Cyanide poisoning: methylene blue
- Digitalis: digoxin immune FAB (Digibind)
- Ethylene poisoning: fomepizole (Antizol)
- Heparin and enoxaparin (Lovenox): protamine sulfate
- Iron: deferoxamine (Desferal)
- Lead: succimer (Chemet)
- Magnesium sulfate: calcium gluconate 10% (Kalcinate)
- Narcotics: naloxone (Narcan)
- Warfarin: phytonadione (vitamin K)

Therapeutic Drug Levels

- Aminophylline: 10–20 mcg/mL
- Carbamazepine: 5–12 mcg/mL
- Digoxin: 0.8–2.0 ng/mL
- Gentamicin: 5–10 mcg/mL
- Lidocaine: 1.5–5.0 mcg/mL
- Lithium: 0.4–1.0 mEq/L
- Magnesium sulfate: 4–8 mg/dL
- Phenobarbital: 10–30 mcg/mL
- Phenytoin: 10–20 mcg/mL
- Quinidine: 2–5 mcg/mL
- Salicylate: 100–250 mcg/mL
- Theophylline: 10–20 mcg/mL
- Tobramycin: 5–10 mcg/mL

Toxic Drug Levels

- Acetaminophen: > 250 mcg/mL
- Aminophylline: > 20 mcg/mL
- Amitriptyline: > 500 ng/mL
- Digoxin: > 2.4 ng/mL
- Gentamicin: > 12 mcg/mL
- Lidocaine: > 5 mcg/mL
- Lithium: > 2.0 mEq/L
- Magnesium sulfate: > 9 mg/dL
- Methotrexate: > 10 mcmol over 24 hr
- Phenobarbital: > 40 mcg/mL
- Phenytoin: > 30 mcg/mL
- Quinidine: > 10 mcg/mL
- Salicylate: > 300 mcg/mL
- Theophylline: > 20 mcg/mL
- Tobramycin: > 12 mcg/mL

Common Drug Class Suffixes

Common Drug Class Suffixes

Suffix	Medication Category
-dipine	Ca+ channel blocker
-afil	Erectile dysfunction
-caine	Anesthetics
-pril	ACE inhibitor
-pam, -lam	Benzodiazepine
-statin	Antilipidemic
-asone, -solone	Corticosteroid
-olol	Beta blocker
-cillin	Penicillin
-ide	Oral hypoglycemic
-prazole	Proton pump inhibitor
-vir	Antiviral
-ase	Thrombolytic
-azine	Antiemetic
-phylline	Bronchodilator
-arin	Anticoagulant
-tidine	Antiulcer
-zine	Antihistamine
-cycline	Antibiotic
-mycin	Aminoglycoside
-floxacin	Antibiotic
-tyline	Tricyclic antidepressants
-pram, -ine	SSRIs

SECTION 1

Management

A. Concepts of Management

1. Leadership: A way of behaving that influences others to respond, not because they have to, but because they want to. Leaders help others to identify and focus on goals and the achievement of them. Leadership is a personal interaction that focuses on the personal development of the members of the group.

    a. Essential components of leadership
       1) Knowledge
       2) Self-awareness
       3) Communication
       4) Energy
       5) Goals
       6) Action

     b. **NURSING INTERVENTIONS**: All nurses will need leadership skills to manage other nurses, assistive personnel, and clients. It is essential to the nursing role to identify and implement effective leadership practices.

2. Management: A problem-oriented process with a focus on the activities needed to achieve a goal; supplying the structure, resources, and direction for the activities of the group. Management involves personal interaction, but the focus is on the group's process. The most effective managers are also effective leaders.

    a. Phases of the management process
       1) Planning
       2) Organizing
       3) Staffing
       4) Directing
       5) Controlling

    b. Management styles
       1) Autocratic
       2) Laissez-faire
       3) Democratic

     c. **NURSING INTERVENTIONS**: Nurses should learn management skills and identify their own personal leadership style. Nurses should know the differences between being an autocratic and democratic leader. The most effective management style in a health care environment is the democratic leader who uses an interdisciplinary approach to encourage open communication and collaboration, which will promote individual autonomy and accountability.

3. Communication: Involves sending, receiving, and interpreting written, face-to-face, and nonverbal information between at least two people

    a. Functional components of communication
       1) Referent
       2) Sender
       3) Message
       4) Channel
       5) Receiver
       6) Environment
       7) Feedback
       8) Interpersonal variables

    b. Therapeutic communication: The purposeful use of communication to build and maintain helping relationships with clients, families, and significant others. Therapeutic communication is client-centered, purposeful, planned, and goal-directed.

    c. Effective communication skills and techniques
       1) Active listening
       2) Open-ended questions
       3) Clarifying techniques
       4) Offering general leads, broad opening statements
       5) Showing acceptance and recognition
       6) Focusing
       7) Asking questions
       8) Giving information
       9) Presenting reality
       10) Summarizing
       11) Offering self
       12) Touch

     d. **NURSING INTERVENTIONS**: Effective communication requires commitment, effort, focus, and cooperation, especially when dealing with complex clinical issues and people who have diverse backgrounds and perspectives. It is essential to understand and use effective communication skills to successfully manage others.

4. Conflict: Arises when there are two opposing views, feelings, expectations, or other divergent issues. It can occur within an individual, between individuals, or between groups and organizations. Conflict can be managed.

    a. Sources of conflict
       1) Lack of resources and/or economics
       2) Differences in values, feelings, beliefs, backgrounds, goals, economic values, and professional values
       3) Struggles for power or influence
       4) Sexual harassment

b. Types of conflict management strategies (optimal goal is creating a win-win solution for all involved)

    1) Avoiding

    2) Cooperating/accommodating

    3) Compromising

    4) Competing

    5) Collaborating

    6) Smoothing

 c. **NURSING INTERVENTIONS**: A nurse manager's role is to identify the source of conflict, understand the issues that have developed, and work toward conflict resolution while maintaining positive regard for each individual. It is essential to address the person with whom there is conflict before going to superiors (use the chain of command). The most important conflict strategy involves collaboration that results in a win-win solution for everyone.

d. SBAR: A communication model utilized in conflict resolution that incorporates the **s**ituation, **b**ackground, **a**ssessment, and **r**ecommendation to improve communication between clinicians

B. Power (the ability, strength, and capacity to do something) vs. Influence (control over people and their actions)

1. Types of power

    a. Reward: the ability to control resources

    b. Coercive: the ability to inflict aversive outcomes or punishment

    c. Legitimate: based on one's position

    d. Referent: based on attractive characteristics

    e. Expert: based on expertise or knowledge

2. Influence tactics

    a. Ingratiation: the ability to manipulate others through flattery and style

    b. Conformity pressure: the pressure to conform to the group; this pressure increases as group size increases to greater than six, or as familiarity with the topic decreases

    c. Foot-in-the-door: a small request followed by a larger request

    d. Door-in-the-face: a large request that is intended to be denied, followed by a smaller request that is intended to be granted

    e. Guilt: the practice of inducing guilt before making a request; granting the request reduces the feeling of guilt

 3. **NURSING INTERVENTIONS**: The power of influence is aimed at accomplishing well-defined goals, preferably as a cohesive team

C. Team Building: Activities or efforts intended to unify people into a team to more effectively accomplish the overall objectives and mission of the organization

1. Components of team building

    a. Clear expectations: Expectations should be clearly defined and communicated to members of the team.

    b. Context: Members should understand why they are participating on the team.

    c. Commitment: Members should feel valuable, excited, and challenged, and should be committed to the success of the team.

    d. Competence: Team should feel like it has the resources, strategies, and support it needs to meet its goals.

    e. Collaboration: Rules of conduct should be followed for conflict resolution and cooperative decision-making.

    f. Communication: There should be a clear, honest, and respectful dialogue between team members.

    g. Creativity: New and innovative ideas should be encouraged and welcomed.

    h. Consequences: Contributions and success should be recognized and rewarded.

 2. **NURSING INTERVENTIONS**

    a. Foster a culture that values collaboration and cooperation.

    b. Communicate that teamwork is expected.

    c. Publicly celebrate team success.

    d. Bring a sense of play and fun to the team.

D. Continuity of Care: Focuses on the experience of the client as the client moves through the health care system; guiding the client through this experience requires coordination, integration, collaboration, and facilitation of all the events along the continuum.

1. Nursing's role in continuity of care

    a. Facilitate the continuity of care provided

    b. Act as a liaison and be a client advocate

    c. Admission, transfer, discharge, and postdischarge

    d. Initiate, revise, and evaluate the plan of care

    e. Report the client's status

    f. Coordinate discharge planning

    g. Facilitate referrals and utilization of community resources

E. Quality

1. **Total Quality Improvement Model (Continuous Quality Improvement)**: A philosophy that doing the right thing, the right way, the first time, with problem-prevention planning (not reactive problem-solving) leading to quality outcomes.

2. **Performance Improvement (Quality Improvement, Quality Control)**: The process used to identify and resolve performance deficiencies focusing on assessment of outcomes to improve delivery of quality care. All employees are involved in this process.

  a. Steps in the Performance Improvement process

    1) A standard is developed and approved by facility committee.

    2) Standards are made available to employees by way of policies and procedures.

    3) Quality issues are identified by staff, management, or risk management department.

    4) An interdisciplinary team is developed to review the issue.

    5) The current state of structure and process related to the issue is analyzed.

    6) Data collection methods are determined.

      a) Quantitative methods

      b) Audits

    7) Data is collected, analyzed, and compared with the established benchmark.

    8) If the benchmark is not met, possible influencing factors are determined. A root cause analysis may be done.

      a) Investigates the consequence and possible causes

      b) Analyzes the possible causes and relationships that may exist

      c) Determines additional influences at each level of relationship

      d) Determines the root cause or causes

    9) Potential solutions or corrective actions are analyzed and one is selected for implementation.

    10) Educational or corrective action is implemented.

    11) The issue is reevaluated at a preestablished time to determine the efficacy of the solution or corrective action.

  3. Nurse's role in performance improvement

F. Variance/Incidence/Occurrence Reports: A variance or incident is an event that occurs outside the usual expected normal events or activities of the client's stay, unit functioning, or organizational processes.

  1. **NURSING INTERVENTIONS**: Incidence or variance reports are not intended to point blame, just document the facts. Their purpose is to identify situations or system issues that contributed to the occurrence and to engage strategies to prevent reoccurrence or to correct the situation. Generally the report is confidential communication and cannot be subpoenaed; however, if it is inadvertently disclosed, it can be subpoenaed. The report should not be placed in the chart.

  2. Reportable incidents include (but are not limited to):

    a. Client injury

    b. Unanticipated client death

    c. Malfunction of equipment

    d. Unanticipated adverse reactions

    e. Inability to meet client needs—system problem, order problem, lack of qualified staff, or client/family refusal of care

    f. Unethical, illegal, or incompetent practice

    g. Client/family complaint about care

    h. Toxic spills, fires, and/or other environmental emergencies

    i. Violent behavior by the client/family

    j. Loss of property

G. Resource Management

  1. Health care reimbursement methods

    a. Retrospective vs. prospective payment

    b. Health-maintenance organizations

  2. Budgeting

    a. Types of budgets

      1) Personnel budget

      2) Operating budget

      3) Capital budget

    b. The budget process

      1) Planning: Assess what the needs are.

      2) Preparation: Develop a plan (time frame).

      3) Modification and approval: Implement (ongoing monitoring and analysis)

      4) Monitoring: Evaluation (revise and modify as needed)

  3. **NURSING INTERVENTIONS**: A nurse manager must be aware of economic issues in health care. Budgetary terms are fundamental to understanding the financial management of facilities. The more information available to the nurse, the better the decisions and input into long-range planning for the facility.

H. Case Management: Case management is a collaborative process of assessment, planning, facilitation, and advocacy for options and services to meet an individual's health needs through communication and available resources to promote quality, cost-effective outcomes.

  1. **NURSING INTERVENTIONS**: A nurse's role in case management is to coordinate services that respond to the hierarchy of the client's individual needs. This system provides care that minimizes fragmentation and maximizes holistic individualized client care.

I. Consultation and Referral

  1. Consultation: A professional provides expert advice in a particular area; a request to determine what treatment or services the client requires

a. Examples of consultation: an orthopedic surgeon for a client with a hip fracture; a psychiatrist for a client whose risk for suicide must be assessed

 b. **NURSING INTERVENTIONS**: Notify the primary care provider of the client's needs, provide the consultant with pertinent information, include consultant's information into the plan of care, and facilitate coordination with other health care providers in order to protect the client from conflicting and potentially dangerous prescriptions.

2. Referral: A formal request for a special service by another care provider so that the client can access the care identified by the primary care provider or consultant. The intervention becomes that specialist's responsibility, but the nurse continues to be responsible for monitoring the client's response and progress.

   a. Examples of referrals (inpatient—physical therapy, wound care nurse; outside of the facility—hospice)

3. Appropriate use of consultation and referral

 4. **NURSING INTERVENTIONS**: The processes of consultation and referral are integral for effective use of services along the continuum, and they establish collaboration with the interdisciplinary team. The nurse should support the client/family with appropriate consultation and referral to contacts in the community.

SECTION 2

Delegation and Prioritization

A. Delegation/Assignment/Supervision/Accountability

1. Definitions

   a. **Delegating:** Transferring the authority to perform a selected nursing task in a selected situation to another team member while maintaining accountability.

   b. **Assigning:** Transferring the authority, accountabilty, and responsibility to another member of the health-care team (e.g., when an RN directs another RN to assess a client, the second RN is already authorized to assess clients in the RN scope of practice)

   c. **Supervising**: Monitoring the progress toward completion of delegated tasks; the amount of supervision required depends on the direction of the delegation, the abilities of the person being delegated to, and the location of the ultimate responsibility for outcomes.

   d. **Accountability**: Moral responsibility for consequences of actions

2. Five rights of delegation

   a. Right person

   b. Right task

   c. Right circumstances

d. Right direction and communication

e. Right supervision and evaluation

 3. **NURSING INTERVENTIONS**: It is essential for a nurse to understand legal responsibilities when managing and delegating nursing care to a wide variety of health care workers. The nurse must delegate activities thoughtfully, taking into account individual job descriptions, knowledge base, and skills demonstrated. Remember, the professional nurse is accountable for determining the extent and complexity of client needs and for assigning work that is consistent with the individual's position, description, and duties.

4. The RN cannot delegate:

   a. Nursing process

   b. Client education

   c. Tasks that require nursing judgment (including care of unstable clients)

B. Roles and Responsibilities for Levels of Staff

1. Assistive personnel (AP) or unlicensed assistive personnel (UAP)

   a. Training is often on the job

   b. An AP may complete a certification program—Certified Nursing Assistant

   c. An AP functions under the direction of the licensed practical nurse (LPN) or RN

   d. Skills

      1) Performs basic hygiene care and grooming

      2) Reports to the LPN or RN

      3) Provides assistance with ADLs such as nutrition, elimination, and mobility

      4) Performs basic skills such as taking vital signs, including pulse oximetry, and calculating I&O

      5) Emphasis is on maintaining a safe environment and recognizing situations to report to immediate superior

2. LPN

   a. May also be called a licensed vocational nurse (LVN)

   b. Education is approximately 12 to 18 months in an accredited program

   c. LPNs must complete and pass the NCLEX-PN® exam for licensure

   d. Supervised by the RN or health care provider.

   e. Scope of practice is determined by the Nurse Practice Act, which varies from state to state (requirements to maintain an active license are determined by each state)

      1) Meets the health needs of clients

      2) Cares for clients whose condition is considered to be stable and/or chronic with an expected outcome

      3) Performs reinforcement teaching

3. RN

    a. May be diploma, associate degree, baccalaureate degree, or higher

    b. Education ranges from 2 to 4 (or more) years

    c. RNs must complete and pass the NCLEX-RN® exam for licensure

    d. Functions under the direction of the health care provider

    e. Advanced clinical skills in caring for the acute client with complex care needs; outcome uncertain

    f. Scope of practice is determined by the Nurse Practice Act, which varies from state to state (requirements to maintain an active license are determined by each state)

4. Advanced practice nurses

    a. May be nondegree or master's degree (or higher)

    b. Education ranges from 18 months to 4 (or more) years (in addition to basic RN program)

    c. Must complete and pass a certification exam (in addition to the NCLEX-RN® exam) applicable to the specialty and practice (adult nurse practitioner, diabetic educator)

    d. Functions vary according to the state practice act, which may be either autonomous or under the direct or indirect supervision of a provider

    e. Skills vary according to the state practice act, and may include the ability to prescribe, diagnose, and treat

5. Health care provider

    a. May be a provider, provider's assistant, or nurse practitioner

    b. In general, only an attending provider has admitting privileges to a facility, although another care provider in the practice may direct the care given to the client

C. Prioritization Principles

Nurses must continuously set and reset priorities in order to safely care for multiple clients.

1. Assessments are completed.

2. Interventions are provided.

3. Steps in a client procedure are completed.

4. Components of client care are completed.

Establishing priorities in nursing practice requires that these decisions be made based on evidence obtained:

1. During shift reports and other communications with members of the health care team

2. Through careful review of documents

3. By continuously and accurately collecting client data

Examples of tasks that can be delegated to LPNs and AP (provided agency policy and state practic guidelines permit)

To LPNs	To AP
• Monitoring client findings (as input to the RNs ongoing assessment of the client)	• Activities of daily living (ADLs)
• Reinforcement of client teaching from a standard care plan	• Bathing
• Tracheostomy care	• Grooming
• Suctioning	• Dressing
• Checking nasogastric tube patency	• Toileting
• Administration of enteral feedings	• Ambulating
• Insertion of a urinary catheter	• Feeding (without swallowing precautions)
• Medication administration (excluding intravenous medications in several states)	• Positioning
	• Bed making
	• Specimen collection
	• Intake and output (I&O)
	• Vital sign (on stable clients)

Prioritization Principles in Client Care

Principle	Examples
Prioritize systemic before local ("life before limb").	Prioritizing interventions for a client in shock over interventions for a client with a localized limb injury
Prioritize acute (less opportunity for physical adaptation) before chronic (greater opportunity for physical adaptation).	Prioritizing the care of a client with a new injury/illness (e.g ., mental confusion, chest pain) or an acute exacerbation of a previous illness over the care of client with a long-term chronic illness
Prioritize actual problems before potential future problems.	Prioritizing administration of medication to a client experiencing acute pain over ambulation of a client at risk for thrombophlebitis
Listen carefully to clients and don't assume.	Recognizing that a postoperative client's report of pain could be due to pain in another location rather than expected surgical pain
Recognize and respond to trends versus transient findings.	Recognizing a gradual deterioration in a client's level of consciousness and/or Glasgow Coma Scale score
Recognize signs of emergencies and complications versus "expected client findings."	Recognizing signs of increasing intracranial pressure in a client newly diagnosed with a stroke versus the clinical findings expected following a stroke
Apply clinical knowledge to procedural standards to determine the priority action.	Recognizing that the timing of administration of antidiabetic and antimicrobial medications is more important than administration of some other medications

A. Ethical Practice

1. Basic ethical principles
    a. Autonomy/self-determination: The right to make one's own decisions
    b. Beneficence/doing good: The obligation to do good for others
    c. Confidentiality/respecting privileged information: The obligation to observe the privacy of another and maintain strict confidence
    d. Fidelity: The obligation to be faithful to an agreement and responsibilities, to keep promises
    e. Justice/treating people fairly: The obligation to be fair to all people (when allocating limited resources)
    f. Nonmaleficence: The obligation not to harm others (Hippocrates states, "First do no harm.")
    g. Paternalism: Assuming the right to make decisions for another
    h. Veracity: The obligation to tell the truth

2. Ethical dilemmas: Ethical dilemmas are problems for which more than one choice can be made and the choice is influenced by the values and beliefs of the decision makers. Ethical dilemmas are very common in health care, and nurses must be prepared to apply ethical theory and decision making.

3. The *American Nurses Association's (ANA) Code of Ethics for Nurses*: Sets guidelines to use when providing client care; outlines the nurse's responsibility to the client and the profession of nursing, and assists the nurse in making ethical decisions.

4. Ethical decision making: A process in which the nurse, the client, the client's family, and the health care team make decisions, taking into consideration personal and philosophical viewpoints, the ANA code for nurses, and ethical principles. Frequently this requires that a balance be struck between science and morality.

5. Advocacy: A process by which the nurse assists the client to grow and develop toward self-actualization. Advocacy is a critical leadership role and emphasizes the values of caring, autonomy, respect, and empowerment.

B. Organ Donation

1. Organ and tissue donation is regulated by state and federal laws. Facilities will have specific policies and procedures to follow during the process.

2. Determination of death

3. Nursing role

4. Family needs

 5. **NURSING INTERVENTIONS**: Nurses have an ethical responsibility to participate in the donation process by presenting the option of organ donation to all suitable clients and families. Families in this situation may be receptive to organ donation because they want something positive to come from their loss. The nurse should be comfortable when discussing this and be able to provide appropriate information about it.

C. Advance Directive: A document in which a client who is competent is able to express wishes regarding future acceptable health care (including the desire for extraordinary lifesaving measures which includes resuscitation, intubation, and artificial hydration and nutrition) and/or designate another person to make decisions when the client becomes physically or mentally unable to do so.

1. Planning guides for seriously ill clients
    a. Living will: Legal document that instructs health care providers and family members about what, if any, life-sustaining treatment an individual wants if at some time the individual is unable to make decisions.
    b. Durable power of attorney for health care: Legal document that designates another person to make health care decisions for the client when the client becomes unable to make decisions independently.

 c. **NURSING INTERVENTIONS**: It is important for a nurse to identify clients who do not have advance directives, to inform them of their rights, and to ensure that clients who have advance directives have copies placed in their charts.

A. Informed Consent: Obtained after a client receives complete disclosure of all pertinent information regarding the surgery or procedure to be performed. In addition, informed consent is obtained only if the client understands the potential benefits and risks associated with having the surgery or procedure.

1. Elements of informed consent
    a. Individual giving consent must fully understand the procedure that will be performed, the risks involved, expected/desired outcomes, expected complications/side effects, and alternate treatments or therapies available.
    b. Consent is given by a competent adult, legal guardian or DPOA, emancipated or married minor, parent of a minor, or a court order.

2. Nurse's role: Witness the client's signature, provide clarification to information already given by physician (do not give new information), and advocate for the client by protecting the client's rights

B. Client Rights

1. Patient Bill of Rights

2. Americans with Disabilities Act

3. Confidentiality: The right to privacy with respect to one's personal medical information

   a. Legislation: Health Insurance Portability and Accountability Act (HIPAA) of 1996

      1) A uniform, federal (national) act that provides privacy protection for health consumers

      2) State laws that may provide additional protections to consumers are not affected by HIPAA

      3) Guarantees that clients are able to access their medical records

      4) Provides clients with control over how their personal health information is used and disclosed

      5) HIPAA outlines limited circumstances in which a client's personal health information can be disclosed without first obtaining consent of the client or the client's family including:

         a) Suspicion of child or elder abuse

         b) When otherwise required by law (such as suspicion of criminal activity due to gunshot wounds)

         c) Incidences of state agencies or health department requirements; reportable communicable disease

C. Legal Responsibilities

1. Sources of law: the Constitution, statutes, administrative agencies, and court decisions

2. Types of laws and courts

   a. Criminal law

      1) Felony—major

      2) Misdemeanor—minor

   b. Civil laws

      1) Tort law

         a) Unintentional torts: negligence, malpractice

         b) Quasi-intentional torts: breach of confidentiality, defamation of character

         c) Intentional torts: assault, battery, falseimprisonment

   c. State laws: Nursing practice is regulated by state law. Each state's board of nursing has rules, regulations, and standards that vary from state to state.

   d. Federal regulations: HIPAA, ADA, MHPA, PSDA, etc.

3. Nurse Practice Act

   a. Varies from state to state

4. Good Samaritan Law

   a. Health care providers are protected from potential liability if volunteering away from their place of employment, as long as the nurses' actions are not grossly negligent.

5. Mandatory reporter of abuse of clients of all ages and communicable diseases

6. Impaired coworker

   a. A nurse who suspects a coworker of using drugs or alcohol while working has the duty to report to the appropriate supervisory personnel according to institutional policy.

7. Malpractice

   a. The failure of a person with professional training to act in a reasonable and prudent manner

8. Negligence

   a. The omission to do something that a reasonable person would do, or doing something that a reasonable person would not do

   b. Standard of professional practice developed by professional organizations—ANA, AACN, AAOHN

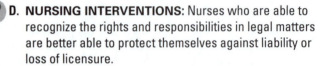 **D. NURSING INTERVENTIONS:** Nurses who are able to recognize the rights and responsibilities in legal matters are better able to protect themselves against liability or loss of licensure.

! POINT TO REMEMBER: One of the most vital and basic functions of a professional nurse is the duty to intervene when the safety or well-being of a client or another person is obviously at risk

SECTION 5
Information Systems and Technology

A. Impact of Technology on the Nursing Profession

1. Allows candidates to test for nursing licensure (NCLEX®) with rapid results

2. Permits verification of licensure online for nurses and other health care professionals

3. Improves communication within and between departments through the use of e-mail, intranet, and the Internet

4. Eases the retrieval of medical histories to optimize decision making

5. Automates medication delivery systems to help prevent error

6. Automates distribution of client-care supplies

7. Facilitates client-centered care with portable and wireless terminals, workstations, and laptops

8. Improves and facilitates client education through the use of multimedia software, including graphics, photographs, videos, and 3-D visuals

9. Supports continuing education with distance learning

   a. Videoconferencing via satellite

   b. Online degrees and certification programs

   c. Computer-mediated instruction

10. Increases client monitoring capabilities

11. Decreases deviation from standards of practice

12. Allows electronic documentation

    a. Bedside charting

    b. Computerized charting

B. Future Impact of Technology

1. Federally mandated electronic transferable medical records

2. Virtual and augmented reality allowing for simulated client teaching activities

C. Data Security

1. Passwords are necessary to prevent improper access to computers and medication systems.

2. Only individuals who have a professional relationship with a client may access the client's personal health information, per HIPAA regulations.

3. Computer terminals must be logged off and locked when not in immediate use.

4. Monitor screens must be shielded or situated so that unauthorized individuals cannot see the information.

! POINT TO REMEMBER: A nurse should not share computer passwords with another person, including coworkers and family members

SECTION 1

The Nurse's Role in Community Nursing

A. Community Nurse Assessment: A comprehensive assessment clarifying the client problem by evaluating:

1. Biological factors
2. Social factors
3. Cultural factors
4. Physical factors
5. Environmental factors
6. Social systems
7. Financial constraints (The client's eligibility for service and situational constraints must also be considered.)

B. Community Nurse Referrals: Assist in linking the community resource with the client to provide holistic care; must have thorough knowledge of resource individuals and organizations.

1. Utilize computerized records, databases, and telecommunication technologies for physical, audio, and visual data
2. Responsible for coordination, providing continuity of care, and evaluating the outcome
3. Examples of community nursing referrals
   a. Psychological services
   b. Support groups
   c. Medical equipment providers
   d. Meal delivery services
   e. Transportation services
   f. Life care planner
4. Examples of community health nurse practice
   a. Home health nurse
   b. Hospice nurse
   c. Occupational health nurse
   d. Parish nurse
   e. School nurse
   f. Case managers
5. **CIRCLE** model of spiritual care (**C**aring, **I**ntuition, **C**aution, **L**istening, and **E**motional support)
6. **Healthy People 2010**—A 10-year national campaign identifying nearly 600 objectives with 1,200 measures to improve the health of all Americans.

SECTION 2

Disaster Planning

A. Disaster: A serious disruption of the functioning of a community that causes widespread human, material, economic, or environmental losses that exceed the ability of the affected community or society to cope with using its own resources

1. Internal disasters are events in the health care facility that threaten to disrupt the care environment.
   a. Structural (fire, loss of power)
   b. Personnel related (strike, high absenteeism)
2. External disasters may be man-made or natural.
   a. Man-made disasters
      1) Transportation-related incidents (e.g., car, train, plane, and subway crashes)
      2) Terrorist attacks, including bombs (e.g., suicide bombs and dirty bombs) and bioterrorism
      3) Industrial accidents
      4) Chemical spills or toxic gas leaks
      5) Structural fires
   b. Natural disasters
      1) Extreme weather conditions, including blizzards, ice storms, hurricanes, tornadoes, and floods
      2) Ecological disasters, including earthquakes, landslides, tsunamis, volcanoes, and forest fires
      3) Microbial disasters such as epidemics and pandemics
      4) A combined internal/external disaster situation can arise when an external disaster, such as a severe weather condition, both causes mass casualties and prevents health care providers from getting to the facility, perhaps due to traffic or road conditions.

B. Disaster Planning

1. Interagency cooperation within the community is essential in a disaster and requires:
   a. Community-wide planning for emergencies and/or hazards that may affect the local area
   b. Coordination between community emergency system and health care facilities
   c. Developing a local emergency communications plan and/or network
   d. Identification of potential emergency public shelters
2. Role of the nurse
   a. In the health care facility
      1) Joint Commission on Accreditation of Healthcare Organizations (JCAHO) mandates specific standards for hospital preparedness
      2) Disaster plans

3) Disaster drills (at least two annually; one involving community-wide resources and actual or simulated clients)

b. In the community

1) Education provided to families about disaster planning

a) A family disaster plan should include:

(1) What to do in an evacuation

(2) Plans for family pets

(3) Where to meet in case of an emergency

b) A family disaster kit should include:

(1) A flashlight with extra batteries

(2) A battery-powered radio

(3) Nonperishable food that requires no cooking (along with a nonelectric can opener)

(4) One gallon of water per person

(5) Basic first-aid supplies

(6) Matches in a waterproof container

(7) Household liquid bleach for disinfection

(8) Emergency blanket and/or sleeping bag and pillow

(9) Rain gear

c. Assess community for risks

C. Disaster Management

1. Emergency management system

a. Provides public access to immediate health care (9-1-1)

b. Dispatch communication center

c. Trained first responders: emergency medical technicians

d. Transportation to medical resources: ground (ambulance) and/or air (helicopter)

2. Declaration of a disaster

a. Disaster area: Local officials request that the governor of the state take appropriate action under state law and the state's emergency plan and declare a disaster area.

b. Federal disaster area: The governor of the affected state requests declaration of a disaster area by the president to qualify the affected area for federal disaster relief.

c. Internal disaster: The nursing or administrative supervisor may declare an internal disaster in case of a facility-related issue.

3. Disaster relief organizations

a. Federal Emergency Management Agency (FEMA)

1) FEMA is part of the U.S. Department of Homeland Security

a) Manages federal response and recovery efforts

b. American Red Cross

1) Not a government agency, but authorized by the government to provide disaster relief

2) The American Red Cross provides:

a) Shelter and food to address basic human needs

b) Health and mental services

c) Food to emergency and relief workers

d) Blood and blood products to disaster victims

3) The American Red Cross also handles inquiries from concerned family members outside the disaster area.

c. Hazardous material response team (HAZMAT)

1) Hazardous materials may be radioactive, flammable, explosive, toxic, corrosive, or biohazardous, or may have other characteristics that make them hazardous in specific circumstances.

2) HAZMAT team members are specially trained to respond to these situations and wear protective equipment.

3) In a toxic exposure disaster, HAZMAT will coordinate the decontamination effort.

D. Role of the Nurse

1. Triage: Process of prioritizing which clients must receive care first

a. Non-mass casualty situation: The nurse prioritizes client care so that clients with conditions of the highest acuity are evaluated and treated first. Emergency services are presented with a large number of casualties; however, they are still functional and able to provide care to victims on all levels. Consists of three levels:

1) Nonurgent: minor injuries that do not require immediate treatment; slightly injured

2) Urgent: major injuries that require immediate treatment

3) Emergent: immediate threat to life; critically injured

b. Mass casualty disaster triage: The field and/or emergency services are presented with a number of casualties and/or ground conditions and are unable to treat everyone; therefore, the staff must provide the greatest good for the greatest number. Consists of four levels:

1) Emergent or Class I (red tag): immediate threat to life; do not delay treatment

2) Urgent or Class II (yellow tag): major injuries that require treatment; can delay treatment 1 to 2 hr

3) Nonurgent or Class III (green tag): minor injuries that do not require immediate treatment, can delay treatment 2 to 4 hr

4) Expectant or Class IV (black tag): expected and allowed to die; prepare for morgue

2. Health care facility disaster plan

a. A nursing or administrative supervisor may implement the disaster plan due to extreme weather conditions or an anticipation of mass casualties.

b. Plans to implement:
   1) Establishment of an incident command center
   2) Premature discharge of clients who are stable from the facility
   3) Transfer of clients who are stable from the intensive care unit
   4) Postponement of scheduled admissions and elective operations
   5) Mobilization of personnel (call in off-duty individuals)
   6) Protection of personnel and visitors
   7) Evacuation plan

c. Role of the charge nurse during a disaster:
   1) Preparation of a discharge list that features clients who can safely and quickly be discharged
   2) Personnel sent to the command center, if required
   3) Off-duty personnel called in, if requested
   4) Disaster victims prepared for admittance

E. Psychosocial Aftermath of a Disaster

1. Crisis intervention

a. Mental health response team employs advanced crisis intervention techniques to help victims, survivors, and their families better handle the powerful emotional reactions associated with crises and disasters.

b. Goals:
   1) Reduce the intensity of an individual's emotional reaction
   2) Assist individuals in recovering from the crisis
   3) Help to prevent serious long-term problems from developing

2. Posttraumatic stress disorder (PTSD): A mental health condition that can develop following any traumatic or catastrophic life experience

a. PTSD symptoms can develop in survivors of a disaster weeks, months, or even years following the catastrophic event

3. Critical incident stress debriefing

a. Health care providers who respond to a highly stressful event that is extremely traumatic or overwhelming may experience significant stress reactions

b. The critical incident stress debriefing process is designed to prevent the development of posttraumatic stress among first responders and health care professionals

1) Defusing: discussion of feelings shortly after the disaster/critical incident (such as at the end of a shift)
2) Formal debriefing: discussion some hours or days after the disaster/critical incident, in a large group setting, with mental health teams of peer support personnel serving as the leaders

SECTION 3
Culturally Competent Care

A. Nursing Process for Culturally Sensitive Care

1. Assessment

a. What is the client's ethnic affiliation?

b. What is its importance in the client's daily life?

c. How well does the client speak, write, read, and understand English?

d. What dietary preferences or prohibitions does the client follow?

e. Are there rituals or customs that the client wishes to keep related to transitions such as birth and death?

f. Does the client want or need to have family involved in his care?

g. Is the client using herbal or other traditional remedies?

 2. **NURSING INTERVENTIONS**

a. Remain sensitive to the client's spiritual beliefs, even if they are in opposition to your personal beliefs.

b. Provide a trained, bilingual interpreter if necessary.

c. Provide a diet that is consistent with the client's customs.

d. Allow family to be involved in the client's care, if desired.

e. Be respectful of the client's cultural preferences for personal space.

f. Be aware of the meaning of eye contact in the client's culture.

g. Check the client's herbal and/or alternative methods to make sure they are not interacting poorly with the medications that the facility is providing.

B. African American

1. African Americans comprise a very diverse population that varies considerably by geographic region, age, and socioeconomic status.

2. Spiritual beliefs

a. Church and religious life are typically very important.

b. Primary religious/spiritual affiliation: Most are Christian, primarily Baptist or from other Protestant sects; or Muslim.

c. Illness may have both natural and supernatural causes.

d. Mental illness may be viewed as a lack of spiritual balance.

e. Some chronic or congenital illnesses may be considered God's will.

3. Practices associated with life transitions

a. Birth

1) May give child a name of African origin, or one that is unique

b. Death

1) The deceased are highly respected.

2) Cremation is avoided.

3) Organ donation is unusual except in the case of an immediate family member.

4. Dietary preferences

a. May prefer cooked and fried foods.

b. Traditional southern cooking may include cooked greens (collard, mustard, turnip) or yams.

5. Cultural variations

a. Language: English with traditional dialects is spoken in Louisiana (Creole) and many parts of the south; "black" English is often spoken in urban areas, primarily inner cities, and is a distinct, expressive dialect with its own rules of grammar and slang.

b. Eye contact: Viewed as a sign of respect and trust.

c. Time orientation: Primarily focused on the present with a flexible time frame.

d. Personal space: Affection is shown by touching, hugging, and being close.

e. Family: Nuclear, extended, frequently matriarchal (women head the household); grandparents often involved in the care and raising of children.

f. Sick role: Attention from family and relatives is expected.

6. Healing practices

a. Home and folk remedies are often used first; usually it is the role of the mother or wife to obtain the remedy from a knowledgeable person.

b. Prayer and visits from a minister may be important.

c. There may be some mistrust of the medical establishment.

7. Health risks

a. Hypertension

b. Coronary artery disease

c. Sickle-cell anemia

d. Diabetes mellitus

e. Prostate, breast, colorectal cancer

f. Renal disease

C. Asian American

1. Asian Americans comprise a very diverse population including ethnic groups of Pacific Islanders, Southeast Asians, Chinese, Japanese, Koreans, and others, each of which have their own customs and practices.

2. Spiritual beliefs

a. Primary religious or spiritual affiliations: Buddhism, Christianity, and Hindu

3. View of illness

a. Chinese traditionally believe that illnesses are caused by imbalances in the yin and yang.

b. External influences block the circulation of vital energy, or chi.

4. Practices associated with life transitions

a. Birth

1) May want female family members at bedside during labor.

2) Breastfeeding is the norm.

3) Genetic defects may be blamed on something the mother did during pregnancy.

4) A new mother may be expected to eat a special diet and remain at home to recuperate for several weeks.

5) Circumcision is a decision that depends on religious and ethnic practice.

b. Death

1) Organ donation is uncommon.

2) An autopsy is discouraged.

5. Dietary preferences

a. Depending on the individual ethnic group, food may be considered important in maintaining a healthy balance, and the client may believe that certain foods are "hot" or "cold."

b. Chinese traditionally believe that food is critical to maintaining the balance of yin (cold) and yang (hot) in the body.

6. Cultural variation

a. Language: Many different dialects exist for most major Asian languages, and English competence varies considerably; use a trained, bilingual interpreter if the client has limited English skills.

b. Eye contact: Avoided with authority figures as a sign of respect.

c. Time orientation: Present oriented; punctuality is not a traditional value, except in Japanese culture where promptness is important.

d. Personal space: Client may be very modest and public display of affection (physical touching) is not typical; the head may be considered to be sacred; therefore, touching someone on the head may be disrespectful.

e. Family: Patriarchal, extended families are common; wife may become a part of husband's family; filial piety (duty and obedience to one's parents and ancestors) is expected.

f. Sick role: People who are sick usually assume a passive role; the client may not ask questions, as this is seen as disrespectful; however, she may nod politely at everything that is said; the client may be stoic in regard to pain.

7. Healing practices

a. May want to use traditional and herbal remedies in addition to medical care.

b. Older adult immigrants may have a strong belief in traditional folk medicine, while second-generation Asian Americans are often more oriented toward Western medicine.

c. Chinese traditionally believe that health is achieved by restoring balance between yin and yang.

d. Other specific health practices may depend on religion or ethnicity.

8. Health risks

a. Hypertension

b. Stomach, cervical, liver cancer

c. Osteoporosis

d. Thalassemia anemia

e. Tuberculosis

D. Hispanic

1. Also known as Latino; comprised of a very diverse population including individuals of Mexican, Cuban, Central American, South American, Spanish, and Puerto Rican heritage

2. Spiritual beliefs

a. Latinos are traditionally very religious.

b. Primary religious/spiritual affiliation is Catholic/Christian.

c. Traditional belief is that health is controlled by fate, environment, and the will of God.

3. Practices associated with life transitions

a. Birth

1) May want female family members present for labor.

2) Most breastfeed.

3) New mother may be expected to eat a special diet and remain at home to recuperate for several weeks.

4) Circumcision is not the traditional practice.

b. Death

1) Extended family may want to tend to the sick and dying.

2) The body is respected and organ donation is discouraged.

3) An autopsy is discouraged.

4) Women who are pregnant may be excluded from attending a funeral.

4. Dietary preferences

a. Traditional diet contains fresh ingredients; processed foods may be distrusted.

5. Cultural variation

a. Language: Majority are bilingual Spanish/English, although English competence varies significantly; use a trained, bilingual interpreter if the client's English skills are limited; considered respectful to address individuals formally until a rapport has been established.

b. Eye contact: Direct eye contact is avoided with authority figures.

c. Time orientation: Primarily oriented in the present with a flexible time frame.

d. Personal space: Handshaking is considered polite, but other touching by a stranger is generally considered inappropriate; embracing is common among family and friends.

e. Family: Family is believed to come first, and members are expected to have a strong sense of family loyalty; most live in nuclear families with extended families and godparents.

f. Sick role: Clients will often assume a passive role and may be stoic with regard to pain.

6. Healing practices

a. Soup and herbal teas may be thought to speed healing process.

b. Siesta is a traditional period of rest after the midday meal thought to be important for maintaining health.

c. The client may seek medical care for severe symptoms while using traditional folk healing measures for chronic or "folk" illnesses.

7. Health risks

a. Diabetes mellitus

b. Childhood obesity

c. Hypertension

d. Vitamin B_{12} deficiency anemia

E. Native American

1. There are 300 or more different Native American tribal groups, each with its own culture, beliefs, and practices.

2. Spiritual beliefs

a. Belief in the Creator; sacred myths and legends provide spiritual guidance.

b. Primary religious/spiritual affiliation: Specific tribes follow rituals referred to in a general way by the tribal name; for example, the Navajo Indians follow "The Navajo Way."

c. Illness results from not living in harmony, or being out of balance with nature.

3. Practices associated with life transitions

   a. Birth

      1) May desire female family members to be present at birth

      2) No circumcision

   b. Death

      1) Organ donation is usually not desired.

      2) An autopsy is usually not desired.

      3) Some tribes avoid contact with a person who is dying (a hospital is preferable to home).

4. Dietary preference

   a. May vary with tribal affiliation, although most are assimilated to U.S.-style diet

5. Cultural variation

   a. Language: Most speak English.

   b. Eye contact: Respect is communicated by avoiding eye contact.

   c. Time orientation: Primarily oriented in the present with a flexible time frame; rushing a client is considered rude and disrespectful.

   d. Personal space: Keep a respectful distance.

   e. Family: Some tribes are matrilineal, meaning they trace ancestral descent through the mother's line instead of the father's line; the mother may be the head of the family or clan.

   f. Sick role: Usually quiet and stoic.

6. Healing practices

   a. A person who is ill may seek both modern medical attention and the services of a traditional medicine man/woman.

   b. Home and herbal remedies may be used.

   c. A medicine bag is a leather pouch that is worn around the neck, and the contents of it are considered sacred; it is improper to ask about the contents of the bag, and every effort should be made not to remove it.

   d. Health practices are intertwined with religious and cultural beliefs.

7. Health risks

   a. Alcoholism

   b. Gallbladder disease

   c. Diabetes mellitus

   d. Coronary artery disease

   e. Tuberculosis

   f. Maternal-infant mortality

   g. Obesity

   h. Hypertension

A. Nursing Process for Spiritually Sensitive Care

1. Assessment

   a. What is the client's religion?

   b. What is its importance in the client's daily life?

   c. What dietary prohibitions does the client follow?

   d. Are there rituals or customs that the client may wish to keep, particularly those related to transitions such as birth and death?

   e. Is there a spiritual leader whom the client wishes to have involved in their care?

   f. Is the client using herbal or other traditional remedies?

   g. Are there any practices that the client may find that will provide comfort or support?

 2. **NURSING INTERVENTIONS**

   a. Remain sensitive to the client's spiritual beliefs, even if they are in opposition to your personal beliefs.

   b. Provide a diet that is consistent with the client's customs.

   c. Provide the client privacy, as desired, for prayer and other rituals.

   d. Allow visits by clergy or supportive members of the client's congregation.

   e. Provide the client with a comfortable and supportive atmosphere that is conducive to religious practices

   f. Check the client's herbal and/or alternative methods to make sure they are not interacting poorly with the medications that the facility is providing

B. Buddhism

1. There are many forms of Buddhism; some sects are based on the country of origin.

2. Spiritual beliefs

   a. Important figure is Siddhartha Gautama.

   b. Spiritual leaders are priests and monks.

   c. Central focus is enlightenment (Nirvana) and the attainment of a clear and calm state of mind.

   d. Illness is a result of karma (cause and effect) and a consequence of actions in this life, or a previous life.

3. Practices associated with life transitions

   a. Birth

      1) Belief in reincarnation

      2) Contraception that prevents conception is acceptable

b. Death

    1) State of mind at the time of death is believed to influence rebirth; therefore, the nurse should ensure a calm, peaceful environment for the client who is dying.

    2) Chanting is common and the family may request a priest to deliver last rites.

    3) Organ donation is encouraged as an act of mercy

    4) Cremation is common.

4. Dietary restrictions

    a. A vegetarian diet is practiced by many

    b. Avoidance of alcohol

    c. Fasting on Holy Day

5. Healing practices

    a. A quiet and peaceful environment is important to allow the client to rest and practice meditation and prayer.

C. Catholicism

1. A form of Christianity; also known as Roman Catholic

2. Spiritual beliefs

    a. Important figures are Jesus Christ and his mother, the Virgin Mary.

    b. Spiritual leaders are priests, nuns, and deacons.

    c. God revealed himself to humanity as the Father to Jesus; the Holy Trinity is the Father, the Son, and the Holy Spirit.

    d. Illness may be God's punishment for sinful thinking or behavior.

3. Practices associated with life transitions

    a. Birth

        1) Contraception, abortion, and sterilization are prohibited.

        2) Baptism is required if an infant's prognosis is grave. If death of an infant is imminent, a nurse (of any religion) can baptize the infant by pouring a small amount of warm water on the infant's head and saying, "I baptize thee in the name of the Father, and of the Son, and of the Holy Spirit."

    b. Death

        1) If death is imminent, a priest should be called to administer the Sacrament of the Sick, otherwise known as "last rites."

        2) Organ donation is acceptable.

        3) Suicide may prevent burial in a Catholic cemetery.

    c. Dietary restrictions

        1) Some Catholics may abstain from eating meat on Ash Wednesday and on Fridays during Lent, which is a 40-day period between Ash Wednesday and Easter.

d. Healing practices

    1) Most Catholic clients who are observant will want to see a priest when they are hospitalized.

    2) A client may request the Eucharist (communion) and/or the Sacrament of Reconciliation (confession) to aid in healing.

    3) A client may wear a cross, medal (symbol of a saint), or scapular (small piece of cloth on a string worn around the neck).

    4) A client may display a statue of Jesus, Mary, or a saint at the bedside, and make use of a rosary (string of prayer beads).

D. Christian Scientist

1. A form of Christianity also known as the Church of Christ, Scientist

2. Spiritual beliefs

    a. Founder is Mary Baker Eddy.

    b. No clergy.

    c. Central beliefs consist of God as divine love; God's infinite goodness heals.

    d. Illness is viewed as a manifestation of human imperfections that can be healed through prayer and spiritual regeneration; no disease is beyond the power of God to heal.

3. Practices associated with life transitions

    a. Birth

        1) Contraception is an individual decision.

        2) Abortion is prohibited.

        3) A client may choose to give birth at home, aided by a midwife, or to minimize hospitalization by going home the same day of the delivery.

    b. Death

        1) Unlikely to seek medical help to prolong life

        2) Organ donation discouraged

4. Dietary restrictions

    a. No requirements, but most abstain from alcohol

5. Healing practices

    a. Most practitioners rely on spiritual healing, but are not completely opposed to medical providers; individuals are free to make their own decisions in each situation.

    b. A client may avoid diagnostic testing to avoid unwanted medical treatment that could violate spiritual beliefs.

    c. Medications and blood products are avoided; immunizations are accepted only to comply with the law.

    d. Full-time healing ministers (Christian Science Practitioners) practice spiritual healing and do not use medical or psychological techniques; the church maintains a directory of Christian Science nurses available to provide medical care in a spiritual atmosphere.

E. Hinduism

1. There are many forms of Hinduism, each with its own practices and customs

2. Spiritual beliefs

   a. No single founder, universally accepted scripture, or religious hierarchy; may be monotheistic (one god), polytheistic (many gods), or atheistic (no god).

   b. Spiritual leaders are priests.

   c. Central belief is that spiritual well-being comes from leading a dedicated life based on nonviolence, love, good conduct, and selfless service.

   d. Illness is a result of karma (cause and effect) and a consequence of actions in this life, or a previous life; illness, accident, or injury may be viewed as a form of purification.

3. Practices associated with life transitions

   a. Birth

      1) Contraception is acceptable.

      2) Abortion may be prohibited.

      3) Noting the exact time of birth is crucial to determining the child's horoscope.

      4) Males are not circumcised.

      5) Traditionally, the child is not named until the 10th day of life.

   b. Death

      1) Belief in reincarnation, and that the soul will reincarnate until its karma is exhausted.

      2) Prolonging life artificially is up to the individual, but allowing a natural death is traditional.

      3) The client may want to lie on the floor while dying.

      4) A thread is placed around the neck/wrist, and family pours water into the mouth and bathes the body.

      5) A nurse should ensure a calm, peaceful environment for the client who is dying.

      6) Organ donation is acceptable.

      7) Prefer cremation and the casting of ashes in a river.

   c. Dietary restrictions

      1) A vegetarian diet is encouraged and practiced by many; of those who eat meat, most abstain from beef and pork.

      2) According to traditional dietary law, the right hand is used for eating and the left hand for toileting and hygiene.

      3) There are several days set aside for fasting during a year; vary by sect.

   d. Healing practices

      1) Personal hygiene is very important and the client may want to bathe daily.

      2) Prayer for health is considered a low form of prayer; therefore, stoicism may be preferred.

      3) Future lives are influenced by how one faces illness, disability, and death.

F. Islam

1. Those who adhere to the Islamic belief are known as Muslims. Sunni Muslims form the worldwide majority and differ from Shi'a Muslims, a worldwide minority, in some matters of faith and practice.

2. Spiritual beliefs

   a. Important figure is the Prophet Mohammed.

   b. Spiritual leaders are Imam.

   c. Central beliefs are one God, Allah; holy text, Qur'an; Judgment Day; Final Day of Resurrection.

   d. Illness, pain, and suffering are manifestations of God's will and are necessary to remove sin.

3. Practices associated with life transitions

   a. Birth

      1) Contraception is acceptable.

      2) After 130 days of gestation (about 18 weeks), the fetus is considered a full human being.

      3) Abortion is permitted under certain circumstances (if the mother's life is in danger), but only if the fetus has not attained personhood.

      4) At birth a prayer is said into the infant's ear.

      5) Circumcision of males is customary.

   b. Death

      1) Any attempt to shorten life is prohibited, but prolonging death by means of futile medical interventions is also prohibited.

      2) The client may want to confess sins prior to death.

      3) The client who is dying may wish to be placed facing Mecca (usually east).

      4) Organ donation is acceptable.

      5) An autopsy is permitted for medical or legal reasons.

      6) Rituals following death include traditional bathing (washed and enveloped with a white cloth) and burial within 24 hr; cremation is prohibited.

4. Dietary restrictions

   a. Food must be halal (lawful).

   b. Pork, alcohol, and some shellfish are prohibited.

   c. Ramadan is a period of fasting that occurs from sunrise to sundown during the ninth lunar month (dates vary from year to year); children, pregnant women, and those who are sick are exempt from fasting.

5. Healing practices

   a. A client may wish to pray five times a day (dawn, midday, midafternoon, sunset, and nightfall) facing Mecca, and may have a prayer rug and Qur'an at the bedside for prayers.

   b. Privacy during prayer is important.

   c. Women are very modest and frequently wear clothes that cover their entire body; during treatment and care, the woman's modesty should be respected as much as possible.

G. Jehovah's Witness

1. A form of Christianity; name is derived from the Hebrew name for God

2. Spiritual beliefs

   a. Founded in the 1870s as the Watchtower Society.

   b. Spiritual leaders are older adults.

   c. Central beliefs include the Bible as the literal word of God, which is historically accurate; all other religions are considered false teachings; conversion of others is important.

   d. Suffering and illness are permitted by God and result from Satan's influence on the world.

3. Practices associated with life transitions

   a. Birth

      1) Contraception is an individual choice.
      2) Abortion is prohibited.
      3) Infants are not baptized.

   b. Death

      1) Organ donation is permitted.
      2) An autopsy is permitted if it is legally required.
      3) May choose burial or cremation.

4. Dietary restrictions

   a. Moderate use of alcohol is permitted, but drunkenness is a sin.

5. Healing practices

   a. Strongly opposed to blood products for transfusion and will refuse even if refusal means death.

   b. Volume expanders are permitted if not derived from blood.

   c. Organ transplantation is permitted if all of the blood is drained from the organ or tissue before being transplanted.

   d. Advocate for a surgery that is bloodless.

   e. Courts have ordered transfusions for very young children; in other cases, they have respected the declared choice of an underage minor who is able to defend his beliefs to the court in a manner that reflects a mature understanding without undue influence from his parents.

   f. The reading of scriptures is believed to comfort the client and leads to mental and spiritual healing.

H. Judaism

1. Predates Christianity, and there are several major divisions with different customs and practices

2. Spiritual beliefs

   a. Spiritual leaders are rabbis.

   b. Central beliefs include one God; a holy text, the Torah (the Old Testament of the Bible); the Messiah has yet to come.

   c. Illness and suffering are not judgments from God, since everyone is mortal.

3. Practices associated with life transitions

   a. Birth

      1) Contraception is considered an individual choice.
      2) Abortion is permitted under certain circumstances.
      3) Ritual circumcision of males is called a Bris, which is performed on the eighth day of life.

   b. Death

      1) An autopsy is discouraged, but not prohibited.
      2) Organ donation is permitted.
      3) Someone stays with the body at all times.
      4) Rituals following death include traditional bathing and burial within 24 hr; cremation is prohibited.
      5) Bereavement does not begin until after burial.

4. Dietary restrictions

   a. Orthodox and observant Jews will observe dietary laws requiring food to be kosher (properly prepared) and may request a kosher food tray.

      1) Complex rules regarding food preparation include a blessing when meat is slaughtered.
      2) Milk and meat cannot be served at the same meal.
      3) Pork and shellfish are prohibited.

   b. Fasting is required on Yom Kippur, the Day of Atonement (in fall, exact date is determined by the Jewish calendar); children, pregnant women, and those who are sick are exempt from fasting.

   c. Lactose intolerance is common among Jews of European origin.

5. Healing practices

   a. Jewish law places the life of the person above all else.

      1) Saving a life overrides nearly all religious obligations.
      2) It is considered to be one of the highest commandments to tend to the sick or dying.
      3) In case of illness, medical care is obligated and health care providers are seen as instruments of God.
      4) Prayers for the well-being of the sick may be said.
      5) Anything that can be done to ease the client's suffering is encouraged.
      6) Males who strictly practice their religion will wear a yarmulke (skull cap) at all times; very observant females may dress modestly and cover their heads at all times.

I. Church of Jesus Christ of Latter-Day Saints

1. Members refer to selves as belonging to The Church or Mormon faith.

2. Spiritual beliefs

   a. Founded by the Prophet Joseph Smith.

   b. Spiritual leaders are priests and older adults.

   c. Central beliefs: God revealed himself to humanity as the Father of Jesus; the Holy Trinity is the Father, the Son, and the Holy Spirit; the holy text is the Book of Mormon.

d. The body is a gift from God and to help keep bodies and minds healthy and strong, God gave a law of health; illness, trials, and adversity are a part of life.

3. Practices associated with life transitions

   a. Birth

     1) Contraception and abortion are forbidden.

     2) Infants are not baptized.

   b. Death

     1) Organ donation is permitted.

     2) An autopsy is permitted.

     3) Life continues beyond death.

4. Dietary restrictions

   a. Alcohol, coffee, and tea are prohibited (some may drink caffeinated soft drinks or herbal teas).

   b. Fasting is required once a month; children, pregnant women, and those who are sick are exempt from fasting.

5. Healing practices

   a. May want to use herbal remedies in addition to medical care.

   b. When blessing the sick, a person is anointed with oil by two older adults.

J. Seventh Day Adventist

1. A form of Christianity also known as Adventist

2. Spiritual beliefs

   a. Central belief includes the Bible as the literal word of God.

   b. Religious leaders are pastors and older adults.

   c. The body is the temple of the Holy Spirit (God) and must be kept healthy.

3. Practices associated with life transitions

   a. Birth

     1) Contraception is an individual choice.

     2) Abortion is acceptable in cases of rape, incest, or if the mother's life is at risk.

     3) Opposed to infant baptism; adults are baptized by total immersion.

   b. Death

     1) An autopsy is acceptable.

     2) Organ donation is acceptable.

4. Dietary restrictions

   a. A vegetarian diet is encouraged.

   b. Alcohol, coffee, and tea are prohibited.

5. Healing practices

   a. Healing can be accomplished both through medical intervention and divine healing.

   b. Prayer and anointing with oil may be performed for a person who is sick.

A. Herbal Medications and Supplements

1. Safety and efficacy

   a. The Dietary Supplement Health and Education Act limits the U.S. Food and Drug Administration's (FDA) control over dietary supplements.

   b. Many herbal drug companies make claims based on their own studies, indicating health benefits from using herbal drugs.

     1) These studies are not approved by the FDA.

     2) Labels on the herbal medications must include a disclaimer, stating that the FDA has not approved the product for safety and effectiveness.

   c. Herbal medications may interact with other medicines and produce serious side effects.

2. Common supplements

   a. Saw palmetto (*Serenoa repens*)

     1) Purported use: treats and prevents benign prostatic hypertrophy (BPH)

     2) Side effects: prolonged bleeding time and altered platelet function

     3) Herb/medication interactions: additive effect with anticoagulants

     4) Studies: several well-conducted studies support the use of saw palmetto for reducing symptoms of BPH

     5) Nursing considerations

       a) Allow 4 to 6 weeks to see effects.

       b) Discontinue use prior to surgery.

   b. Valerian root

     1) Purported uses: insomnia, migraines, and menstrual cramps

     2) Side effects: drowsiness, anxiety, hepatotoxicity (long-term use)

     3) Herb/medication interactions: additive effect with barbiturates and benzodiazepines

     4) Studies: several studies support the use of valerian for mild to moderate sleep disorders and mild anxiety

     5) Nursing considerations

       a) Advise the client against driving or operating machinery.

       b) Advise the client against long-term use.

       c) Discontinue valerian at least 1 week prior to surgery.

   c. St. John's wort (*Hypericum perforatum*)

     1) Purported uses: depression, seasonal affective disorder, and anxiety

2) Side effects: headache, sleep disturbances, hepatotoxicity (long-term use), and constipation
3) Herb/medication interactions: may reduce the effects of many medications
   a) Theophylline (Theo-Dur)
   b) HIV protease inhibitors and non-nucleoside reverse transcriptase inhibitors
   c) Cyclosporine (Neoral)
   d) Diltiazem (Cardizem) and nifedipine (Procardia)
4) Studies: several well-conducted studies support the use of St. John's Wort for mild to moderate depression
5) Nursing considerations
   a) St. John's wort has many medication interactions and should not be taken with other medications.
   b) Should not be used to treat severe depression.
   c) Should only be used with medical guidance.

d. Echinacea (*Echinacea purpurea*)
   1) Purported uses
      a) Prevents and treats the common cold
      b) Stimulates the immune system
      c) Promotes wound healing
   2) Side effects: headache, epigastric pain, and constipation
   3) Herb/medication interactions
      a) May reduce the effects of immunosuppressants
      b) May increase serum levels of alprazolam (Xanax), calcium-channel blockers, and protease inhibitors
   4) Studies: well-conducted studies have conflicted as to the effectiveness of echinacea in the treatment of the common cold
   5) Nursing considerations
      a) Long-term use may cause immunosuppression

e. Ginkgo (*Gingko biloba*)
   1) Purported uses: improves cerebral circulation to treat dementia and memory loss
   2) Side effects: dizziness and palpitations
   3) Herb/medication interactions
      a) May increase the effects of MAOIs, anticoagulants, and antiplatelet aggregates
      b) May reduce the effectiveness of insulin
   4) Studies: studies conflict as to the effectiveness of gingko in all purported uses
   5) Nursing considerations
      a) Discontinue 2 weeks prior to surgery.
      b) May cause seizures with overdose.
      c) Keep out of the reach of children.

f. Ginseng (*Panax Quinquefolius*)
   1) Purported uses: improves strength and stamina and prevents and treats cancer and diabetes mellitus
   2) Side effects: insomnia and nervousness
   3) Herb/medication interactions
      a) May decrease the effectiveness of anticoagulants and antiplatelet aggregates
      b) May increase the effectiveness of antidiabetic agents and insulin
   4) Studies: conflict as to the effectiveness of ginseng in all purported uses
   5) Nursing considerations
      a) Ginseng is contraindicated for women who are pregnant and/or lactating.

g. Glucosamine (2-Amino-2-deoxyglucose)
   1) Purported uses: relieves osteoarthritis and promotes joint health
   2) Side effects: itching, edema, and headache
   3) Herb/medication interactions: may increase resistance to antidiabetic agents and insulin
   4) Studies: several studies support the use of glucosamine in reducing the symptoms of osteoarthritis in the knees
   5) Nursing considerations
      a) Use glucosamine with caution in clients who have a shellfish allergy.
      b) Monitor glucose frequently in clients who have diabetes mellitus.
      c) Allow extended time to see the effects of glucosamine.
      d) Use it often in combination with chondroitin.

h. Chondroitin sulfate
   1) Purported uses: relieves osteoarthritis
   2) Side effects: headache, hives, photosensitivity, hypertension, and constipation
   3) Herb/medication interactions: may increase the effects of anticoagulants
   4) Studies: several studies support the use of chondroitin sulfate in reducing the symptoms of osteoarthritis in the knees
   5) Nursing considerations
      a) Do not give chondroitin sulfate to women who are pregnant or breastfeeding.
      b) It is often used in combination with glucosamine.
      c) Allow extended time to see its effects.

i. Omega-3 fatty acids
   1) Purported uses: improves hypertriglyceridemia and helps to maintain cardiac health
   2) Side effects: nausea, diarrhea, hypotension
   3) Herb/medication interactions: may increase the risk of vitamin A or D overdose

4) Studies: several well-conducted studies support the use of omega-3 fatty acids in reducing blood triglyceride levels, preventing cardiovascular disease in clients with a history of a heart attack, and slightly reducing blood pressure

5) Nursing considerations

   a) Omega-3 fatty acids are found in fish oils, nuts, and vegetable oils.

   b) Some fish contain methylmercury and polychlorinated biphenyls (PCBs) that can be harmful in large amounts, especially in women who are pregnant or nursing.

j. Melatonin

  1) Purported uses: treats insomnia and jet lag

  2) Side effects: morning grogginess, lower body temperature, vivid dreams

  3) Herb/medication interactions: beta blockers, warfarin, and steroids

  4) Studies: several studies support antioxidant effects

  5) Nursing considerations: Pregnant or nursing women should not take melatonin.

B. Nursing Assessments for Herbal Medications

1. Ask the client specifically about herbal medications, vitamins, or other supplements during the client interview

2. Over-the-counter medications are often not considered medications by the client

 3. **NURSING INTERVENTIONS**

  a. Instruct the client that herbal medications and supplements are not regulated by the FDA, often interact with other medications, and may cause serious side effects.

  b. Instruct the client that it is important for him to use herbal medications and supplements cautiously and with medical supervision.

  c. Discourage use in pregnant mothers, nursing mothers, infants, young children, and older adults (with cardiovascular or liver disease).

C. Alternative and Complementary Therapies

1. Nonbiomedical therapy

  a. Covers a wide range of healing practices and philosophies that mainstream Western medicine (biomedical model) does not commonly use, study, or advocate.

  b. While some scientific evidence exists regarding some of these therapies, for most, there are key questions that are yet to be answered through well-designed scientific studies, such as whether they are safe and whether they work for the diseases or medical conditions for which they are used.

  c. Studies show that up to 50% of Americans include alternative and complementary therapies in maintaining their health.

d. Nonbiomedical therapies are usually not covered by health insurance.

e. Practitioners may not be licensed or regulated.

2. Common Complementary and Alternative Medicine (CAM) therapies

  a. National Center for Complementary and Alternative Medicine (NCCAM)

    1) Complementary and Alternative Medicine Domains

     a) Mind-body therapy is the most commonly used CAM therapy and uses a variety of techniques designed to enhance the mind's capacity to affect bodily function and symptoms.

      (1) Prayer (most common)

      (2) Meditation: focusing the mind upon a sound, phrase, object, or visualized image to promote relaxation

      (3) Journaling

      (4) Imagery

      (5) Music

      (6) Animal-assisted therapy

      (7) Biofeedback: A method of treatment that uses monitors to "feed back" physiological information (of which clients are normally unaware). By watching a monitor, clients can learn by trial and error to adjust their mental processes to control involuntary bodily processes, such as heart rate.

     b) Biologically based therapies use substances such as herbs, foods, vitamins, and other natural, but as yet unproven, substances.

      (1) Aromatherapy: ancient therapy that uses plant and essential oils

      (2) May be inhaled, placed in compresses, or applied to the skin

      (3) Special diets: macrobiotic, vegan

      (4) Herbal supplements

     c) Manipulative and body-based therapies use manipulation and/or movement of one or more parts of the body.

      (1) Chiropractic: manipulation of the vertebrae to relieve pressure on the nerves and return the body to balance

      (2) Therapeutic massage: a range of therapeutic approaches involving the practice of kneading or manipulating an individual's muscles and soft tissues

      (3) Hydrotherapy: practice of physiotherapy in a pool (typically heated)

(4) Tai Chi: an ancient Chinese practice designed to exercise body, mind, and spirit, improving the flow of chi, the vital life energy that sustains health and calms the mind
  (a) Described as meditation in motion; participants perform a defined series of postures or movements in a slow, graceful manner
  (b) Scientific studies have shown that Tai Chi:
    1. Improves muscle flexibility and builds muscle strength
    2. Reduces falls in older adults and those with balance disorders

d) Energy therapies involve the use of energy fields; their existence has not been scientifically proven.
  (1) Reiki: a Japanese technique for stress reduction and relaxation
    (a) Administered by the laying on of hands
    (b) Based on the idea that an unseen life-force energy flows through us and is what causes us to be alive
  (2) Therapeutic touch
  (3) Electromagnetic fields
  (4) Yoga and dance

e) Traditional or folk medicine
  (1) Traditional Chinese therapies
    (a) Acupressure: placing physical pressure by hand or elbow onto certain points of the body (acupoints) to stimulate the flow of chi, the vital life energy
    (b) Acupuncture: placing very thin needles into certain points of the body (acupoints) to stimulate the flow of chi, the vital life energy; often used to eliminate or reduce pain
    (c) Herbs (ginger, green tea)
  (2) Native American therapies
  (3) Various cultural folk remedies

b. Assessments
  1) Ask the client about the use of alternative, complementary, or folk remedies.

 c. **NURSING INTERVENTIONS**
  1) Assist the client with using the chosen therapy appropriately.
  2) Provide client teaching, which includes safety and contraindications of complementary therapies.
  3) Refrain from endorsing products.

INDEX

beclomethasone dipropionate, 216*t*

behaviorist model of mental health treatment, 94

beneficence, 247

benzodiazepines
    for alcohol withdrawal, 108
    antidote/reversal agent, 239
    for bipolar disorder, 105
    for phobic disorders, 99
    for suicidal patient, 106

benztropine, 234
    for Parkinson's disease, 77

beta-2 adrenergic agonists, 215–216

beta-adrenergic blockers (sympatholytics), 212–213
    in amputation treatment, 45
    for angina, 58
    for hypertension, 61
    for hyperthyroidism, 51
    for myocardial infarction, 59
    for phobic disorders, 99

beta-interferon, for multiple sclerosis, 77

betamethasone, 129*t*, 216*t*

betamethasone sodium phosphate, 216*t*

bethanechol, 226*t*

bethanechol chloride, for urine retention, 71

biguanides, 218*t*

bilirubin, 145
    in laboratory profile, 31

binge, 113

binge eating, 110

binuclear family, 152*t*

biofeedback, 263

biological modifiers, for chemotherapy, 81

biophosphonates, for osteoporosis, 44

biophysical profile (BPP), 119*t*

biopsy, kidneys, 66

bipolar disorder, 104–105
    medications, 232

birth
    African-American practices, 255
    Asian-American practices, 256
    Buddhist practices, 257
    Catholic practices, 258
    Christian scientist practices, 258
    Church of Jesus Christ of Latter Day Saints practices, 260–261
    Hindu practices, 259
    Hispanic practices, 256
    Islamic practices, 259
    Jehovah's Witness' practices, 260
    Jewish practices, 260
    Native-American practices, 257
    Seventh Day Adventist practices, 261

bisacodyl, 225*t*

bisphosphonates, 229

blackout, 113

bladder
    overactive, anticholinergics for, 226–227
    postpartum care, 136
    removal, 71

blended family, 152*t*

bleomycin, for chemotherapy, 81

blocking, 101

blood cholesterol, 15*t*

blood coagulation tests, 56

blood disorders, 54–56

blood glucose, 15*t*, 90

blood lipid levels, 90

blood pressure, 15*t*
    guidelines for children, 155*t*
    of newborn, 138*t*
    in pregnancy, 122

blood products, administration, 221*t*

bloodstream infection, central venous catheters and, 211*t*

body fluids, 18

body image changes
    in adolescent, 165
    in preschooler, 162
    in school-age child, 163
    in toddlers, 160

body mass index (BMI), 15*t*

body mechanics, 9–10

bonding, postpartum, 136

bone marrow, and anemia, 55

bone scan, 41

borderline personality, 106–107

bowel, postpartum care, 136

brachtherapy, 82

bradycardia, sinus, 57

brain. *See also* neurosensory disorders
    MRI of, 73

Braxton-Hicks contractions, 117*t*

breast-feeding, 140, 158
    medications and, 209

breasts
    cancer, 149
    clinical exam, 15*t*
    development, 155
    postpartum, 135

bromocriptine, for Cushing's, 49

bromocriptine mesylate
    for acromegaly, 46
    for Parkinson's disease, 77

bronchial asthma, 193

bronchiolitis, in children, 188–189

bronchitis, chronic, 24

bronchodilators, 200
    for chronic bronchitis, 24
    for laryngotracheobronchitis, 188
    for pneumonia, 25

bronchoscopy, 22

Buddhism, religious competent care, 257–258

budesonide, 216*t*

budgeting, 244

Buerger's disease, 63

bulimia, 111

bumetanide, 225*t*
    for hypertension, 61

BUN, 66

buprenorphine, for opioid withdrawal, 107

bupropion, for nicotine withdrawal, 107

burns, 84–86, 85*t*
    care for children, 190–191
    preventing
        for adolescent, 166
        for infants, 158

        for preschooler, 162
        for school-age child, 164
        for toddlers, 160–161

buspirone, 231

C

C-reactive protein, 56

calcitonin, for phantom limb pain, 45

calcium
    diet for alterations, 89
    healthy eating guidelines, 87
    imbalance, 20*t*
    laboratory values, 90
    supplements for osteoporosis, 44

calcium channel blockers, 211
    for angina, 58
    for hypertension, 62
    for myocardial infarction, 59
    after myocardial infarction, 59

calcium gluconate, 129*t*

calcium gluconate, for hypoparathyroidism, 51

calcium IV, for acute renal failure, 68

cancer
    breast, 149
    cervical, 148
    in children, 201–203
    disease-related consequences, 81
    endometrial, 149
    laryngeal, 25–26
    lungs, 26
    management, 81–82
    ovarian, 149
    overview, 81
    pain management in, 82
    pancreatic, 40
    prostate, 71

candidiasis (thrush), 146

cane, 11

CAPD (continuous ambulatory peritoneal dialysis), 70

captopril, 211
    for heart failure in child, 176
    for hypertension, 62

carbamazepine, 234, 235*t*
    for alcohol withdrawal, 107
    for delirium tremens, 108
    for seizure, 74
    therapeutic level, 239

carbidopa, 234
    for Parkinson's disease, 77

carbohydrates, healthy eating guidelines, 87

carbon dioxide, toxicity, 24

cardiac catheterization, 57–58
    for child, 175–176

cardiac disease, in pregnancy, 122–123

cardiac glycosides, 213

cardiogenic shock, 64

cardiopulmonary resuscitation (CPR), 64–65
    guidelines for children and infants, 203

cardiovascular system, 56–65
    cardiac disorders, 58–63
    diagnostic procedures, 56–58
    pharmacology for, 211–215

case management, 244–245

community nursing, 252
comorbidity, 113
compensation, 96
competence, in team building, 243
complex seizure, 74
compulsion, 113
computed tomography (CT scan), 73
computerized adaptive testing, 2
concrete thinking, 113
condom, 237t
condyloma, 147
confabulation, 113
confidentiality, 247, 248
conflict, 242–243
conformity, 243
congenital aganglionic megacolon, 182, 183t
  collaborative care, 184t
congenital anomaly in children, 175–182
  cerebral palsy, 181–182
  club foot, 177–178
  developmental dysplasia of hip, 178
  gastrointestinal system disorders, 182
  heart disease, 175–177
  hydrocephalus, 179–180
  neural tube defects, 180–181
  scoliosis, 164, 165, 179, 194
conjunctiva, of children, 154
Conn's Syndrome (hyperaldosteronism), 49
conscious, 92
conscious defense mechanisms, 97
consequences, in team building, 243
consultation, 244–245
contact transmission-based precautions, 12
context, in team building, 243
continuity of care, 243
continuous ambulatory peritoneal dialysis
  (CAPD), 70
contraception, 145
contraceptives, 236–237
contraction stress test, in pregnancy
  diagnosis, 118–119
conversion disorders, 100
conversion factors, 208
COPD (chronic obstructive pulmonary
  disease), 23–24
coronary artery bypass graft (CABG), 64
corpus luteum, 116
corrosives, accidental injestion, 191
corticosteroids
  for glomerulonephritis, 67
  for gouty arthritis, 42
  for laryngotracheobronchitis, 188
  for lupus erythematosis, 84
  for osteoarthritis, 41
  and peptic ulcer disease, 34
  for rheumatoid arthritis, 42
cortisone, for Addison's disease, 48
cough suppressants, for pneumonia, 25
coumadin, for thrombophlebitis, 62
countertransference, 113
CPR (cardiopulmonary resuscitation), 64–65
  guidelines for children and infants, 203
cranial nerves, 72
creatinine, 66

and kidney failure, 69
creatinine phosphokinase MB, 57
creativity, in team building, 243
CRIES Neonatal Postoperative Scale, 170t
criminal law, 248
crisis, 113
crisis intervention, 98, 254
critical incident stress debriefing, 254
Crohn's disease, 35
croup, 188
crutches, 11
CT (computed tomography) scan, 72
cultural/social crisis, 98
culturally competent care, 254–257
cultures, 210
curare, antidote/reversal agent, 239
Cushing's disease, 48
Cushing's syndrome, 48
CVA (cerebrovascular accident), 75
cyanide poisoning, antidote/reversal agent, 239
cyclophosphamide, 202
  for chemotherapy, 81
  for nephrosis, 68
cyclosporine, St. John's wort interaction, 262
cyclothymia, 105
cystic fibrosis, 198, 200–201
cystitis, 67
cystoscopy, 66

D

dabigatran, 223
  for thrombophlebitis, 62
dactinomycin, for chemotherapy, 81
data security, 249
deafness, 80
death and dying
  African-American practices, 255
  Asian-American practices, 256
  Buddhist practices, 257–258
  Catholic practices, 258
  of children, 172–175
  child's response to, 173t
  Christian scientist practices, 258
  Church of Jesus Christ of Latter Day
    Saints practices, 260–261
  Hindu practices, 259
  Hispanic practices, 256
  Islamic practices, 259
  Jehovah's Witness' practices, 260
  Jewish practices, 260
  Native-American practices, 257
  Seventh Day Adventist practices, 261
decerebrate posturing, 72
decision making, ethical, 247
declaration of disaster, 253
decongestants, 218t
  for respiratory infection, 187
decorticate posturing, 72
defense mechanisms, 96–97, 113
delegation, 245
delirium, 109
delirium tremens, 108–109
delivery. See labor and delivery
delusions, 101, 113

dementia, 109
democratic leader, 242
democratic parenting style, 152t
denial, 96, 113
dental assessments, 15t
dentition
  of children, 155
  of infant, 157
Denver Developmental Screening Test, 156
depressive disorders. *See also* antidepressants
  major, 103–104
  postpartum, 137t
dermatitis, atopic, 192
desensitization, 113
desioratadine, 218t
desmopressin, 220
desmopressin acetate (DDAVP), for diabetes
  insipidus, 47
detached retina, 79
developmental disorders, pervasive, 101–103
developmental dysplasia of hip, 178
DEXA (dual-energy X-ray absorptiometry)
  scan, 41
dexamethasone, 221
  for Ménière's disease, 80
  for spinal cord injury, 76
dextroamphetamine
  for ADHD, 103
  and amphetamine, 233t
dextrose, 18
diabetes insipidus, 47
diabetes mellitus, 52–53
  in pregnancy, 125
  Type 1, in children, 194–197
diabetic, 197
diabetic ketoacidosis, 53
dialectical behavior therapy (DBT), 106
dialysis, 69
diarrhea
  in children, 186
  medications, 36xx, 225
diavalproex sodium, for seizure, 74
diazepam, 231
  for alcohol withdrawal, 107, 108
  for children, 185
  for delirium tremens, 108
  for status asthmaticus, 75
  for suicidal patient, 106
diclofenac, 230t
dictatorial parenting style, 152t
dideoxycytidine, for AIDS, 83
Dietary Supplement Health and Education
  Act, 261
diets, therapeutic, 87–89
digitalis
  antidote/reversal agent, 239
  for heart failure, 60
digoxin, 213
  for heart failure in child, 176
  monitoring, 90
  therapeutic level, 239
  toxic level, 239
  for valvular disorders, 61
dilation, 127

diltiazem, 211
    after myocardial infarction, 59
    St. John's wort interaction, 262
dinoprostone cervical gel, 237
diphenhydramine, 218*t*
diphenhydramine HCl, 192
dipyridamole, 223
    for transient ischemic attacks (TIA), 75
disaster
    management, 253
    planning, 252–254
    psychosocial aftermath, 254
disease-modifying antirheumatic drugs
        (DMARDs), 230*t*
    for rheumatoid arthritis, 42
disease prevention, 15
diskectomy, 79
disorganized schizophrenia, 101
displacement, 96
dissociation, 114
distributive shock, 64
disulfiram, 233
    for alcohol abstinence, 107
    for aversion therapy, 108
diuretics, 225–226
    for cirrhosis, 38
    for SIADH, 48
    for valvular disorders, 61
diverticular disease, 36
DMARDs (disease-modifying antirheumatic
        drugs), 230*t*
    for rheumatoid arthritis, 42
dobutamine, for shock, 64
dobutamine hydrochloride, for heart failure, 60
docusate sodium, 225*t*
donepezil, for Alzheimer's disease, 110
door-in-the-face, 243
dopamine agonist, for Parkinson's disease, 77
dopamine, for shock, 64
dornase alfa, for cystic fibrosis, 200
dosage, calculations for, 208
doxazosin mesylate, 212
doxepin, 231*t*
doxorubicin hydrochloride
    for chemotherapy, 81
    toxicity, 82
doxycycline calcium, 228*t*
drag-and-drop/ordered response questions, 3
drain cleaner, accidental injestion, 191
dravastatin sodium, 215
droplet transmission-based precautions, 12
drowning prevention
    for adolescent, 166
    for infants, 158
    for preschooler, 162
    for school-age child, 164
    for toddlers, 161
drugs. *See also* pharmacology
    abuse in pregnancy, 142
dual-energy X-ray absorptiometry (DEXA)
        scan, 41
duloxetine, 231*t*
durable power of attorney for health care, 247

dwarfism, 46–47
dyhydration, from gastroenteritis, 186
dysfunctional grief, 104, 173
dysreflexia, 76
dystocia, 133

E

ears
    auditory assessment, 80
    of children, 154
    of newborn, 139*t*
eating disorders, 110–111
    in adolescence, 166
ECG, 57
echinacea, 262
echolalia, 101, 114
echopraxia, 101, 114
eclampsia, 123
ectopic pregnancy, 127
eczema, 192
edrophonium, 234
efavirenz, for AIDS, 83
effacement, 127
ego, 92
ego defense mechanism, 96
elation, 105
electroconvulsive therapy, for depressive
        disorder, 104
electroencephalogram (EEG), 73
electrolytes
    depletion from gastroenteritis, 186
    imbalance, 19–21
electromyography (EMG), 41
elimination habits, of newborn, 141
embolism
    amniotic fluid, 133
    pulmonary, 26–27
emergencies
    childbirth, 133
    respiratory, 27
emergency contraception, 236*t*
emergency management system, 253
Emergency Medical Treatment and Active
        Labor Act (EMTALA), 131
emotional abuse, 111, 191, 192
emotional neglect, 191, 192
emotional status, postpartum, 136
empathy, 96
emphysema, pulmonary, 23–24
enabling, 114
enalapril, 211
    for heart failure in child, 176
    for hypertension, 62
enalaprilat, 211, 213
end-of-life care, 86–87
endocrine system, 45–54
    adrenal gland, 48–50
    disorders in children, 194–197
    pancreas, 52–54
    parathyroid gland, 51–52
    pharmacology for, 218–221
    pituitary gland, 45–48
    thyroid gland, 50–51

endometrial cancer, 149
endometriosis, 150
endoscopy, 31
energy therapies, 264
engorgement, postpartum, 135
enoxaparin, 222
    antidote/reversal agent, 239
    after myocardial infarction, 59
enteral feeding tubes, 33
enteric transmission-based precautions, 12
enterococci infection, vancomycin-resistant
        (VRE), precautions required, 14*t*
environmental safety, 9
ephedrine, 218*t*
epidural block, in labor and delivery, 130
epidural hematoma, 76–77
epiglottitis, 187–188
epinephrine
    adrenal medulla production of, 48
    aerosol, for children, 188
    for shock, 64
episiotomy, 134
eplerenone, for Conn's Syndrome, 49
epoetin alfa, 222*t*
epoetin alfa/erythropoietin, for chronic renal
        failure, 69
epogen, for acute renal failure, 68
ergonomics, 9–10
Erikson, Erik, 93
    autonomy vs. shame and doubt, 159
    industry vs. inferiority, 163
    trust vs. mistrust stage, 157
erythrocyte sedimentation rate (ESR), 56
erythromycin, 228*t*
erythropoietin, 54
escitalopram, 231*t*
esmolol HCl, 213
esomeprazole, 224
esophagogastroduodenoscopy (EGD), 32
estrogens, 116
    adrenal cortex production of, 48
    for chemotherapy, 81
eszopiclone, 233
etanercept, 230*t*
ethambutol, for tuberculosis, 25
ethical issues, 247
ethinyl estradiol, 236*t*
ethinyl estradiol vaginal ring, 236*t*
ethylene poisoning, antidote/reversal agent, 239
etonogestrel, 236*t*
exanthem subitum (roseola), 204*t*
expectation, in team building, 243
expectorants, 217*t*
expert power, 243
extended family, 152*t*
external fixation device, 44
extrapyramidal reaction, 114
extravasation, IV infusion and, 210*t*
eyes
    children's characteristics, 154
    common problems, 79–80
    of newborn, 139*t*
ezetimibe, 215

F

face, children's characteristics, 153
Faces, Legs, Activity, Cry, and Consolability (FLACC) Postoperative Pain Tool, 170t
falls, 8
    preventing for infants, 158
    preventing for toddlers, 161
family abuse, 111–112
family-centered care, 152
family disaster kit, 253
family response to hospitalization of child, 166
family therapy, 95
famotidine, 224
fasting blood glucose, 195
fat
    foods with increased levels of, 87t
    healthy eating guidelines, 87
fear
    irrational, 98–99
    of strangers, 157
Federal Emergency Management Agency, 253
female reproductive organs, 116
fentanyl, 235
    for children, 170
fertilization, conditions necessary for, 116
fetal alcohol syndrome (FAS), 142
fetus
    age, 120
    assessment of, 120
    distress, 132
    heart tones, 122
    lie of, 127–128
fever, in children, 182, 186
fexofenadine, 218t
FFP, 221t
fibrillation, 57
fidelity, 247
figan, for children, 186
filgrastim, 222t
fill-in-the-blank questions, 3
finger foods, for infants, 158
finger to nose test, 156
fire response procedures, 9
flight of ideas, 114
fluconazole, 229t
fludrocortisone acetate, 221
fludrocortisone, for Addison's disease, 48
fluid volume deficit (FVD), 18
fluids, 18–22
    intravenous, 18t
fluorouracil (5-FU), for chemotherapy, 81
fluoxetine, 231t
    for anorexia nervosa, 110
    for multiple sclerosis, 77
    for OCD, 99
    for suicidal patient, 106
fluphenazine, 232
fluroquinolones, 228t
fluticasone propionate, 216t
fluvastatin, 215
fluvoxamine, 231t
    for OCD, 99
folic acid antagonists, 202

folic acid deficiency anemia, 55
follicle-stimulating hormone (FSH), 46
fontanel, 156
foot care, diabetes and, 196
foot-in-the-door, 243
forceps, in delivery, 134
formoterol, 215t
formula feeding, 141
formula, iron-fortified, 158
fosinopril, 211
foster family, 152t
Fowler's position of client, 10t
fractures, 44
    basilar skull, 76
    care for children, 191
Freud, Sigmund, 92, 100
full-liquid diet, 88
furosemide, 225t
    for cirrhosis, 38
    for heart failure in child, 176
    for hypertension, 61
    for nephrosis, 68
    for nephrotic syndrome, 199t

G

gabapentin, 234, 235t
    for bipolar disorder, 105
    for multiple sclerosis, 77
galantamine, for Alzheimer's disease, 110
gallbladder, diseases, 39
gallium nitrate, for hyperparathyroidism, 52
gasoline, accidental injestion, 191
gastric aspirate, laboratory profile, 31
gastroenteritis, in children, 186
gastroesophageal reflux (GER), 182, 183t
    collaborative care, 184t
gastrointestinal reflux disease, 33
gastrointestinal system, 31–41
    disorders, 33–36
        congenital anomaly in children, 182, 183–185t
        diagnostic procedures, 31–33
        therapeutic procedures, 32–33
    parasites, laboratory profile, 32
    pharmacology for, 224–225
    surgical procedures, 37
gastrointestinal tubes, 32t
gate-control theory of pain, 129
gay/lesbian family, 152t
generalized anxiety disorder (GAD), 98
generalized seizures, 74
genital herpes, 147t
genital warts, 147
genitalia, of children, 156
genitalia, of newborn, 139t
genitourinary system disorders, 65–71
    diagnostic tests, 65
gentamicin
    therapeutic level, 239
    toxic level, 239
gentamicin sulfate, 228t
German measles (rubella), 205t
gestational age, assessment of, 140–141
gestational diabetes mellitus, 125

gestational hypertension, 123
gigantism, 46
Gingko biloba, 262
    for memory enhancement, 110
ginseng (*Panax Quinquefolius*), 262
glaucoma, 80
    medications, 235
glipizide, 218t
gliptins, 218t
glomerulonephritis, 67, 199–200t
gloves, 13t
glucagon, 52, 219
glucocorticoids, 216–217, 230t
    adrenal cortex production of, 48
    inhaled, 215
glucosamine (2-amino-2-deoxyglucose), 262
glucose
    conversion to glycogen, 52
    laboratory values, 90
glucose tolerance test, in pregnancy, 125
glyburide, 218t
glycemic agent, 219
glycosylated hemoglobin, 195
goggles, 13t
gonadotropic hormones, 46
gonorrhea, 147t
Good Samaritan law, 248
Goodell's sign, 117t
gout, medications for, 231t
gouty arthritis, 42
grandiosity, 114
granulocytes, pheresed, 221t
graphic option for questions, 3
gravidity, 120
great vessels, transposition of, 177t
grief, 104, 114
    in children, 172
    symptoms of normal, 173
group therapy, 94–95, 106
growth and development
    of adolescent, 164–165
    of infants, 156–159
    of preschooler, 161–162
    of school-age child, 163
    of toddlers, 159–161
growth hormone
    hypersecretion of, 46
    hyposecretion of, 46
GTPAL, 120
guaifenesin, 217t
guanfacine, 212
    for Asperger's syndrome, 102
    for hypertension, 62
Guillain-Barré syndrome, 78
guilt, 243

H

hair, of children, 153
half-life for medication, 210
hallucinations, 101, 114
haloperidol, 232
    for delirium tremens, 108
    for end-of-life care, 86
hand hygiene, 11

mouth, of newborn, 139t
MRI (magnetic resonance imaging), 41
MRSA (methicillin-resistant staphylococcus aureus), precautions required, 14t
mucolytic agents, 217t
    for chronic bronchitis, 24
mucosal healing agents, for irritable bowel syndrome, 34
mucosal protectants, 225
mucositis, as chemotherapy side effect, 82
multigeneration antibiotics, 228t
multigravida, 120
multipara, 120
multiple-choice questions, 3
multiple response questions, 3
multiple sclerosis (MS), 77
mumps, 204t
Munchausen syndrome by proxy (MSBP), 191, 192
musculoskeletal disorders, 41–45
    amputation, 45
    arthritis, 41–42
    in children, 194
    diagnostic tests, 41
    fractures, 44
    osteomyelitis, 44
    osteoporosis, 43–44
    total joint arthroplasty, 44–45
musculoskeletal system
    of children, 155–156
    of newborn, 139t
    pharmacology for, 229–231
myasthenia gravis, 78
Mycobacterium tuberculosis, 25
myelomeningocele, 180
myocardial function, impaired, in children, 175–177
myocardial infarction (MI), 59–60
myoclonic seizure, 74
myomas (uterine fibroids), 149
myopia, 79

N

Nagele's rule, of delivery date calculation, 118
nails, of children, 153
naloxone HCl, 129t
naltrexone, for alcohol abstinence, 107
naphazoline, 218t
naproxen, 230t
narcissism, 114
narcotics
    antidote/reversal agent, 239
    in preoperative care, 28
Nasogastric tube, 32t
natalizumab, for ulcerative colitis, 35
nateglinide, 218t
Native-American client, culturally competent care of, 256–257
natural disasters, 252
nausea
    as chemotherapy side effect, 82
    as postoperative complication, 30t

NCLEX®
    communication questions, 5
    exam day, 6
    information about, 2
    item types, 3
    priority setting questions, 5–6
    registration process, 2–3
    test plan, 2–3
    test-taking strategies, 4–6
neck, children's characteristics, 154
negative punishment, 94
negative reinforcement, 94
neglect, 111
negligence, 248
neologisms, 101, 114
neomycin, for cirrhosis, 38
neonate
    Erikson's development stage, 93
    Hirschsprung's disease and, 190
    response to medication, 171
neostigmine, 234
    for myasthenia gravis, 78
nephroblastoma, 202
nephrosis, 67
nephrotic syndrome, 199–200t
nerve conduction studies, 41
nervous system, pharmacology for, 231–235
neural tube defects, 180–181
neuroblastoma, 202–203
neurogenic shock, 64
neuroleptic malignant syndrome, 114
neurologic disorders, chronic, 234
neurological system
    assessment, 71–72
    of children, 156
neurosensory disorders, 71–80
    common surgical procedures, 79
    diagnostic procedures, 72–73
    sensory assessment, 79–80
newborn
    care of, 138–141
    complications, 142–145
    physical assessment, 139–140t
    preterm, 144
nicardipine, 213
nicotine withdrawal, medications for, 107
nifedipine, 211, 238t
    for hypertension, 62
    for myocardial infarction, 59
    for Raynaud's syndrome, 63
    St. John's wort interaction, 262
nightmares, suppressing, 100
nitrates, for angina, 58
Nitro-Bid, 214
Nitro-Dur, 214
nitrofurantoin, 228t
nitroglycerin, 213
    for angina, 59
    after myocardial infarction, 59
nitrolingual, 214
nitrostat, 214
nizatindine, 224
non-stress test, in pregnancy diagnosis, 118
non-weight bearing ambulation devices, 11

nonbiomedical therapy, 263
Noncommunicating Children's Pain Checklist, 170t
nonmaleficence, 247
nonviral hepatitis, 39
noreigestromin, 236t
norepinephrine, adrenal medulla production of, 48
norepinephrine levarterenol, for shock, 64
nose, of children, 154
nose, of newborn, 139t
NSAIDS, 230t
    for gouty arthritis, 42
    for joint replacement, 44
    for lupus erythematosis, 84
    for osteoarthritis, 41
    and peptic ulcer disease, 34
    for rheumatoid arthritis, 42
nuchal cord, 132
nuclear family, 152t
nulligravida, 120
nullipara, 120
nurse/client relationship, in mental health treatment, 95–96
Nurse Practice Act, 245, 246, 248
nursing assistant, roles and responsibilities for, 245
nutrition
    for adolescent, 165–166
    for diabetic child, 196
    foods with increased levels of fat and water-soluble vitamins, 87t
    for infants, 158
    for preschooler, 162
    for school-age child, 164
    therapeutic diets, 87–89
    for toddlers, 160

O

obesity
    morbid, bariatric surgery for treating, 37
    in school-age child, 164
object permanence, 157
obsession, 114
obsessive-compulsive disorder (OCD), 99
obstretics, assisted/operative, 134
obstructed airway, in children, 203
occurrence reports, 244
ocreotide, for acromegaly, 46
olanzapine, 232
    for schizophrenia, 101
    for suicidal patient, 106
older adult
    Erikson's development stage, 93
    medications in, 209
omega-3 fatty acids, 262–263
omeprazole, 224
oncology nursing. See cancer
ondansetron, 225t
open-ended statements, 96
ophthalmologic medications, 235
opioid analgesics, 235–236
    for children, 170
    for chronic pancreatitis, 40

spinal cord injury, 76
spinal fusion, 79
spine of children, 156
spironolactone, 225*t*
    for cirrhosis, 38
    for hypertension, 61
splitting, 97, 114
SSRIs (selective serotonin reuptake
        inhibitors), 231*t*
    for Asperger's syndrome, 102
    for depressive disorder, 104
St. John's wort (*Hypericum perforatum*),
        261–262
    avoiding, in heart failure, 60
    for depressive disorder, 104
stable angina, 58
staff, roles and responsibilities for levels, 245–246
stairs, walking with assistive devices, 11
staphylococcus aureus, methicillin-resistant
        (MRSA), precautions required, 14*t*
statins, 215
    for angina, 58
station in labor, 128
status asthmaticus, 23, 193
status epilepticus, 75
sterile technique (surgical asepsis), 11
steroids
    for inflammatory bowel disease, 35
    for nephrosis, 68
stimulant medications, for ADHD, 103
stone, kidney (urolithiasis), 68
stool softeners, 225
    for irritable bowel syndrome, 34
    for peptic ulcer disease, 34
stranger fear, 157
strategies for test-taking, 4–6
streptokinase, for myocardial infarction, 59
streptomycin, 228*t*
    for tuberculosis, 25
stress incontinence, 71
stroke, 75
subdural hematoma, 77
sublimation, 96
substance abuse, 107–109
    in pregnancy, 142
    preventing for adolescent, 166
    preventing for school-age child, 164
substance dependence, 107
sucking and rooting reflex, 139*t*
sucralfate, 225
suctioning, 28
sudden infant death syndrome (SIDS), 159
suffocation prevention
    for infants, 159
    for toddlers, 161
suicide, 105–106, 166
sulfonamides, 228*t*
    for cystitis, 67
sulfonylureas, 218*t*
summarizing, 96
superego, 92
supervision, 245

supine position of client, 10*t*
surgical asepsis (sterile technique), 11
surgical procedures for children, 189–190
sympatholytics (alpha adrenergic blockers), 212
sympatholytics (beta adrenergic blockers),
        212–213
    for hypertension, 62
sympathomimetics, for respiratory infection, 187
syndrome of inappropriate secretion of anti-
        diuretic hormone (SIADH), 47–48
syphilis, 148*t*

T

tabeprazole sodium, 224
tachycardia, 57
tadalafil, 227
Tai Chi, 264
talipes equinovarus, 177
tamoxifen citrate, for chemotherapy, 81
tamsulosin, 226*t*
tardive dyskinesia, 114
team building, 243
technology, impact on nursing profession, 248–249
teeth, of children, 155
teletherapy, 82
temazepam, 233
temper tantrums, 160
temperature
    conversions, 208
    guidelines for children, 155*t*
    hypothalamus regulation, 74
    of newborn, 138*t*
tenecteplase, 224
terbutaline, 129*t*, 215*t*
terbutaline sulfate, 238*t*
terminally-ill children, 174*t*
termination phase, in nurse/client
        relationship, 96
tertiary prevention, 15*t*
test-taking
    and anxiety, 6
    strategies, 4–6
testing, computerized adaptive, 2
tetanus (*Clostridium tetani*), 205*t*
tetracyclines, 228*t*
tetralogy of Fallot, 177*t*
thalassemia, 56
theophylline, 216
    monitoring, 90
    St. John's wort interaction, 262
    therapeutic level, 239
    toxic level, 239
therapeutic communication, 242
therapeutic diets, 87–89
therapeutic drug levels, 239
therapeutic massage, 263
therapeutic medication monitoring, 90
therapeutic play, 168
thiazide, and digoxin, 213
thiazide diuretics, 225*t*
thiazide-hydrochlorothiazide, for
        hypertension, 61

thiazolidinediones, 218*t*
thiothixene, 232
thoracentesis, 23
thoracic injury, 76
thorax, of children, 155
threapeutic drug monitoring, 209
throat, of children, 154–155
thromboangiitis obliterans (Buerger's disease), 63
thrombocytopenia, as chemotherapy side
        effect, 82
thromboembolic disorder, postpartum, 137
thrombolytics, 224
    for myocardial infarction, 59
    for pulmonary embolism, 27
thrombophlebitis, 62
    IV infusion and, 210*t*
    as postoperative complication, 31*t*
thyroid gland, 50–51
thyroid hormone, 219–220
thyroid hormone antagonist, 220
thyroidectomy, 51
thyrotropic hormone (TSH), 46
ticlopidine, 223
    for transient ischemic attacks (TIA), 75
time limits for exam, 2
time, preschoolers and, 161
timolol maleate, 235
tiotropium, 216
tobacco, as newborn complication, 142–143
tobramycin
    therapeutic level, 239
    toxic level, 239
tocolytics, 238*t*
toddlers
    caring for terminally ill, 174*t*
    cognitive development, 159
    Erikson's development stage, 93
    expected growth and development, 159–161
    hospitalization age-related interventions, 167*t*
    hospitalization impact, 167*t*
    moral development, 160
    motor skills, 159*t*
    play while hospitalized, 168
    response to death/dying, 173*t*
    self-concept development, 160
toilet training, 160
tolterodine
    for multiple sclerosis, 77
    for urge incontinence, 71
tonic-clonic seizure, 74
tonic neck reflex, 139*t*
tonsillectomy, 189
topical analgesics, for osteoarthritis, 41
topiramate, for bipolar disorder, 105
tort law, 248
total joint arthroplasty, 44–45
total parenteral nutrition (TPN), 33, 210–211
Total Quality Improvement model, 243
toxic drug levels, 239
tracheostomy care, 28
traction, 44
traditional nuclear family, 152*t*

transference, 114
transferring clients, 9
transient hyperglycemia, 54
transient ischemic attacks (TIA), 75
transitional crisis, 98
transmission-based infection control, precautions, 11–12
transposition of the great vessels, 177*t*
tranylcypromine, 231*t*
Trendelenburg position of client, 10*t*
Trendelenburg sign, 178
triage, 253
triamcinolone, 192
triamcinolone acetonide, 216*t*
triamterene, 225*t*
    for hypertension, 61
trichomoniasis, 146, 148*t*
tricyclic antidepressants, 231*t*
    for depressive disorder, 104
trihexyphenidyl, for Parkinson's disease, 77
trimethoprimsulfamethoxazole, 228*t*
troponin, 57
trough levels of medication, 210*t*
trycyclic antidepressants, for stress incontinence, 71
tuberculosis (TB), 25
    precautions required, 14*t*
    test indicating exposure, 22
tumors, 81. *See also* cancer
TURP (transurethral resection of prostate), 71
turpentine, accidental injestion, 191

U

ulcerative colitis, 35
ultrasonography, 146
    in pregnancy diagnosis, 118
umbilical cord, 116, 138
    care of, 141
    compression, 132
unconscious, 92
unconscious mechanisms, 96
undifferentiated schizophrenia, 101
undoing, 97
unstable angina, 58
uracil mustard, for chemotherapy, 81
urethral meatus, 156
uric acid, 66
urinalysis, 65–66
urinary retention/hesitancy
    alpha-adrenergic blockers for, 226
    as postoperative complication, 30*t*
urinary system
    indwelling catheter, 67
    infection as postoperative complication, 31*t*
    pharmacology affecting, 225–227
    surgical procedures, 70–71

urine retention, 71
urolithiasis, 68
uterus
    disorders, 149–150
    fibroids, 149
    hyperstimulation, 133
    labor contractions, 127
    postpartum, 135–136

V

vacuum extraction, 134
vagina, 156
    infection, 146–148
    secretions, 116
valacyclovir, 229*t*
valarian root, 261
valproic acid, 234, 235*t*
    for bipolar disorder, 105
    for seizure, 74
valsartan, 211
valvular disorders, 60–61
vancomycin, 228*t*
vancomycin-resistant enterococci (VRE) infection, precautions required, 14*t*
vardenafil, 227
variance reports, 244
variant angina, 58
varicella (chickenpox)
    precautions required, 13*t*
    vaccine, 238
varicose veins, 62–63
vasodilators, 213
    myocardial infarction and, 59
vasopressin, for diabetes insipidus, 47
vasospasm, in pregnancy, 123
vein stripping, 63
venous spasm, IV infusion and, 210*t*
ventricular dysrhythmias, 57
ventricular fibrillation, 57
ventricular septal defect (VSD), 176*t*
ventricular tachycardia, 57
veracity, 247
verapamil, 211
    and digoxin, 213
    for hypertension, 62
    for myocardial infarction, 59
vinblastine, for chemotherapy, 81
vincristine, for chemotherapy, 81
vincristine sulfate, 202
    toxicity, 82
visual acuity, evaluation, 79
Visual Analog Scale (VAS), 170*t*
vital sign guidelines, for children, 155*t*
vitamin B_{12}, anemia from lack of intake or absorption, 55
Vitamin D supplements, for osteoporosis, 44

vitamins
    for delirium tremens, 108
    foods with increased levels of water-soluble, 87*t*
    supplements for cirrhosis, 38
vomiting
    as chemotherapy side effect, 82
    by children, 186
VRE (vancomycin-resistant enterococci) infection, precautions required, 14*t*

W

walker, 11
walking on stairs, with assistive devices, 11
warfarin, 223
    antidote/reversal agent, 239
    after myocardial infarction, 59
    for transient ischemic attacks (TIA), 75
water, body weight percentage, 18
water-soluble vitamins, foods with increased levels of, 87*t*
waxy flexibility, 114
weaning, 158
weight bearing ambulation devices, 11
weight, of infant, 156
Wernicke-Korsakoff syndrome, 108
Wharton's jelly, 116
Whipple procedure, 40
whooping cough (pertussis), 204*t*
Wilms' tumor, 202
word salad, 114
working phase, in nurse/client relationship, 95
World Health Organization, highly active antiretroviral therapy guidelines (HAART), 83
wound, postoperative complications
    dehiscence/evisceration, 31*t*
    delayed healing, 31*t*
    hemorrhage, 30*t*
    infection, 31*t*

Y

young adult, Erikson's development stage, 93

Z

zalcitabine, for AIDS, 83
zatirlukast, 217
zidovudine, 229*t*
    for AIDS, 83
zileuton, 217
ziprasidone, 232
    for schizophrenia, 101
zoledronate, 229
zolpidem tarate, 233